The Biology of the Intervertebral Disc

Volume I

Editor

Peter Ghosh, B.SC., Ph.D., A.R.I.C., F.R.A.C.I.

Director
Raymond Purves Research Laboratories at
Royal North Shore Hospital of Sydney
and
Associate Professor,
Department of Surgery
University of Sydney
St. Leonards, N.S.W.
Australia

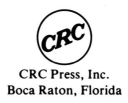

CRC Press, Inc.
Boca Raton, Florida

Library of Congress Cataloging-in-Publication Data

The Biology of the intervertebral disc.

Includes bibliographies and indexes.
1. Intervertebral disk displacement.
2. Intervertebral disk. I. Ghosh, P. (Peter),
1940-   . [DNLM: 1. Intervertebral Disk.
WE 740 B615]
RD771.I6B56   1988   617'.375   87-21781

ISBN 0-8493-6711-5 (v. 1)
ISBN 0-8493-6712-3 (v. 2)

Direct all inquiries to CRC Press, Inc., 2000 Corporate Blvd., N.W., Boca Raton, Florida, 33431.

© 1988 by CRC Press, Inc.

International Standard Book Number 0-8493-6711-5 (v. 1)
International Standard Book Number 0-8493-6712-3 (v. 2)

Library of Congress Card Number 87-21781
Printed in the United States

Dedicated to my wife Nancy, for her support,
encouragement, and understanding during
the difficult times.

FOREWORD

Some long-standing facts, positive recent developments, and certain recent circumstances have set the stage for this timely contribution to the literature. First, one third of all orthopedic referrals are for complaints pertaining to the spinal column. Second, in Western societies, derangements of the intervertebral disc associated with aging, degeneration, and prolapse are the major causes of back pain and allied symptoms. Third, spinal diseases and disorders are the principal cause of physical handicap and activity limitation in the young. In older age groups, they rank third after heart disease and arthritis. Fourth, recent times have seen quantum leaps of knowledge in connective tissue biology — the structure and function of the major macromolecular components collagen(s) and proteoglycan(s), their synthesis and catabolism, and the mechanisms controlling these processes.

Similar (though perhaps less spectacular) advances have been made in ultrastructural research and spinal biomechanics. *Pari passu* with these events has come the clear need for multidisciplinary research. Connective tissues have a ''connecting'' function which holds implicit connotations for mechanical properties. Now, as perhaps never before, the natural corollaries for connective tissue research are correlative studies. A glance at the cited references in these volumes attests to this.

Nothing is more daunting to a chemist than an uncharacterized mixture, let alone an inability to solubilize its components without their degradation. That, in short, is the situation with which research workers were confronted not so long ago. So the mystery of the collagen molecule could be likened to two equations with three unknowns. The key to proteoglycan structure and its functions started to turn only when it became possible to extract these giant molecules from tissues in their native form, and to purposefully disaggregate them and study their interaction with hyaluronic acid. The technology to unravel the complexities of connective tissue biology is already here, but it would indeed be a great shame if research in molecular biology and applied science in diseases and disorders of the musculoskeletal system became separated. The late Dame Honor Fell often referred to ''the unnatural divorce of biochemistry and morphology'' and no one attempted reconciliation more than she. Such wise counsel equally applies to biomechanics, morphology, and related areas. To this end, those interested in this ''recalcitrant gristle'' should take stock of the common clinical problems, where on the basis of existing knowledge, it is reasonable to look towards endeavor in applied research using more than one tool and involving more than one discipline.

To produce this book the editor assembled a group of distinguished scientists, each of whom has made valuable, and original, contributions each in his own field. For this first edition, congratulations are in order. The patent need to assemble such knowledge between the covers of a book assuredly means it will not be the last.

T. K. F. Taylor D.Phil(Oxon), F.R.C.S., F.R.C.S.(Edin), F.R.A.C.S.
Professor of Orthopaedics and Traumatic Surgery
The University of Sydney

PREFACE

While none would deny the importance of the intervertebral disc for normal activity and function, few have earnestly striven to unlock its secrets. The elegant pathoanatomical studies by Püschel, Junghanns, Schmorl, and Hirsch provided early insights into the complexity of this structure, the morphological variations with aging, and frequency of failure in man. Although more than 50 years have elapsed since the observations of Mixter and Barr that disc degeneration and protrusions could be the cause of sciatica, it is only now that some of the enzymes responsible for the turnover of disc matrix components have been identified and a means of their control indicated. It is perhaps because of this paucity of basic knowledge that major advances in the treatment of disc disorders have not been forthcoming. It might be argued by some that chemonucleolysis has provided one solution. However, it must be recognized that we are still uncertain of the manner by which this procedure provides symptomatic relief. Such a situation highlights the need to reappraise the intervertebral disc in the light of our present knowledge and provide new directions for research in the future.

I was therefore delighted to be given the opportunity by CRC Press to bring together the experience and views of some of the leading authorities on disc biology and function in a single treatise. Contributors were selected on the basis of their expertise and were requested to provide an up-to-date review of their area which would be of value to both researchers in the field as well as the uninitiated. The liberal use of prints and line drawings was especially encouraged for we believed that these invarably assist in the interpretation of complex information and ideas. The outcome of this approach has been the production of a two-volume set which covers the disc in terms of its anatomy, growth, assembly, biomechanical function, nutrition, biochemistry, pathology, and response to a variety of therapeutic modalities, including chemonucleolysis. A chapter on the recently developed technique of nuclear magnetic resonance imaging, as applied to the disc, was included because of the strong interest in this subject and its obvious potential for both clinical and research applications.

All contributors were aware of the inadequacies in our knowledge of the disc and were united in their desire to stimulate in others a greater interest in this unique structure. If this review requires revision within the next few years, we will have achieved our objective.

Peter Ghosh
Editor

THE EDITOR

Peter Ghosh, Ph.D. is the Director of the Raymond Purves Research Laboratories at the Royal North Shore Hospital of Sydney, and Associate Professor in the Department of Surgery, the University of Sydney, N.S.W., Australia. Dr Ghosh graduated B.Sc. with Honors from the University of London in 1962. After a year's research in industry, he commenced Ph.D. studies at the University of East Anglia, Norwich, Norfolk, U.K. On Graduating in 1966, Dr. Ghosh was appointed Research Fellow in the Department of Medical Chemistry, John Curtin School of Medical Research, Australian National University, Canberra, A.C.T., Australia. Here he developed strong interests in the mode of action of immunosuppressive and antiinflammatory drugs. This research subsequently led to his appointment to the staff of the Riker Research Institute, Sydney, where he became Head of the Department of Medical Chemistry in 1969. His entry into connective tissue research, particularly the intervertebral disc, commenced in 1971 when he took up the position of National Health and Medical Research Council (NHMRC) Senior Research Officer in the Department of Surgery (Orthopaedic and Traumatic) at the University of Sydney with Professor Thomas Taylor, D.Phil., F.R.C.S. The establishment of Orthopaedic Research Laboratories at the Royal North Shore Hospital of Sydney through a generous donation from the Raymond E. Purves Foundation provided the facilities for an expansion of Dr. Ghosh's activities in connective tissue research and he was appointed as the first Director of the Laboratories in 1973. He was elected Fellow of the Royal Australian Institute of Chemistry in 1975 and awarded the title of Associate Professor, University of Sydney in 1986. He was treasurer of the Connective Tissue Society of Australia and New Zealand from 1976 to 1984 and President from 1984 to 1985. He is a Trustee and scientific advisor to Spinecare, the Children's Spinal Research Foundation, Scientific assessor/advisor for the NHMRC and Medical Research Council of New Zealand, reviewer for *Journal of Rheumatology, Rheumatology International* and *Australian Journal of Biological Sciences,* and consultant for several drug companies. Dr. Ghosh is author or coauthor of 24 book chapters, editorials, review articles, and 125 research publications. He is an active member of several scientific societies including the Orthopaedic Research Society (U.S.), Australian Rheumatism Association, Australian Biochemical Society, Australian Society of Experimental Pathology, and the Australian and New Zealand Society for Cell Biology.

CONTRIBUTORS

Michael A. Adams, Ph.D.
Research Fellow
Department of Anatomy
University of Bristol
Bristol, United Kingdom

Richard M. Aspden, Ph.D.
Research Associate
Department of Medical Biophysics
University of Manchester
Manchester, United Kingdom

Nikolai Bogduk, Ph.D.
Senior Lecturer
Faculty of Medicine
University of Newcastle
Newcastle, Australia

Wallace F. Butler, Ph.D.
Lecturer
Department of Anatomy
School of Veterinary Science
Bristol, United Kingdom

Henry V. Crock, M.D., F.R.A.C.S.
Consultant Spinal Surgeon
Cromwell Hospital
London, England

David R. Eyre, Ph.D.
Ernest M. Burgess Professor of
  Orthopaedic Research
Departments of Orthopaedics and
  Biochemistry
School of Medicine
University of Washington
Seattle, Washington

Peter Ghosh, Ph.D., F.R.A.C.I.
Director
and Associate Professor
Raymond Purves Research Laboratories
The University of Sydney at The Royal
  North Shore Hospital of Sydney
St. Leonards, Australia

Miron Goldwasser, M.D., F.R.A.C.S.
Orthopaedic Surgeon
Sacred Heart Hospital
Coburg, Australia

D. Stephen Hickey, Ph.D.
Research Associate
Department of Medical Biophysics
University of Manchester
Manchester, United Kingdom

David W. L. Hukins, Ph. D.
Senior Lecturer
Department of Medical Biophysics
University of Manchester
Manchester, United Kingdom

William D. Hutton, D. Sc.
Professor
Department of Mechanical Engineering
South Australian Institute of Technology
The Levels, Pooraka
Adelaide, South Australia

Alice Maroudas
Pearl Milch Professor in Biomedical
  Engineering Sciences
Technion-Israel Institute of Technology
Technion City
Haifa, Israel

Cahir A. McDevitt, Ph.D.
Head, Section of Biochemistry
Department of Musculoskeletal Research
The Cleveland Clinic Foundation
  Research Institute
Cleveland, Ohio

James Melrose, Ph.D.
Research Fellow
Raymond Purves Research Laboratories
The University of Sydney at The Royal
  North Shore Hospital of Sydney
St. Leonards, Australia

James R. Taylor, M.D., Ph.D.
Associate Professor
Department of Anatomy and Human
  Biology
The University of Western Australia
Nedlands, Australia

Lance T. Twomey, Ph.D.
Professor and Head
Department of Physiotherapy
Curtin University of Technology
Shenton Park, Australia

**Barrie Vernon-Roberts, M.D., Ph.D.,
  F.R.C.P.A., F.R.C.Path.**
Professor of Pathology
University of Adelaide
Head of Division of Tissue Pathology
Institute of Medical and Veterinary
  Science
Adelaide, Australia

Hidezo Yoshizawa
Professor of Orthopaedic Surgery
Fujita-Gakuen University
School of Medicine
Toyoake, Japan

TABLE OF CONTENTS

Volume 1

Volume 2

Chapter 1

DISC STRUCTURE AND FUNCTION

David W. L. Hukins

TABLE OF CONTENTS

I. INTRODUCTION

The spine can be considered, to a first approximation, as a column of relatively rigid vertebrae connected by the flexible intervertebral discs. Because of their flexibility, the discs allow the spine to twist and bend so that the body is able to assume a wide range of postures. It is sometimes supposed that their primary function is to act as shock absorbers — there is considerable evidence against this supposition. First, the disc does not act as a shock absorber during in vitro mechanical tests.[1] Second, shock absorption is normally achieved by the musculature.[2] Third, there is no reason why the spine needs to be regularly punctuated by shock absorbers any more than do the other long bones. Finally, the intervertebral discs form joints which are clearly responsible for conferring the flexibility that is essential for the spine to perform its function as the main component of the axial skeleton.

An intervertebral disc also has to withstand compression. Most of this compression arises from muscular contraction during movement. When the muscles contract, they exert forces which have an appreciable component along the axis of the spine and hence tend to compress the disc. For example, the external and internal oblique muscles of the abdomen are tilted by about 40° with respect to the axis of the spine; contraction of these muscles causes twisting.[3] A tensile force F generated in these muscles during twisting will then exert an axial compression of about F cos 40° = 0.8F on the intervertebral discs in the lumbar (low back) region of the spine. The common assumption that upright stance is responsible for most of the compressive loading on human discs is incorrect. Nachemson[4] has shown that when the human body is supine, the compressive load on the third lumbar disc is 300 N which rises to only 700 N when upright stance is assumed. However, bending forward by only 20° increases this load to a much higher value of 1200 N[4].

There are 23 discs in the human spine which account for 20 to 30% of its length.[5,6,7] Apart from the fused vertebrae of the sacrum and coccyx, the only vertebrae not connected by intervertebral discs are the two cervical vertebrae at the cranial extremity of the spine (the atlas and the axis) which pivot at the specialized atlanto-axial joint; the atlas and the base of the skull articulate at the specialized occipito-atlantal joint[8] which also does not contain a disc. Other mammals have differing numbers of vertebrae, and the tail does not closely resemble the human coccyx, but the structures of their intervertebral discs in corresponding regions of the spine are often remarkably similar. (Further details on comparative anatomy are given in Chapter 3).

The disc is not the only structure connecting the vertebrae. Figure 1 shows two vertebrae connected to form a so-called "motion segment". The vertebral bodies or centra are connected by the anterior and posterior longitudinal ligaments, parallel to the axis of the spine, as well as by the disc.[8] Further ligaments connect the vertebral arches of adjacent vertebrae, e.g., the two ligamenta flava, the interspinous ligament, and the supraspinous ligament occur in most of the lumbar region.[8,9,10] Also projecting from the neural arch are the superior and inferior processes which terminate in flattened facets. The facets of adjacent vertebrae articulate (superior of one with inferior of next) in the facet joints (also known as apophyseal or zygapophyseal points). Facet joints are conventional synovial joints in which the capsular ligaments confer further stability on the spine.[11-15] All of these structures assist the intervertebral disc in maintaining stability during movement of the spine[16] and in its response to compression.[17]

The aim of this chapter is to describe the structure of the disc and to discuss how this structure is related to mechanical stability during twisting, bending, and compression of the intervertebral joint. The first section of the chapter is concerned with structure (gross anatomy and ultrastructure), but ignores specialized topics such as vascularity (see Chapter 4), nerve supply (see Chapter 5), and the cells.[18,19] Although cells are essential for controlling the growth, repair, and metabolism of the disc, its mechanical function can be explained largely

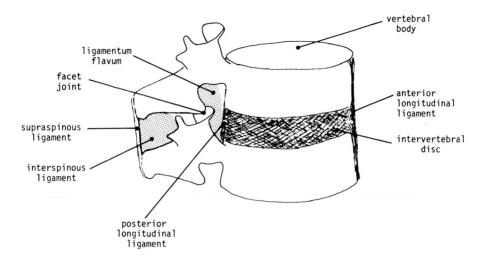

FIGURE 1. Sketch of a typical "motion segment" of the spinal column consisting of two vertebrae linked by an intervertebral disc, facet joints, and various ligaments.

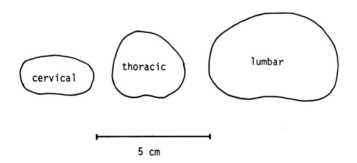

FIGURE 2. Typical disc shapes in transverse section for (a) cervical, (b) thoracic, and (c) lumbar regions of the human spine.

in terms of the properties of the extracellular matrix. These properties are reviewed in the second part of the chapter in order to relate disc structure to function in the third part. Disc structure is so complicated that it is not possible to relate every observable detail to function — differences occur along the length of the spine, during aging, and between individuals. Indeed, a discussion which attempted this task would obscure the essential features and so be pointless. Finally, the chapter concludes by discussing how the disc functions in the intact spine.

II. STRUCTURE

A. Gross Anatomy

An intervertebral disc is roughly cylindrical. However, its cross-sectional shape is not perfectly circular, and it does not usually have the same height posteriorly as anteriorly. Figure 2 shows some typical disc shapes in transverse section. These sections tend to be roughly elliptical in the cervical region, to resemble a rounded triangle in the thoracic region, and to resemble an ellipse in the lumbar spine. There are detailed differences within each region and between individuals which have been described for lumbar discs by Farfan.[20] Cross-sectional shape can be quantified by a shape index, S, defined by

$$S = 4\pi A/C^2 \tag{1}$$

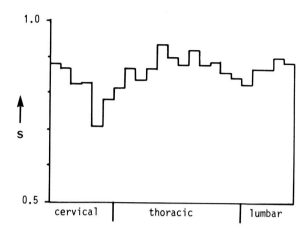

FIGURE 3.   The distribution of the shape index, S, defined in Equation 1, for discs along the length of the human spine; the lower the value of the index, the greater the deviation from a circular transverse section. (Data from reference 7.)

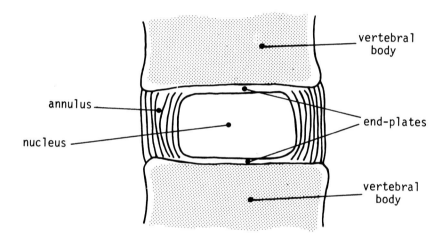

FIGURE 4.   Diagrammatic representation of a sagittal section of a human lumbar disc showing the attachments of the annular lamellae to the vertebrae and end-plates; the thickness of the end-plates has been exaggerated for clarity.

where A is the area and C the circumference of the cross section. S has a maximum value of unity for a circular cross section; the lower its value the more the shape departs from a circle. Figure 3 shows how S varies for the discs along the length of the spine; it is clear that the discs of the midthoracic spine have the most nearly circular cross sections, while those of the midcervical have the least circular cross sections.[7] Cross-sectional area increases almost linearly from the cranial to the caudal extremity of the spine.[7] Most discs appear roughly wedge shaped in sagittal section (Figure 4), because the anterior height is greater than the posterior. Figure 5 shows posterior height divided by anterior height for all the discs of the human spine; the nearer the value of this ratio to unity, the less wedge shaped is the disc. This figure clearly shows that thoracic discs are less wedge shaped than either cervical or lumbar discs.[7] Unlike cross-sectional area, disc height does not vary regularly along the length of the spine, but is greatest in the midthoracic region.

The intervertebral disc has a soft inner region, the nucleus pulposus (or nucleus) surrounded by the lamellae of the tough outer region, the annulus fibrosus (or annulus). Figure 6 is a

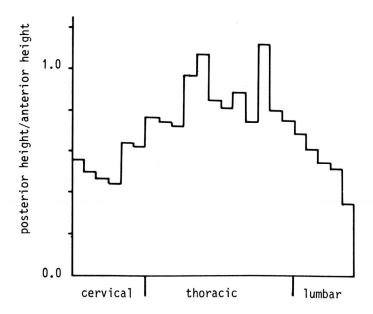

FIGURE 5. Posterior height divided by anterior height for discs along the lengths of the human spine; the lower the number the more wedge-shaped the disc. (Data from reference 7.)

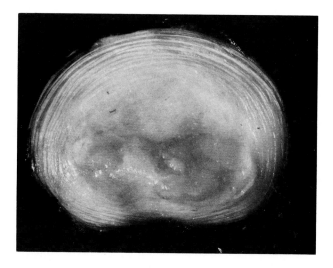

FIGURE 6. Transverse section of a human lumbar disc (16-year-old female) showing the nucleus surrounded by the lamellae of the annulus.

transverse section which clearly shows these regions. Typically, the annulus consists of about twelve coaxial lamellae (thickness about 1 mm in human discs) which form a tube enclosing the nucleus. In the anterior annulus these lamellae can be clearly distinguished, although they are not always easy to separate — especially in older discs. Posteriorly the annulus is thinner and the lamellae tend to merge together. Although the annulus and the nucleus are quite different in texture, their boundary is not clearly defined. Indeed, Peacock[21] described the annulus as an outer zone of fibrocartilage and a transition zone separating it from the nucleus. Sometimes short lengths of laminated structure can be seen in the nucleus.[22] The most realistic description consists of the conventional division into nucleus and annulus

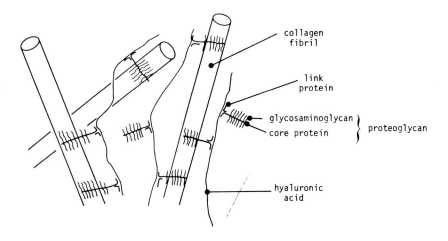

FIGURE 7. Schematic diagram of possible macromolecular interactions which can occur in the disc (not to scale).

while recognizing that there is a gradual transition from the mucoid texture of one to the laminated structure of the other.

Superior and inferior surfaces of the disc are coated with hyaline cartilage end-plates as shown in Figure 4. End-plates are thin compared with the total thickness of the disc. For example, human lumbar discs typically have a thickness of around 1 cm as compared to 1 mm for each end-plate. There is no consensus as to whether end-plates should be considered a part of the disc or as parts of a vertebra. However, the question is of no functional importance because the vertebral bodies and discs are firmly attached so that they act together as an intact anterior spinal column.[23]

Inner lamellae of the annulus are attached to the end-plates to form a closed vessel containing the nucleus, as shown in Figure 4; in complete contrast the outer lamellae are attached to the bone of the vertebral bodies.[21,24,25] This difference in attachment suggests that there may be some difference in function between the inner and outer regions of the annulus, as described later in this chapter.[23]

Changes occur in the appearance of the disc during aging. The boundary between the nucleus and annulus becomes even less distinct while the nucleus itself becomes more fibrous and desiccated.[21,26] Some of the nucleus can protrude into the vertebral body through fissures in the end-plates to form features called Schmorl's nodes. These nodes are often supposed to be a result of trauma. However, Hansson and Roos[27] distinguished two kinds of protrusion. One kind, with an irregular appearance, could be reproduced by compression of cadaveric motion segments and, therefore, appeared to have a traumatic origin. The other, more regular, kind of protrusion could not be reproduced in this way; as a result they considered that it was congenital or developmental in origin — in agreement with an earlier proposal by Ball.[28] Most of the aging changes which occur in the disc can be better appreciated at the ultra-structural level and so will be described in the remainder of Section II, which deals in turn with details of the nucleus, annulus, and end-plates.

B. Nucleus

The nucleus consists of a highly hydrated gel of proteoglycans containing some collagen. In children and young adults, water accounts for over 80% of the weight of the nucleus.[29] This high water content arises because of the macromolecular composition of the nucleus. The proteoglycans consist of sulfated glycosaminoglycan side-chains (chondroitin and keratan sulfates) covalently bound to a protein core as shown in Figure 7.[30] Because the negatively charged sulfate groups are part of this very high molecular weight structure, they are not free to diffuse out of the nucleus and so they attract water by the mechanism described later in this chapter in Section III.A.[31,32] Furthermore, some of the proteoglycans form ''aggregates'' as a result of the presence of hyaluronic acid in the nucleus.[30,33] In these aggregates the protein core is bound to hyaluronic acid by a specific interaction which is stabilized by ''link proteins''.[30,34-37] Hyaluronic acid is a nonsulfated glycosaminoglycan with a much longer chain length than the sulfated glycosaminoglycans which form the side-chains of the proteoglycans.[30,35] Further interactions probably occur between the sulfated glycosaminoglycans and the collagen fibrils of the nucleus. These glycosaminoglycans interact with collagen molecules in dilute solution[38] and so also presumably interact with the surface of collagen fibrils.[39] However, the behavior of individual molecules in dilute solution may not be a good model for what happens in a tissue where the collagen molecules are assembled into fibrils.[40] Figure 7 summarizes the kinds of interactions which can occur between the macromolecular components of the nucleus; further details of some of these interactions appear in Chapter 6, which is concerned with disc proteoglycans.

Collagen accounts for only about 5% of the weight of the nucleus.[41] It is present as individual fibrils with a diameter of around 30 nm, which are randomly dispersed and not organized into any more complex structure.[25,42,43] Chapter 7 gives a detailed account of the collagen of the disc; most of the collagen in the nucleus is the same genetic type (type II) that occurs in hyaline cartilage.[44]

Changes occur in the composition of the nucleus during aging — the most remarkable is the loss of water, which accounts for the changes, described already in Section II.A, in its gross appearance.[29,45,46] The water content of the nucleus decreases linearly with age [29] (linear correlation coefficient, r = −0.79). It has also been claimed that the annulus loses water as well as the nucleus,[29] but the figures published in support of this claim show no correlation between annular water content and age (r = 0.17). Changes in the glycosaminoglycan content of the nucleus are implicated in the loss of water because they lead to a decrease in the number of sulfate groups which attract water into the tissue.[31,32,47] Other changes occur in the nucleus at the ultrastructural level. Sometimes banded fibers appear in the aging human nucleus[48] which are reminiscent of the large-diameter collagen fibrils observed in amianthoid degeneration of aging hyaline cartilage.[49,50]

Nuclear magnetic resonance (NMR) shows that the chemical environment of the water molecules changes during aging and, more especially, during degeneration of the disc.[51] This technique is discussed in more detail in Chapter 13. This method can be used to image the disc in vivo so that the nucleus and annulus can be clearly distinguished, as shown in Figure 8. An image like Figure 8 consists typically of 256×256 picture elements or ''pixels'' whose intensity depends on the magnitude of the NMR signal. The signal obtained from the nucleus of a degenerate disc is less than that from normal adjacent discs;[52] a similar, although less marked, reduction of signal intensity appears to be associated with aging.[53]

Signal intensity depends on a number of factors,[54,55] each of whose contributions can be separated numerically to form different kinds of images.[56] More specifically, the intensity, I, depends on the residual magnetization, M_∞ which is a measure of the number of hydrogen nuclei per unit volume, and two relaxation times — T_1 and T_2. The spin-lattice relaxation time, T_1, is a measure of the time taken for an excited hydrogen nucleus to transfer its energy to the molecules of the surrounding medium, while the spin-spin relaxation time, T_2, involves other mechanisms by which the energy of the excited nucleus is dissipated to other nuclei.[54,55] Values of T_1 and T_2 depend on the environment of the excited hydrogen nucleus. Signal intensity depends on how the images are recorded. Two conventional techniques involve the use of pulsed microwaves to record the NMR signals. In the ''spin-echo'' technique the signal intensity is given by

$$I = M_\infty \exp(-2\tau/T_2)\{1 - 2\exp(-[T_r - \tau]/T_1) + \exp(-T_r/T_1)\} \qquad (2)$$

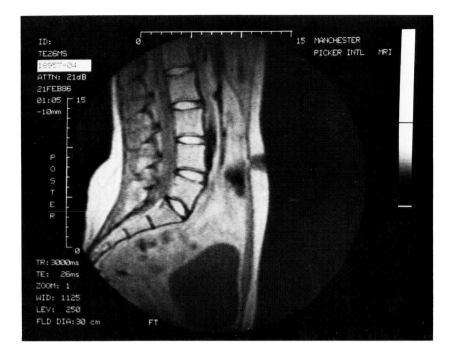

FIGURE 8.   Nuclear magnetic resonance image of the human lumbar spine (21-year-old female) in which the annulus and nucleus of each disc can be clearly distinguished.

where τ is the time period between pulses and T_r is the repetition time of the sequence.[54,56] In the "saturation recovery" technique the signal intensity is given by[56,57]

$$I = M_\infty \exp(-2\tau/T_2)\{1 - \exp(-T_r/T_1)\} \tag{3}$$

There are robust numerical techniques which allow T_1 and T_2 to be computed from the signal corresponding to each pixel in the raw NMR image.[56] Both T_1 and T_2 decrease with age; also there is a highly significant difference in T_1 values between normal and degenerate discs at all ages. For example, degenerate discs have T_1 = 421 ± 28 ms (mean ± SE), which is appreciably lower than for the oldest normal discs investigated (age range 61 to 70 years), which yield a value of 563 ± 33 ms, and very much lower than for the youngest age group (11 to 20 years), where the value was 951 ± 39 ms.[51] Thus the structural changes in the nucleus which accompany aging and degeneration occur even at the molecular level.

C. Annulus

Collagen fibrils in the annulus aggregate into crimped fibers whose appearance is reminiscent of the fibers which occur in tendon. The crimped structure has been demonstrated most clearly in fibers teased from the annulus and examined by scanning electron microscopy (SEM).[58]

Figure 9 is a schematic representation of the structure of the annulus. Two adjacent lamellae are represented as coaxial cylindrical sheets; in this figure the inner lamella has been displaced upwards along the spinal axis to produce an exploded view in which its structure can be clearly seen. In each lamella the fibers are parallel and tilted with respect to the axis of the spine; the direction of tilt alternates in successive lamellae as shown in Figure 9. As a result, the nucleus is contained by layers of fibrocartilage in which the bands of fibers cross over each other in successive layers. This pattern of tilted fibers can be observed by dissection of the disc, since individual fibers can be distinguished with the naked eye,[59] as well as by

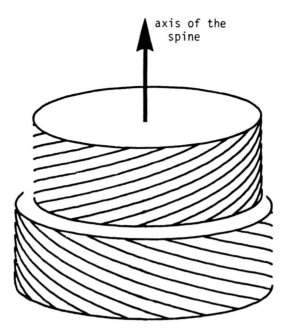

axis of the
spine

FIGURE 9.   Exploded view of two adjacent annular lamellae,
in which the inner lamella has been displaced upwards so that
its structure can be seen. Each lamella contains parallel collagen
fibers which are tilted with respect to the spinal axis direction;
the direction of tilt alternates from one lamella to the next.

light microscopy[22] and SEM.[25,60-62] Advantages and disadvantages of various techniques for measuring the orientations of collagen fibrils in tissues have been discussed elsewhere.[63]

The most convenient technique for measuring the fiber angle precisely is X-ray diffraction. High-angle X-ray diffraction patterns, like Figure 10, can be readily recorded from excised portions of human annulus and from the intact discs of small mammals. The most obvious feature of this pattern is an intense cross; the angle at which the fibers of the annulus are tilted, with respect to the direction of the spinal axis, is given by half the obtuse angle between the arms of the cross.[64] High-angle X-ray diffraction patterns like Figure 10 have been widely used to measure the tilt angle in adult,[42,43,64,65] fetal,[66] and aging human annulus[67] as well as in the annulus of other mammals.[67-69] The technique has also been used to demonstrate reorientation of fibers during compression,[70] bending, and torsion[71] of intact rabbit discs and so provides confirmation of theories relating disc structure to function[72] which are described later in this chapter. An advantage of X-ray diffraction for many of these studies is that fully hydrated tissues can be examined.[73] Similar measurements can be made on low-angle X-ray diffraction patterns[74] but high-angle diffraction experiments are more convenient to perform because it does not take so long to record the patterns.[63] As a result of all these experiments, it is now well established that the annular fibers are tilted by about 60 to 70° with respect to the spinal axis direction. Recent measurements indicate that discs from the thoracic and lumbar regions of the human spine have tilt angles of 70 $\pm$ 2° (mean $\pm$ standard deviation), which are slightly higher than those of 65 $\pm$ 2° (significant at the $p = 0.001$ level) from the cervical region.[7]

There is a steady increase in the proportion of collagen from the inner to the outer annulus;[30,41,75] there is also a variation in the genetic type of collagen present. Inner annulus contains mainly the same type II collagen which occurs in hyaline cartilage; the outer lamellae of both human and pig discs contain appreciable proportions of the type I collagen which occurs predominantly in tendon and fibrous cartilage.[76-78] This difference in composition

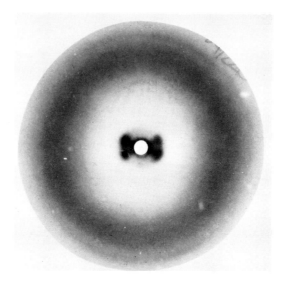

FIGURE 10.   High-angle X-ray diffraction pattern recorded from a sample of human annulus with copper K_α X-rays (wavelength 0.154 nm). The sample was kept fully hydrated during exposure to X-rays.

may reflect the need of the inner and outer regions of the annulus to blend into very different tissues while maintaining the strength of the structure. Outer lamellae, which like tendon attach to bone, contain type I collagen — as does bone itself.[79] Type II collagen predominates in hyaline cartilage[79] — the material of the end-plates into which the inner lamellae merge. However, it may be that type I collagen arises from the repair of the outer lamellae, since scars contain type I collagen[80] and small scars occur in the outer annulus of degenerate discs.[81]

Annular fibers do not consist of collagen alone, but like the fibers in tendon, consist of a mixture of components; as a result they are presumed, like other connective tissues, to function as composite materials.[39] Although the presence of elastic fibers has been controversial in the past, it has now been clearly established by light[82] and electron microscopy.[67,83,84] Elastic fibers consist of two components — the rubber-like protein elastin and the elastic fiber microfibrils which are composed of glycoprotein.[85] During the early stages of development, microfibrils form the bulk of the fibers so that they have an obviously fibrous appearance in the electron microscope,[85] which can be clearly seen in micrographs of human fetal annulus.[84] During development the proportion of elastin increases[85] and so elastic fibers appear more amorphous in micrographs of adult human annulus.[67] It has been proposed that the function of elastic fibers is to confer resilience on the annular fibers, i.e., to make them less susceptible to suddenly applied forces;[86] this proposal will be discussed in more detail in Section III.B. Furthermore, Johnson et al.[82] have shown that elastic fibers only occur in those regions of the annulus close to its attachments with the vertebrae and end-plates.

Collagen fibrils in the annular fibers are surrounded by a layer of hydrated proteoglycan gel, as shown in Figure 11. This gel also forms the bulk of the nucleus as described in Section II.B. However, proteoglycans which cannot form aggregates with hyaluronic acid are concentrated in the nucleus,[30] whereas those of the annulus tend to aggregate and so be more firmly bound within the tissue. Aggregation may be less important within the nucleus, because it is contained within a closed vessel of inner lamellae and end-plates from which the high molecular weight proteoglycans are unlikely to diffuse. However, it would appear

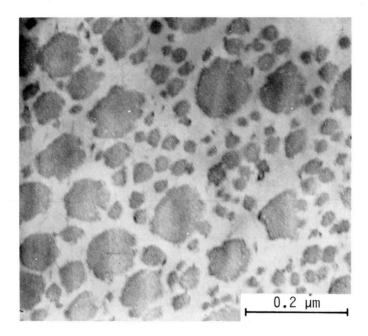

FIGURE 11. Transmission electron micrograph of a section of human annulus showing the collagen fibrils, in transverse section. The space between fibrils is considered to be occupied by a proteoglycan gel.

more important to protect the periphery of the disc, i.e., the annulus, from the possible effects of proteoglycan loss by the formation of aggregates.

The main structural change which occurs in the annulus during aging is the appearance of larger-diameter collagen fibrils.[67] Figure 12 compares the distribution of collagen fibril diameters in the annulus of a 16-year-old and an 86-year old human disc. In the younger specimen, there is a single peak centered at 30 nm and the narrow distribution of diameters closely resembles that measured from fetal material.[84] The older specimen differs from the younger in two important respects. First, the major peak, although still centered near 30 nm, is broader. Second, and even more importantly, an appreciable number of larger-diameter fibrils has appeared.[67] Whether these larger fibrils are aggregates of smaller ones, or whether they are a result of growth during aging, or whether they consist of new collagen, is unknown.

Perhaps the increase in the proportion of type I collagen during aging of the annulus is implicated in the appearance of these larger-diameter fibrils, since type I fibrils are generally thicker than those of type II collagen.[76] Appearance of wide, banded structures in the aging nucleus, which may be collagen fibrils,[48] has already been noted in Section II.B, as has the possible similarity with aging changes in hyaline cartilage.[49,50] Formation of large-diameter collagen fibrils possibly features in the aging of nucleus, annulus, and hyaline cartilage.

The characteristic pattern of tilted fibers shown in Figure 9 does not change during aging, and the tilt angle remains the same as in the fetus.[67] It had been suggested that fiber tilt decreases during aging in the anterior annulus of the human disc.[42] However, this suggestion was based on measurements of only a few discs, including one fetal specimen which was measured to have an abnormally low tilt of 45° by polarized light microscopy — normally the value for fetal discs is identical to those for adults.[66]

More recently, the tilt angle has been measured in anterior, lateral, and posterior samples of annulus from ten human lumbosacral discs covering an age range of 0 to 86 years. Figure 13 shows, as an example, the spread of values obtained from the anterior samples; there is no correlation between fiber tilt and age in these (linear correlation coefficient r = 0.24)

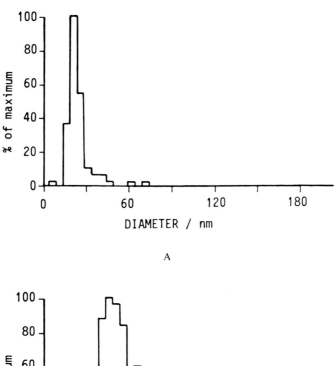

A

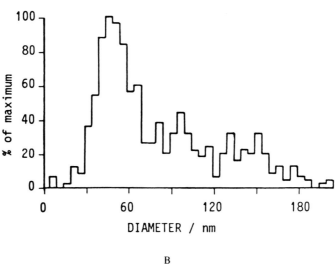

B

FIGURE 12.   Histogram showing the distribution of collagen fibril diameters in (A) 16-year-old (female) and (B) 86-year-old (female) annulus. (Data from reference 67.)

or the other samples.[67] Genetic and environmental differences between individuals might lead to a wide spread of values in a human population, which could cause slight aging changes to be imperceptible. Therefore, the experiment was repeated on specimens from 36 mice of the same strain, specially reared for aging research. Figure 14 shows that no significant change occurs in the fiber tilt of the ventral annulus during aging (corresponding to the anterior annulus in the human disc); a similar absence of change was noted in the dorsal and lateral annulus.[67] Thus, the overall structure of the annulus does not change during aging, although there are some changes in chemical composition[30,36,44] and in the distribution of collagen fibril diameters.

D. End-Plates

The end-plates are composed of hyaline cartilage, which is a clear "glassy" tissue lacking the obviously fibrous appearance of the fibrocartilage which forms the annulus. Nevertheless,

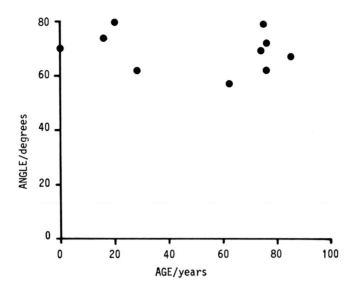

FIGURE 13.   Collagen fiber tilt measured from the anterior annulus of ten human discs (age range fetal to 86 years). (Data from References 67 and 84.)

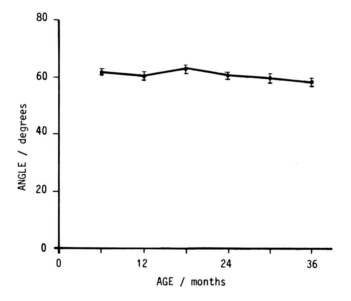

FIGURE 14.   Collagen fiber tilt measured from the anterior annulus of the discs from 36 mice of the same strain; each point represents the mean of six measurements and the error bars represent the standard error of the mean. (Data from reference 67.)

hyaline cartilage also consists of a hydrated proteoglycan gel reinforced by collagen fibrils.[8] Thus, end-plates are reminiscent of the articular cartilage of synovial joints. However, in complete contrast to articular cartilage, which is firmly attached to the subchondral bone by its collagen fibrils,[87,88] there are no collagenous connections directly anchoring the end-plates to the bone of the underlying vertebral bodies.[25]

End-plates are directly connected to the lamellae which form the inner one-third of the annulus,[24,25] as shown schematically in Figure 4 and by the scanning electron micrograph of Figure 15. The micrograph clearly shows that there is not a sharp discontinuity between

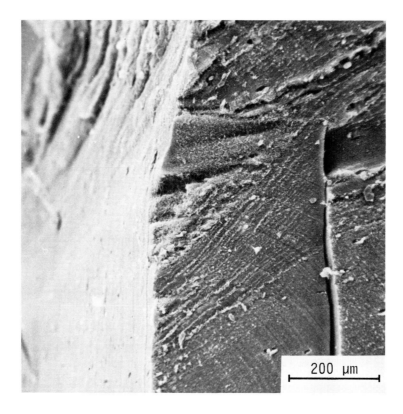

FIGURE 15.   Scanning electron micrograph showing the inner lamellae of the annulus merging into an end-plate of a human disc.

annulus and end-plate, despite their differing textures, but that one structure gradually merges into the other. Indeed lamellae can be distinguished in some scanning electron micrographs of the end-plate, as shown in Figure 16, which may account for the parallel "fibers" observed by Peacock[21] using the light microscope. Figure 16 shows that the wider true fibers in the end-plates have diameters of around 200 nm, which are too small to be resolved by the light microscope, and are probably individual collagen fibrils. These collagen fibrils tend to be oriented parallel to the surface of the end-plates, i.e., roughly horizontally in Figure 4.[24,25]

III. PROPERTIES OF THE COMPONENTS

A. Swelling Pressure

The extracellular matrix, whose structure is shown schematically in Figure 7, has a high density of fixed negative charges because of the proteoglycans which it contains.[31,32,89] Proteoglycans consist of glycosaminoglycans covalently bound to a protein core. Glycosaminoglycans contain carboxylate ($-CO_2^-$) and, except for hyaluronic acid, sulfate ($-SO_4^-$) groups which are not free to diffuse out of the matrix, because they are part of a complex, high molecular weight polymer.[34,37] Indeed aggregation of proteoglycans (described in Section II.B) to form a macromolecular network containing negatively charged polymers makes diffusion out of the tissue even more unlikely. These conclusions are supported by experiments on articular cartilage in which proteoglycans were chemically removed from the tissue. The remainder of the matrix was found to be not appreciably charged at physiological pH.[31,90] Furthermore, the fixed-charge density of cartilagenous tissues measured by physical-chemical techniques corresponds with expectations based on their glycosaminoglycan contents.[91,92]

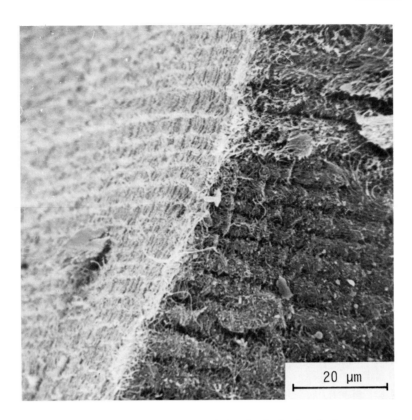

FIGURE 16. Scanning electron micrograph showing laminations in the structure of human end-plate.

Because of its fixed negative charge density, the matrix attracts water.[31,32] The fixed negative charges associated with the polyanionic glycosaminoglycans will be electrostatically balanced by mobile cations, e.g., Ca^{2+}. Although the polyanions cannot diffuse out, mobile anions, e.g., PO_4^{3-}, can diffuse into the tissue from the surrounding fluids. These mobile anions must be electrically balanced by further mobile cations which can also diffuse into the tissue. As a result, the matrix has a higher concentration of mobile ions than its surroundings and so has a higher osmotic pressure. Because of its enhanced osmotic pressure, the extracellular matrix attracts water. Since the tendency to attract water depends on the fixed charge density, it also depends on the proportion of glycosaminoglycans in a tissue. As a result, the nucleus of a healthy disc attracts more water than the annulus because it contains a higher proportion of glycosaminoglycans.[47] The distribution of water in the disc has been measured by chemical analysis,[41,47] but more recently it has been determined by computing M_∞ in of Equations 2 and 3, for each pixel in an NMR image.[93] As a result, an image like Figure 17 is obtained in which the contrast can be directly related to the water content of each part of the disc; a densitometric trace across the image then yields the distribution of water, e.g., corresponding to a sagittal section in Figure 17.

The extracellular matrix tends to swell because it attracts water by osmosis; as a result, it exerts a "swelling pressure" which enables it to support an applied load.[31,32,89,92] This explanation for swelling pressure has been tested by extracting proteoglycans from intervertebral disc and other cartilagenous tissues. They were then redissolved in "physiological saline" at comparable concentrations to those encountered in vivo and the osmotic pressures of the solutions measured. These measured osmotic pressures were in good agreement with those predicted by the mechanism described above.[94] As a result, it is argued that the fixed-charge density of the proteoglycans leads the matrix to exert an osmotic swelling pressure

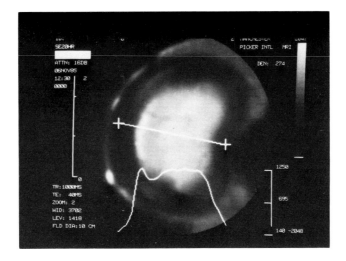

FIGURE 17.   Nuclear magnetic resonance image computed from M_x values for a transverse section of a human (16-year-old female) disc; the densitometer trace along the midline is a measure of the hydration of the disc in sagittal section.

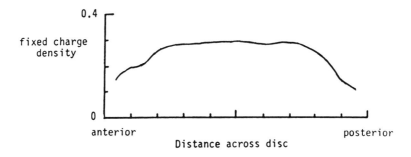

FIGURE 18.   Fixed-charge density across a sagittal section of a human disc (28-year-old). (Data from reference 94.)

which can support an applied load,[31,32,89,92] in much the same way as air pressure in a tire supports the weight of a car.

A consequence of this argument is that most of the compressive load acting on a healthy disc, along the direction of the spinal axis, is balanced by the nucleus.[86] Figure 18 shows that the nucleus of a healthy disc has a fixed-charge density which is about twice as great as the average value for the annulus — accounting for the distribution of water shown in Figure 17.[47] Thus, if the average annular swelling pressure is p, the nuclear swelling pressure is 2p. In order to estimate the forces exerted by these two regions of the disc, when subject to axial compression, it is necessary to calculate their cross-sectional areas. Both the disc as a whole and the nucleus are roughly elliptical in transverse section. For a human lumbar disc, typical semi-minor and semi-major axes would be 1.70 and 2.45 cm; corresponding values for the nucleus are 1.20 and 1.95 cm.[20] The force exerted by the nucleus (cross-sectional area × pressure) is then

$$1.20 \times 1.95\pi \times 2p = 4.68\pi p \qquad (4)$$

Similarly the force exerted by the annulus is

$$\{(1.70 \times 2.45) - (1.20 \times 1.95)\} \pi \times p = 1.83\pi p \qquad (5)$$

so that the force exerted by the intact disc is

$$(4.68 + 1.83)\pi p = 6.51\pi p \qquad (6)$$

Thus, the relative force exerted by the nucleus, expressed as a percentage of the total for an intact disc is

$$100(4.68\pi p/6.51\pi p) = 72\% \qquad (7)$$

i.e., the nucleus supports about 70% of the compressive force acting on a disc along the axis of the spine.

This view of the function of the nucleus was first clearly postulated by Naylor et al.,[64] but has been consistently challenged by Farfan.[20] Experimental evidence is conflicting. Injection of extra fluid into the nuclei of cadaveric discs increases their stiffness, thus emphasizing the importance of the fluid content of the nucleus in supporting applied load.[95,96] More directly, it has been shown that removal of the nucleus from living baboon discs changes the response of the spine to oscillatory compression.[97] In contrast, measurements on human cadaveric discs have suggested that removal of the nucleus has little influence on the response of the disc to compression.[98] Measurements of pressure distribution under discs during in vitro compression are conflicting[99,100] The interpretation of these experiments has, furthermore, ignored the perturbing influence of the pressure transducers, which could lead to serious systematic error.[101] Some measurements of nuclear pressure in vitro indicate its importance in withstanding axial compression[4,102] while others do not.[103,104] Similar in vivo measurements of pressure in the nucleus emphasize its importance in the response of the disc to applied load.[4,102]

On balance, it appears that the nucleus plays the major part in withstanding axial load on the healthy disc. However, the role of the annulus is not negligible, and the nucleus may not act so effectively in the aging disc when its water content is much reduced. The relatively fluid appearance of the nucleus in Figures 6 and 17 suggests a tissue which is well suited to transmitting compression — a function similar to that of brake fluid in a car. In contrast, the laminated structure of the annulus suggests some form of container. This suggestion is emphasized by the way in which the inner lamellae merge into the end-plates to completely enclose the nucleus, as shown in Figures 4 and 16. Calculations presented above indicate that the annulus must directly withstand some of the axial load transmitted to the disc, but that its contribution is not so great as that of the nucleus. Indeed, a clear distinction in function is not to be expected since there is no sharp boundary between the nucleus and annulus (see Section II.A). The gradual transition from one to the other is emphasized by the water content plotted in Figure 17, which undergoes a gradual transition from the high value in the nucleus to the low value in the outer annulus. During aging, the water content of the nucleus, but not of the annulus, falls dramatically in human discs as described in Section II.B. This fall in water content is a result of decreased fixed-charge density.[47] It has been argued, however, that it is more profitable to consider young discs when trying to understand the functions of their different regions.[86] The human nucleus does not become completely fibrotic until about 40 years of age[21] (which is relatively late in life), suggesting that, like wrinkles in the skin which appear at about the same age, the fibrotic nucleus confers no functional advantage. Thus it seems reasonable to suppose that the relatively fluid nucleus with its high fixed-charge density has the function of supporting axial load.

When the body is supine, the swelling pressure does not lead to axial expansion of the spine because of tension in the ligaments and muscles.[32] Although the swelling pressure tends to push two adjacent vertebrae apart, the axial resultant of these tensions tends to pull them together again. Thus the system is in equilibrium, at least in the axial direction, provided that the tensile forces are sufficient to balance the internal pressure. It has been shown that, in the young human spine, the ligamentum flavum is stretched so that it is in tension even when the muscles are relaxed; the restoring force, which can be as high as 15 N, is adequate to balance a swelling pressure of about 0.07 MN m^{-2} which is comparable to that measured in cadaveric spines.[105]

There are two reasons why consideration of swelling pressure alone is inadequate for understanding the stability of the disc when it is subjected to compressive forces. First, compression creates shear stresses within a material (see, for example, Reference 106). Axial compression of a mucoid tissue, like the nucleus, would simply squeeze it sideways, unless it were effectively contained. Second, the pressure in a fluid is isotropic — it acts radially as well as axially. Once again, effective containment is essential if the swelling pressure is not simply to lead to leakage of fluid. To return to the analogy drawn earlier, the brake fluid in a car is contained within pipes; the force applied to the pedal will not be transmitted to the brakes if fluid can leak out. Figure 4 shows that the nucleus is contained within the annulus and the end-plates. Actually the disc is more complicated than this simple analogy suggests because some fluid is lost during sustained compression,[107] presumably in order to dissipate some of the potentially damaging energy stored by the compressed structure. Energy dissipation will be discussed further in subsequent sections. Nevertheless, the nucleus remains contained by the annulus during compression of the disc. In order to understand how the annulus can contain the radial component of the swelling pressure, it is necessary to consider its structure shown schematically in Figure 9. However, it will first be necessary to understand something of the properties of its fibers which are an essential feature of this structure.

B. Fiber Tension

Fibers reinforce biological and engineering structures because they can withstand tension.[89,106,108-110] Muscles generate tension because they actively contract, pulling their points of attachment closer together; in contrast, collagenous fibers are passive components which become stretched by the forces acting on them.[3,86] When a collagen fiber is stretched, the restoring stress in the stretched fiber is able to balance an applied force.[109] Thus their function resembles that of the steel cables supporting a suspension bridge; the weight of the bridge is balanced by the tension in the stretched cables. The similarity of annular fibers to tendon, in both composition and structure, has already been noted in Section II.C. Tendons have negligible flexural or torsional stiffness and simply buckle under directly applied axial compression. However, they are stiff and strong when subjected to axial tension which tends to stretch them.

Collagen fibers can then only reinforce a tissue if they are oriented so that they tend to be stretched by an applied force.[63,109,110] If they are not stretched in their axial direction, they cannot generate a restoring force and are ineffective. Exactly the same principles apply to engineering structures which rely on ropes (rigging of sailing ships) steel cables (suspension bridges), etc.,[106] and in synthetic materials which are reinforced by glass, polymer, or carbon fibers.[108] A simple example is provided by guy ropes which will only hold up a tent if they point in the right directions, i.e., if they are properly oriented.

The importance of correct orientation of reinforcing fibers in tissues indicates that the annulus is not directly responsible for withstanding much of the pressure applied to the disc. Axial compression of the annulus tends to compress its fibers, if they are not subjected to any other forces. When fiber-reinforced materials are compressed, their fibers tend to buckle either cooperatively, as shown in Figure 19a, or noncooperatively, as shown in Figure 19 b.[108] Each fiber simply buckles like a tendon — the surrounding material (proteoglycan gel

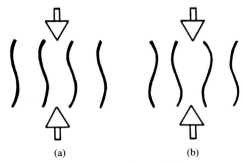

FIGURE 19. (a) Cooperative and (b) noncooperative buckling of the fibers in a composite material subjected to compression in the fiber axis direction.

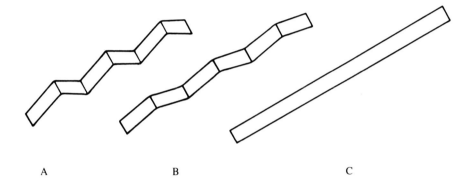

FIGURE 20. Appearance of a crimped fiber (a) unstretched; (b) in an intermediate stage of stretching, showing partial removal of the crimp; and (c) stretched sufficiently to remove the crimp.

in the annulus) may influence the mode of buckling (cooperative or noncooperative), but does not prevent it.[108] Thus, the annulus does not have a suitable structure for withstanding directly applied compression. However, we have already seen, in Section III.A, that the nucleus of a healthy disc has a high internal pressure and so supports most of the compressive load. We shall see, in Section IV.C, that in an intact disc the radial component of this pressure places the fibers of the annulus in tension, so that they are stretched when the disc is compressed. As a result they do not tend to buckle.

Many of the mechanical properties of annular fibers have not been investigated, and the results of those experiments which have been performed tend to be inconclusive. Results of tensile strength measurements parallel to the spinal axis direction vary widely.[111] Other measurements of tensile strength and stiffness[112] appear to be unreliable,[113] perhaps because of the way in which fiber orientation was allowed for in their interpretation.[69] Allowance for fiber orientation is complicated because reorientation occurs when strips of annulus are subjected to tensile stress in the testing experiments.[114]

Nevertheless, many of the properties of annular fibers can be inferred from the properties of tendons which they closely resemble. In both tissues, the collagen fibrils aggregate into fibers with an obvious crimped appearance shown schematically in Figure 20a.[58] On average, the proportion of collagen in the annulus is only about half that of tendon (compare References 112 and 115), but it increases from the inner to the outer lamellae.[41] In the initial stages of stretching, a tendon is relatively extensible because the crimp has to be removed before the tissue develops its maximum stiffness.[116] Figure 20b shows an intermediate stage of crimp removal, and Figure 20c shows a straightened fiber which is much stiffer. Figure 21 then shows the stress (force/cross-sectional area) required to develop a given strain

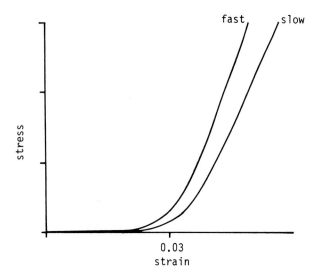

FIGURE 21. Schematic diagram showing the stress (force/cross-sectional area) required to develop a given strain (fractional increase in length) during fast and slow stretching of a tendon.

(fractional increase in length) in a tendon.[116-122] The steepness of the curve, which is a measure of the stiffness of the material, gradually increases until the crimp is removed at a strain of around 0.03 to 0.04.[116] Figure 21 also shows that a tendon is stiffer if it is stretched rapidly than if it is stretched slowly;[120] this behavior is typical of a viscoelastic material.

Viscoelastic materials have time-dependent mechanical properties, because they do not store all of the energy which is transferred to them when they are deformed by an applied force.[123] For example, when a material is stretched, its energy increases. An elastic material stores this deformation energy so that it recoils immediately to its original dimensions when the deforming force ceases to be applied. The other extreme of mechanical behavior is exemplified by a liquid which is sheared by an applied force and does not store any of its deformation energy — as a result, it cannot return itself to its original position once the applied force has been removed. Liquids have some resistance to flow which is termed "viscosity". A viscoelastic material is intermediate in its mechanical properties — it dissipates some of the energy used to deform it and so may not return immediately to its original dimensions when the deforming force is removed. Viscoelasticity of collagenous tissues is discussed in more detail elsewhere.[109,110] All of the properties described in this paragraph are demonstrated by tendon[117,118,120-122] and so, presumably, by annular fibers.

Dissipation of deformation energy by viscoelastic materials protects them against fracture, but this protective mechanism can fail during cyclic loading. If excessive energy is supplied to a fiber-reinforced composite material, like a collagenous tissue, the material can fracture in a variety of ways which are effectively damaging mechanisms for dissipating energy.[108] Viscoelastic materials have alternative mechanisms, which are not damaging, for dissipating this energy. However, it takes a finite time for energy to be dissipated and, when the deforming force ceases to be applied, a viscoelastic material may return to its original dimensions gradually. As a result, a tendon which is subject to successive cycles of stretching and relaxing becomes stiffer and, after about 50 cycles dissipates very little of the energy supplied to it.[117,120,122] Under such conditions, fatigue failure may occur where the material fractures at a lower stress that it would normally be able to support.[108]

Changes occur in the mechanical properties of tendons at strains of about 0.03 to 0.04 which may be potentially damaging. It has been reported that rat tail tendons which are

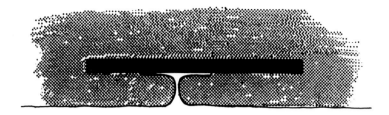

FIGURE 22.   Deflection of a crack in a proteoglycan gel by a collagen fibril.

stretched to strains above 0.04 retain a residual strain when the stretching force is removed.[120] I have previously interpreted this result as implying that the tendon is damaged — in the sense that it has undergone an irreversible change.[109] However, an alternative explanation is that, at such high strains, a tendon simply takes much longer to return to its original length. Such an interpretation still implies that these high strains are potentially hazardous because, if the tendon takes so long to relax, it could be damaged by further loads being applied before its energy dissipation mechanisms have recovered. The distinction between a permanent deformation and slow recovery is perhaps not important in vivo where biological mechanisms exist to repair damaged tissues. The extent to which these mechanisms may operate in the annulus has been discussed elsewhere.[11,86,124]

Ultimately, the mechanical properties of the annular fibers depend upon their composition. Each fiber consists of collagen fibrils surrounded by proteoglycan gel (see Section II.C) and is, therefore, itself a fiber-reinforced material. By analogy with the behavior of synthetic composite materials,[108] it appears that tensile stress tends to shear the interface between the collagen fibrils and the surrounding gel. The fibrils reinforce the tissue because they tend to be stretched by these shear forces.[39] The result is a fiber which is stiff and strong in tension whose viscoelastic properties, at least in the case of tendon, can be explained in terms of the properties of the proteoglycan gel and the collagen fibrils.[125] In tendon, and presumably in annular fibers, the crimp arises because the individual collagen fibrils are crimped.[126] When a fiber is stretched, the fibrils will be straightened by shear of the gel phase before they are directly stretched themselves.[39,127] The fiber does not, therefore, acquire its maximum stiffness until the crimp is removed at strains of 0.03 to 0.04.[116] Shear forces can lead to propagation of cracks across the proteoglycan gel. Once again, by analogy with the properties of synthetic materials,[108] the collagen fibrils are expected to protect the fiber against fracture by preventing cracks from spreading. Figure 22 shows a crack propagating through the proteoglycan gel, perpendicular to the axis of the fiber — the direction in which it would form under tension.[128] Eventually, it encounters a collagen fibril. Because the fibril is much stronger than its interface with the gel,[39,125] the interface is sheared and the crack deflected. If the fibril is sufficiently long, the crack will not continue around its ends so that catastrophic failure is averted.

It has been suggested that the elastic fibers provide protection against the potentially damaging effects of sudden loading on the annular fibers.[86] Materials have been formulated for engineering applications in which a few fibers with high strength but low stiffness are incorporated into a conventional fiber-reinforced composite material. Incorporation of these low-stiffness fibers confers extra resilience on the material.[108] Since elastic fibers are much less stiff than collagen fibrils, they may have a similar effect on the properties of annular fibers.

IV. MECHANICAL FUNCTION

A. Twisting

It is clear from the preceding section that torsion of the disc must stretch the collagen

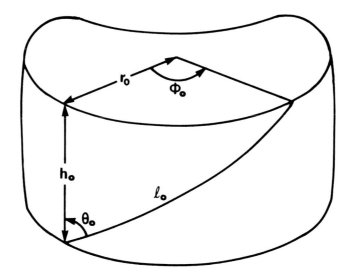

FIGURE 23.   Schematic diagram of a fibril in a single lamella of the annulus, defining fiber length, ℓ, tilt, θ, and azimuthal span, ϕ. The lamella has local height, h, and radius of curvature, r, for its transverse section in the region of the fiber.

fibers of the annulus if they are to provide reinforcement; only then will the disc be stable during twisting of the spine. This section is concerned with a model for the relationship between the structure and mechanical function of the disc, which explains how torsion leads to fiber strain.[72,129] In the next four paragraphs the mathematical details of the model are developed. These four paragraphs may be ignored without loss of continuity, by those readers who are not interested in the mathematical details — the mathematical paragraphs are followed by a qualitative discussion of the implications of the model.

Figure 23 shows a fiber in a single lamella of the annulus, in order to describe its geometry. This fiber has length, ℓ, and is tilted by an angle, θ, with respect to the spinal axis direction. It has an azimuthal span, φ, in a region of the lamella whose transverse section has a radius of curvature, r; the disc height in this region is h. Suppose that, when no external forces are applied to the intervertebral joint, the resting disc is described by the set of values $\{\ell_0, \theta_0, \varphi_0, r_0, h_0\}$ and in some general state by $\{\ell, \theta, \varphi, r, h\}$. Relationships between these values can be derived by simple geometry:

$$\ell_0^2 = h_0^2 + r_0^2\varphi_0^2 \quad \ell^2 = h^2 + r^2\varphi^2 \tag{8}$$

$$r_0\varphi_0 = h_0\tan\theta_0 \quad r\varphi = h\tan\theta \tag{9}$$

$$h_0 = \ell_0\cos\theta_0 \quad h = \ell\cos\theta \tag{10}$$

$$r_0\varphi_0 = \ell_0\sin\theta_0 \quad r\varphi = \ell\sin\theta \tag{11}$$

The fiber strain resulting from deforming the geometry of the disc from its resting state is defined by

$$\epsilon = (\ell - \ell_0)/\ell_0 = (\ell/\ell_0) - 1 \tag{12}$$

Thus the condition that the fiber shall reinforce the deformed disc is that ℓ/ℓ_0 is greater than

posterior

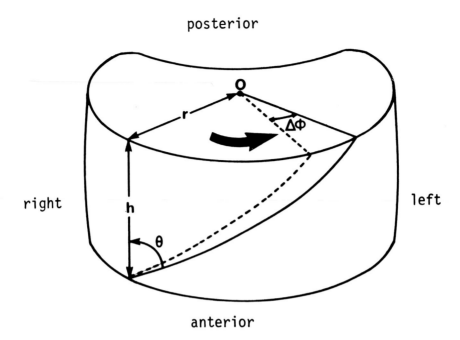

anterior

FIGURE 24. Effect of torsion, in the direction indicated by the curved arrow, on the fiber of Figure 23; the original locus of the fiber (dashed line) moves to a new position (continuous line) with consequent changes in its tilt and azimuthal span.

unity, i.e., that ϵ exceeds zero. Combining and rearranging the conditions of Equation 8 yields:

$$\frac{\ell}{\ell_0} = \left\{ 1 + \frac{(h^2 + r^2\varphi^2)}{\ell_0^2} - \frac{(h_0^2 + r_0^2\varphi_0^2)}{\ell_0^2} \right\}^{1/2} \tag{13}$$

Substituting this expression for ℓ/ℓ_0 from Equation 13 into Equation 12 gives:

$$\epsilon = \left\{ 1 + \frac{(h^2 + r^2\varphi^2)}{\ell_0^2} - \frac{(h_0^2 + r_0^2\varphi_0^2)}{\ell_0^2} \right\}^{1/2} - 1 \tag{14}$$

which will be used to consider fiber strain arising from torsion and bending (Section IV.B) of the disc.

Figure 24 shows the effect of torsion of the disc on the fiber of Figure 23. If the ends are effectively anchored, the original locus of the fiber (dashed line) will be displaced to the new locus (continuous line). Pure torsion of the disc, in the direction of the curved arrow of Figure 24, is supposed to increase the azimuthal span of the fiber by $\Delta\varphi$ while leaving the disc height and local radius of curvature unaffected; thus the condition for pure torsion can be expressed by

$$\varphi = \varphi_0 + \Delta\varphi, \quad h = h_0 \quad r = r_0 \tag{15}$$

Substituting the condition of Equation 15 into the expression for fiber strain of Equation 14 yields:

$$\epsilon = \left\{ 1 + \frac{2r_0^2}{\ell_0^2} \varphi_0 \Delta\varphi + \frac{r_0^2}{\ell_0^2} (\Delta\varphi)^2 \right\}^{1/2} - 1$$

$$= \left\{ 1 + \frac{2r_0^2}{\ell_0^2} \varphi_0 \Delta\varphi \right\}^{1/2} - 1 \quad \Delta\varphi \ll \varphi_0 \tag{16}$$

The small angle approximation is valid since, for the disc structure described in Section II.C, $\varphi_0 \approx 60°$ while for physiological torsion of the disc $\Delta\varphi \approx 3°$.[20] Substituting expressions for φ_0, from Equation 9, and ℓ_0, from Equation 11, in Equation 16 gives

$$\epsilon = \left\{ 1 + \frac{2r_0}{h_0} (\sin\theta_0 \cos\theta_0)\Delta\varphi \right\}^{1/2} - 1$$

$$= \left\{ 1 + \frac{r_0}{h_0} (\sin2\theta_0)\Delta\varphi \right\}^{1/2} - 1 \tag{17}$$

This paragraph is concerned with the assumptions underlying Equation 17. Note that $\Delta\varphi$ is only identical to a true torsion angle (the angle through which the intact disc is twisted) when the torsion axis (parallel to the axis of the spine) passes through O (Figure 24), the center of curvature of the transverse section of the lamella in this region. The exact position of the torsion axis is uncertain, but it appears to pass slightly posterior to the geometric center of the disc.[20,101] If the torsion axis does not pass exactly through O, torsion might have some small effect on r but this is not expected to be appreciable, given the position of the axis and the low values of $\Delta\varphi$ achieved in practice. Indeed intervertebral discs do not appear to change shape when twisted in vitro. In practice the disc can never be subjected to pure torsion because the axial component of muscular contraction (Section I) and the restoring forces generated by the stretched collagen fibers[20] will compress it slightly at the same time. Mechanical integrity of a fiber, i.e., the assumption that it is effectively anchored at both ends, need not imply that the individual collagen fibrils are continuous throughout its length — for reasons which are discussed elsewhere.[39]

In this paragraph the implications of Equation 17 will be discussed. It is clear from this equation that ϵ must exceed zero whenever $\Delta\varphi$ is positive, i.e., fibers tilted in the direction shown in Figure 24, but not those tilted in the opposite direction, can reinforce the disc in torsion in the direction shown. Furthermore, if h_0 is assumed constant across the thickness of the annulus and given that θ_0 does not vary, the fibers of the outer lamellae will be subjected to higher strains than those of the inner lamellae since they have higher values of r_0. In some regions of the disc, h_0 does increase with r_0. Then ϵ will be distributed more evenly between inner and outer lamellae than would be the case if h_0 remained constant.[72] However, the increase in h_0 is not sufficiently great, nor is this feature sufficiently general, to discount the conclusion that the fibers of the outer lamellae provide more reinforcement during torsion of the disc.

The underlying assumption of this model, that the annular fibers have the mechanical integrity required to provide reinforcement, has been verified by experiment. Figure 24 shows that if a fiber is stretched, i.e., if its ends are effectively anchored, θ_0 increases to a new value θ. This reorientation has been observed during in vitro torsion of fully hydrated rabbit discs by measuring θ, before and after the intervertebral disc was twisted, by X-ray diffraction.[71] The measured reorientation was consistent with that predicted by geometry.

It appears that only half the total number of annular fibers can reinforce the disc during torsion in a given direction, and that most of the reinforcement is provided by the fibers of the outer lamellae. Fibers tilted in the direction shown in Figure 24 will be stretched when a person twists to the left, as indicated by the curved arrow. However, they will not be stretched when twisting to the right because they are tilted in the wrong direction, reinforcement can then only be provided by fibers which are stretched because they have the alternative tilt direction — like those in the lamellae adjacent to that shown in Figure 24 (see Figure 9). For a disc which is roughly cylindrical in shape, fibers will be stretched more in the outer than in the inner lamellae of the annulus; thus the outer lamellae provide most of the strength in torsion.

Annular fibers are capable of withstanding the kinds of strain imposed upon them by normal twisting of the disc, which is limited to a few degrees by the facet joints.[14,20] Substituting reasonable values for r_0, h_0, and θ_0 (1 cm, 1 cm, and 65°, respectively) into Equation 17 indicates that $\Delta\varphi$ can attain a value of about 5° before the fiber strain exceeds a potentially hazardous value of around 0.03 (see Section III.B). Using $\Delta\varphi$ as a rough measure of the angular twist imparted to the disc, this result implies that the fibers can provide reinforcement during physiological twisting of around 3°.[14,20] However, if the facet joints are asymmetric, or in some way damaged, torsion may injure the disc.[11,12,20,81] Initial injury takes the form of cracks between the lamellae of the annulus[12,20,81] which resemble[69,86] delamination fractures in synthetic laminated fiber-reinforced composite materials.[108]

Finally, lumbar and cervical discs have cross-sectional shapes which do not suit them for strength in torsion. A disc which was circular in transverse section would have an even distribution of the stress arising from torsion around its circumference.[20] Although a typical thoracic disc, as shown in Figure 2, has a roughly circular cross-section, the lumbar and cervical discs do not — as exemplified by their values of S being considerably less than unity in Figure 3. Indeed, a simple electrical analogue shows that lumbar discs and, presumably, also cervical discs which have a similar cross-sectional shape (Figure 2) are subject to posterior and posteriolateral stress concentrations as a result of torsion.[20,81] These stress concentrations could lead to local areas of high energy which were potentially damaging for the disc. However, the shapes of lumbar and cervical discs do have some functional advantages which are discussed in the next section.

B. Bending

The disc will only be able to contribute to mechanical stability of the intervertebral joint during bending of the spine if its collagen fibers are stretched and so provide reinforcement. The human spine can bend forwards (flexion) much further than it can bend backwards (extension) or sideways (laterally). Thus, most of the remarks of this section are addressed directly to flexion because it places the greatest demands on the disc in bending. Nevertheless, the principles involved apply to lateral bending and extension too. Flexion of the spine involves bending of the intervertebral joints with the result that the posterior annulus is stretched[130-132] as shown in Figure 25. The next two paragraphs are concerned with the mathematical development of the model relating disc structure to mechanical function so that it includes bending;[72,129] these two paragraphs may be omitted without loss of continuity.

Figure 25a shows a sagittal section along the midline of a single lamella in the disc which is shown flexed, through an angle α, in Figure 25b. Here, h_0 is the initial posterior height of the lamella at the midline and R is the distance of the lamella from the flexion axis, which passes through the nucleus pulposus or the inner region of the anterior annulus[133,134] so that flexion stretches the posterior annulus.[130-132] As a result, the posterior height of the lamella under consideration acquires a new value, h, so that the flexed state is defined by

$$\left. \begin{array}{l} h = h_0 + \Delta h = h_0 + R \tan\alpha \\ \varphi = \varphi_0 \quad r = r_0 \end{array} \right\} \tag{18}$$

assuming that the posterior radius of curvature of the lamella, in transverse section, and the azimuthal span of a posterior fiber remain unchanged by flexion. Some slight changes are

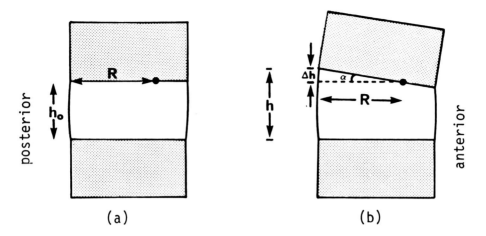

FIGURE 25.   Schematic sagittal section along the midline of a single lamella in a disc shown (a) unflexed and (b) flexed through an angle, α, about an axis at a distance, R, from the posterior margin of the lamella.

expected in the values of these parameters, but they are not expected to be so great as to influence the general argument. Substituting the condition for flexion of Equation 18 into the general expression for fiber strain of Equation 14, yields

$$\epsilon = \left\{ 1 + \frac{2h_0\Delta h + (\Delta h)^2}{\ell_0^2} \right\}^{1/2} - 1$$

$$= \left\{ 1 + \frac{2h_0 R\,\tan\alpha}{\ell_0^2} + \frac{R^2\,\tan^2\alpha}{\ell_0^2} \right\}^{1/2} - 1 \tag{19}$$

assuming that the ends of the fiber are effectively anchored (see Section IV.A). From Equations 10 and 19 the expression for posterior fiber strain becomes

$$\epsilon = \left\{ 1 + \frac{2R}{h_0}\cos^2\theta_0\tan\alpha + \frac{R^2}{h_0^2}\cos^2\theta_0\tan^2\alpha \right\}^{1/2} - 1 \tag{20}$$

Equation 20 then shows that the strain in the posterior fibers is always positive, i.e., they can reinforce the annulus during flexion of the disc, given that $\theta_0 \simeq 65°$ and that $0°\leqslant\alpha<90°$. Furthermore, this strain increases with distance from the bending axis so that the outer lamellae of the annulus are responsible for most of the strength of the disc during flexion — provided, once again, that θ_0 is constant across the thickness of the annulus and that h_0 increases less rapidly than R. It appears that h_0 does not increase from the inner to the outer lamellae of the posterior annulus, so this simple interpretation of Equation 20 appears valid, although it may be complicated by the curvature of some posterior lamellae as observed in sagittal section.

The fiber reorientation which the model predicts has been measured experimentally and shown to be in good agreement with theory. According to Equation 9

$$\frac{\tan\theta}{\tan\theta_0} = \frac{r\varphi}{r_0\varphi_0} \cdot \frac{h_0}{h} \tag{21}$$

Assuming that r_0 and φ_0 remain unchanged during bending, the condition of Equation 18 may be combined with Equation 21 to give

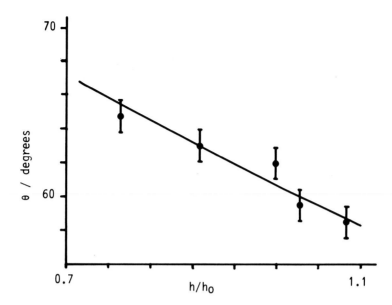

FIGURE 26. Dependence of fiber tilt, θ, on h/h_o during bending of a rabbit intervertebral disc from an extended ($h/h_o < 1$) to a flexed ($h/h_o > 1$) position.

$$\theta = \tan^{-1}\left\{ \frac{h_o}{h} \cdot \tan\theta_o \right\} \qquad (22)$$

which shows how the posterior fiber tilt decreases as the posterior height increases during flexion. This predicted reorientation of the posterior fibers has been measured experimentally during in vitro bending of an intact, fully hydrated intervertebral disc from a rabbit. In this experiment, the disc was moved, in stages, from an extended to a flexed position. At each stage the posterior disc height was measured with a travelling microscope and the fiber tilt determined by X-ray diffraction.[71] Figure 26 shows that the fiber tilt decreases as posterior height increases, in the manner predicted by Equation 22. Thus the annular fibers have the mechanical integrity to reinforce the disc as expected.

It appears that only those fibers which are posterior to the bending axis position can reinforce the annulus during flexion of the disc, and that most of the reinforcement is provided by the fibers of the outer lamellae. Anterior fibers will, of course, provide reinforcement during extension while lateral fibers are stretched considerably by lateral bending. But both of these movements involve much smaller bending angles than does flexion, and so the demands which they place on the system of reinforcing fibers are much less. Flexion, and indeed any form of bending, resembles torsion in that most of the stability which the disc provides to the intervertebral joint arises from stretching the fibers of the outer lamellae of the annulus.

The shapes of lumbar and cervical discs appear well suited to providing stability during flexion of the spine. Figure 2 shows typical shapes for lumbar and cervical discs, which, unlike the roughly circular cross-sections of some thoracic discs, place a large proportion of reinforcing fibers posterior to the bending axis.[7,72] Thus, if some fibers should be damaged by flexion, there are plenty in reserve to guard against catastrophic failure of the posterior annulus. It has been proposed, therefore, that the roughly elliptical shapes of cervical and lumbar discs help to confer stability during flexion,[72] but they are less stable than circular cross sections during torsion (Section IVA). Thus, there appear to be conflicting criteria for strength in torsion and strength in flexion, although the reasoning underlying this view has

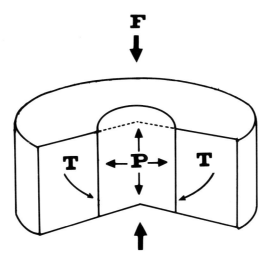

FIGURE 27.   An internal pressure, P, in the nucleus is balanced axially by an applied compressive force, F, and radially by a circumferential tensile force, T, in the annulus.

been questioned.[101] Thoracic discs adopt a shape which is stronger in torsion because they are subjected to a more limited range of flexion-extension than lumbar discs.[7] Consequently, disc shapes can be related to differing requirements for mechanical stability in different regions of the human spine.[7] Nevertheless, lumbar discs can be damaged in vitro by offset compression intended to simulate the effects of hyperflexion. As a result, hyperflexion is supposed to be a cause of disc prolapse.[135]

C. Compression

The disc is able to support compressive loads acting along the axis of the spine, because the proteoglycan gel of the nucleus pulposus, and to some extent of the annulus itself, exerts a swelling pressure as described in Section III.A. However, the system is only stable if the annulus is reinforced so that it can contain the nucleus (preventing it from being sheared laterally), and so that it can withstand the radial component (perpendicular to the axis of the spine) of the swelling pressure. Once again this problem has already been discussed in Section III.A. Figure 27 then summarizes the forces acting on the disc in which the internal pressure, P, is balanced axially by an applied compressive force, F, and radially by the tension, T, acting circumferentially within the annulus. Thus, the disc is supposed to act rather like a pressure vessel in which the internal pressure tends to stretch the walls of the container. The restoring force in the stretched walls then balances this pressure when the system is in equilibrium.[106,136] In a cylindrical pressure vessel the greater tension acts circumferentially[106,136] as illustrated by the structures of wooden barrels which are reinforced by steel hoops around their circumference — hence the circumferential stress is sometimes called "hoop stress". The question which then arises is whether tension in the system of tilted collagen fibers in the annulus is able to balance the internal pressure of the disc. This question is answered, mathematically, in the next three paragraphs which are followed by a qualitative discussion of the conclusions.

A simple model for fiber-reinforcement of the annulus, when subjected to the internal pressure of the disc, can be most easily derived from the geometry of a cylinder with a circular cross section, although the results are more general and apply to any cross-sectional shape.[72,129] The volume, V, enclosed by a single lamella with a circular cross section is given by:

$$V = \pi r^2 h \tag{23}$$

Substituting expressions for r, from Equation 11, and for h, from Equation 10, into Equation 23 gives:

$$V = \pi \left(\frac{\ell \sin\theta}{\varphi} \right)^2 \ell \cos\theta$$

$$= (\pi\ell^3/\varphi^2)\sin^2\theta \cos\theta \tag{24}$$

Compression of the disc is expected to impose changes on the values of the variables in Equation 24; for small changes

$$\frac{\delta V}{V} = \frac{\delta\ell}{\ell^3} \cdot \frac{\partial}{\partial\ell} (\ell^3) + \frac{\delta\varphi}{(1/\varphi^2)} \cdot \frac{\partial}{\partial\varphi} \left(\frac{1}{\varphi^2} \right)$$

$$+ \frac{\delta\theta}{(\sin^2\theta \cos\theta)} \cdot \frac{\partial}{\partial\theta} (\sin^2\theta \cos\theta) \tag{25}$$

When the derivatives of Equation 25 have been evaluated, it takes the form:

$$\frac{\delta V}{V} = \frac{3}{\ell} \delta\ell - \frac{1}{\varphi} \delta\varphi + \left\{ \frac{2\cos^2\theta - \sin^2\theta}{\sin\theta \cos\theta} \right\} \delta\theta \tag{26}$$

Application of this result to any stage of compression assumes that the disc passes through a series of states in which it always has cylindrical geometry. Now suppose that the azimuthal span of a fiber is unchanged by compression and that the volume of the disc is conserved, i.e.,

$$\delta\varphi/\varphi = 0 \quad \delta V/V = 0 \tag{27}$$

In reality volume is not conserved during sustained compression because some fluid tends to flow from the nucleus.[107] However, only about 1% of the fluid is lost during axial compression of a cadaveric disc over a 4-hr period.[107] Since it takes a finite time to squeeze liquid from the disc, the constant volume condition can be considered to apply when the compressive load is first applied. Substituting the conditions of Equation 27 into Equation 26 gives:

$$\frac{3\delta\ell}{\ell} = \left\{ \frac{\sin^2\theta - 2\cos^2\theta}{\sin\theta \cos\theta} \right\} \delta\theta \tag{28}$$

Fibers can only reinforce the disc if they tend to be stretched, i.e., when

$$\delta\ell/\ell > 0 \tag{29}$$

According to Equation 28, Equation 29 can only be satisfied when:

$$\sin^2\theta > 2\cos^2\theta \quad \cos\theta \neq 0 \quad \sin\theta \neq 0$$

$$\Rightarrow \tan\theta > \sqrt{2}$$

$$\Rightarrow \theta > 54.7° \quad 0 \leq \theta \leq 90° \tag{30}$$

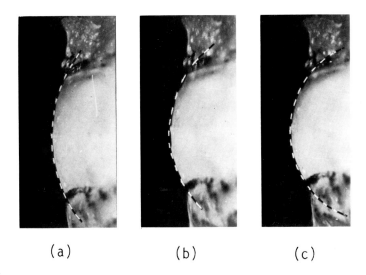

(a)   (b)   (c)

FIGURE 28.   Profile of the anterior annulus of a rabbit lumbar intervertebral disc (a) slightly compressed, (b) compressed, and (c) compressed near to failure with an arc of a circle superimposed on the anterior margin.

Thus collagen fibers of the annulus can provide reinforcement during compression of the disc since $\theta_0 \simeq 65°$ and so exceeds the critical value of Equation 30. Experimental evidence for fibers reinforcing the annulus in this way is provided by X-ray diffraction studies of fiber reorientation during compression of fully hydrated rabbit discs in vitro.[70] Equation 22 applies to compression of the disc, as well as to height changes occurring during bending. Its predictions were found to be in good agreement with the changes in fiber orientation observed experimentally.[70]

In practice, the disc does not remain cylindrical but bulges slightly during compression as shown in Figure 28. This bulging can be taken into account in more sophisticated theories of fiber reinforcement of the annulus during compression of the disc.[137,138] Figure 28 shows that, at various stages of compression, the bulge profile can be represented by an arc of a circle. This result is expected because the surface area of a lamella is then minimized for a given volume contained. The length of a fiber is then given by:

$$\ell = \int_{-\varphi_0/2}^{+\varphi_0/2} \{x^2 + [(\varphi_0/h)^2 - (\omega/f)^2]^{-1}\}^{1/2} d\omega$$

$$x = r_0 + \{f^2 - (h\omega/\varphi_0)^2\}^{1/2} - \{f^2 - (h/2)^2\}^{1/2}$$

(31)

where f is the radius of curvature of the bulge.[138] Provided ℓ, calculated from Equation 31, exceeds ℓ_0 the fiber will be able to reinforce the disc. However, not all the volume displaced by compression can be accommodated in the annular bulge; the remainder of the displaced volume must be contained by the end-plates bulging into the cancellous bone of the vertebrae.[23,138] The way in which volume is redistributed affects the critical value of θ, which must be exceeded if collagen fibers are to reinforce the annulus. For the volume redistribution observed in practice, θ needs to be about 65°, which is very close to observed values (Section II.C).[138]

Most of the reinforcement during compression is expected to be provided by collagen fibers of the inner lamellae of the annulus. Consider a cylindrical pressure vessel of internal radius, r_i, and external radius, r_e, containing a fluid which exerts a pressure, P. This pressure is balanced by a circumferential stress, σ_c, and a radial stress, σ_R, in the wall of the vessel; these stresses are related to the pressure by:

$$\left.\begin{array}{l} \sigma_c(r) = r_i^2 P\{1 + (r_e/r)^2\}/(r_e^2 - r_i^2) \\[2mm] \sigma_R(r) = r_i^2 P\{1 - (r_e/r)^2\}/(r_e^2 - r_i^2) \\[2mm] r_i \leqslant r \leqslant r_e \end{array}\right\} \qquad (32)$$

(See, for example, Reference 136). Note that, for a given value of r, σ_c is always greater than σ_R, i.e., the circumferential stress plays the greater part in balancing the internal pressure. Also both stresses take their lowest values on the outer surface of the vessel (r = r_e) where the radial stress is zero; the thicker the wall (i.e., the higher the value of r_e) the lower is the circumferential stress. Comparing the annulus with a thick-walled pressure vessel, it would appear that the inner lamellae are more important than the outer lamellae for containing the swelling pressure of the disc. Experiments confirm that the fibers of the outer lamella provide little, if any, reinforcement during compression.[59,138]

In summary, compression of the disc raises the pressure in the nucleus (Section II.A) and, as a result, the collagen fibers of the inner lamellae of the annulus are stretched, as are the collagen fibrils reinforcing the cartilage end-plates. Since collagen fibrils tend to be oriented parallel to the surfaces of the end-plates (Section II.D), the fibrils will be stretched when increased nuclear pressure causes the end-plates to bulge into the cancellous bone of the vertebral bodies.[24] Although it has been argued that end-plate bulging is negligible,[139] radiographs indicate that it occurs during in vitro compression of intervertebral joints.[140] Blood flow from the bone during such experiments is consistent with this conclusion as is the observation that the annular bulge cannot accommodate all the volume displaced.[23,138,140] Thus, increased nuclear pressure arising from axial compression of the disc can be balanced by tension in the end-plates and inner lamellae of the annulus, which enclose the nucleus (Section II.A) and are suitably reinforced by collagen.

V. CONCLUSIONS

Collagen fibers of the annulus fibrosus provide reinforcement because they are stretched when the intervertebral disc is twisted, bent, and compressed. The disc is then able to confer stability on the intervertebral joint during twisting and bending of the spine. Criteria for strength in torsion and flexion are conflicting and, as a result, discs in different regions of the spine have differing cross-sectional shapes. For example, thoracic discs tend to have a roughly circular cross section which would be expected to distribute torsional stress more evenly than the elliptical cross sections of lumbar and cervical discs, which appear less likely to be damaged by flexion. Contraction of the muscles which twist and bend the spine also leads to compression of the discs. The disc is able to withstand such compressive forces, acting along the axis of the spine, because of the swelling pressure exerted by proteoglycan gel, a component of the extracellular matrix of both the annulus and nucleus. Simple calculations suggest that the gelatinous nucleus plays the greater part in directly withstanding the compressive load. The annulus serves mainly to contain the nucleus, preventing it from being sheared laterally (perpendicular to the axis of the spine) by applied loads and its own internal swelling pressure, because its pattern of tilted collagen fibers provides the necessary reinforcement. Indeed the inner lamallae of the annulus merge into the vertebral end-plates to form a vessel which completely encloses the nucleus.

There appears to be some specialization of function within the annulus — the outer lamellae provide strength during twisting and bending while the inner lamellae are mainly responsible for strength in compression. Since compression of the disc arises as a result of twisting and bending the spine, this specialization need not lead to an uneven distribution of stress between the inner and outer lamellae. Specialization arises because the collagen fibers of the outer lamellae will be stretched most whenever the disc is twisted or bent. However, the inner lamellae will have to provide most of the circumferential stress required to balance the internal swelling pressure exerted by the nucleus — by analogy with the mechanics of thick-walled pressure vessels. Although this functional specialization was proposed on mechanical grounds, it is consistent with some features of the anatomy of the disc. The attachment of the inner lamellae to cartilage end-plates to form a vessel enclosing the pressurized nucleus has already been mentioned. In contrast, the outer lamellae of the annulus are attached to the vertebral bodies so that their fibers will be stretched directly when one vertebra moves relative to another during twisting and bending of the spine. Furthermore, the outer lamellae contain a type of collagen not found in the inner lamellae which may reflect some difference in function.

Differing attachments of the inner and outer lamellae emphasize that the structure and function of the intervertebral disc cannot be considered completely in isolation from the rest of the spinal column. The alternating arrangement of discs and vertebral bodies, together with the longitudinal ligaments (Figure 1), form the anterior spinal column. Flexion of the spine tends to stretch the posterior longitudinal ligaments, while extension stretches the anterior longitudinal ligaments.[16] Since these ligaments consist of crimped collagen fibers with mechanical properties reminiscent of tendon,[141,142] they can then assist the disc in providing stability during flexion and extension of an intervertebral joint.[16]

It appears that the cancellous bone, which forms the interior of the vertebral bodies, is also compressed by the axial component of the forces generated by muscular contraction. Indeed, the vertebral end-plates may bulge into the vertebral bodies indicating that the nucleus, when contained by the annulus, is less compressible than the cancellous bone.[23,138,140] Compression of intervertebral joints to failure in vitro invariably leads to fracture of the vertebral bodies and cracking of the end-plates, rather than to damage of the annulus,[98,111,140,143] similar fractures occur in vivo[144] and lumbar vertebrae somtimes show signs of trabecular microfractures.[145,146] During in vitro compression of intervertebral joints, blood is squeezed from the bone through the perivertebral sinuses.[140] Blood flow in vivo might then provide a mechanism for dissipating some of the energy stored by a compressed spine and, hence, help to protect against fracture.[23,140] This suggestion is consistent with the considerable capacity of vertebral veins, which "must be considered emissary veins rather than nutrient veins draining the blood,[147] and with their absence of valves, so that blood can flow back into the vertebrae to restore their mechanical properties.[23]

Finally the posterior bony structures of the vertebrae, which form the neural arch surrounding the spinal cord, together with their associated ligaments and facet joints, also influence the mechanical stability of the spinal column. In particular, the facet joints limit torsion in the lumbar spine and so help to protect its discs from injury.[14] Capsular ligaments of the facet joints also help to confer stability on the spinal column.[11-16] Although the interspinous and supraspinous ligaments exhibit high strains during in vitro flexion,[16] they do not appear to be sufficiently stiff and seem far too flimsy, at least in some mammals, to provide reinforcement during flexion of the spine.

It is the combination of the mechanical properties of all its parts which leads to mechanical stability of the spine. Nevertheless, the discs are the major structures of the intervertebral joints, which are mainly responsible for conferring flexibility along most of the spinal column. They enable the spine to adopt the wide range of postures essential for it to function satisfactorily as the main component of the axial skeleton.

ACKNOWLEDGMENTS

Many of the ideas in this chapter were developed in collaboration with Richard Aspden, Steve Hickey and Jeremy Klein; the experiments, on which these ideas are based, were performed in collaboration with them, Karen Davies, and Jagtar Pooni. I am grateful to Karen Davies for preparing the illustrations and to Celia Hukins for help with the literature, as well as to Pat Mellor and Peggy Burt for typing the manuscript.

REFERENCES

1. **Smeathers, J. E.,** Some time dependent properties of the intervertebral joint when under compression, *Eng. Med.,* 13, 83, 1984.
2. **Smeathers, J. E. and Biggs, W. D.,** Mechanics of the spinal column, in *Engineering Aspects of the Spine,* Institution of Mechanical Engineers, London, 1980, 103.
3. **Farfan, H. F.,** Muscular mechanism of the lumbar spine and the position of power and efficiency, *Orthop. Clin. N. Am.,* 6, 135, 1975.
4. **Nachemson, A.,** Lumbar intradiscal pressure, in *The Lumbar Spine and Back Pain,* 2nd ed., Jayson, M. I. V., Ed., Pitman Medical, Tunbridge Wells, England, 1980, chap. 12.
5. **Todd, W. T. and Pyle, I. S.,** A quantitative study of the vertebral column by direct and roentgenographic methods, *Am. J. Phy. Anthropol.,* 21, 321, 1928.
6. **Taylor, J. R.,** Growth of the human intervertebral disc and vertebral bodies, *J. Anat.,* 120, 49, 1975.
7. **Pooni, J. S., Hukins, D. W. L., Harris, P. F., Hilton, R. C., and Davies, K. E.,** Comparison of the structure of human intervertebral discs in the cervical, thoracic and lumbar regions of the spine, *Surg. Radiol. Anat.,* 8, 175, 1986.
8. **Warwick, R. and Williams, P. L.,** *Gray's Anatomy,* 35th ed., Longman, London, 1973.
9. **Rissanen, P. M.,** The surgical anatomy of the supraspinous and interspinous ligaments of the human spine with special reference to ligament ruptures, *Acta Orthop. Scand.,* Suppl. 46, 1960.
10. **Ramsey, R. H.,** The anatomy of the ligamenta flava, *Clin. Orthop. Relat. Res.,* 44, 129, 1966.
11. **Farfan, H. F., Cossette, J. W., Robertson, G. H., Wells, R. V., and Kraus, H.,** The effects of torsion on the lumbar intervertebral joints: the role of torsion in the production of disc degeneration, *J. Bone Jt. Surg.,* 52A, 468 1970.
12. **Farfan, H. F.,** A reorientation in the surgical approach to degenerative joint disease, *Orthop. Clin. N. Am.,* 8, 9, 1977.
13. **Cyron, B. M., and Hutton, W. C.,** Articular tropism and stability of the lumbar spine, *Spine,* 6, 168, 1980.
14. **Adams, M. A. and Hutton, W. C.,** The relevance of torsion to the mechanical derangement of the lumbar spine, *Spine,* 6, 241, 1981.
15. **Adams, M. A., and Hutton, W. C.,** The mechanical function of the lumbar apophyseal joints, *Spine,* 8, 327, 1983.
16. **Panjabi, M. M., Goel, V. K., and Takata, K.,** Physiologic strains in the lumbar spinal ligaments. An *in vitro* biomechanical study, *Spine,* 7, 192, 1982.
17. **Shah, J. S., Hampson, W. G. J., and Jayson, M. I. V.,** The distribution of surface strain in the cadaveric lumbar spine, *J. Bone and Jt. Surg.,* 60B, 246, 1978.
18. **Pritzker, K. P. H.,** Aging and degeneration in the lumbar intervertebral disc, *Orthop. Clin. N. Am.,* 8, 65, 1977.
19. **Ghadially, F. N.,** Fine structure of joints, in *The Joints and Synovial Fluid,* Vol. 1, Sokoloff, L., Ed., Academic Press, London, 1978, chap. 3.
20. **Farfan, H. F.,** *Mechanical Disorders of the Low Back,* Lea & Febiger, Philadelphia, 1973.
21. **Peacock, A.,** Observations on post-natal structure of intervertebral disc in man, *J. Anat.,* 86, 162, 1952.
22. **Walmsley, R.,** The development and growth of the intervertebral disc, *Edinburgh Med. J.,* 60, 341, 1953.
23. **Klein, J. A. and Hukins, D. W. L.,** Functional differentiation in the spinal column, *Eng. Med.,* 12, 83, 1983.
24. **Aspden, R. M., Hickey, D. S., and Hukins, D. W. L.,** Determination of collagen fibril orientation in the cartilage of vertebral end plate, *Connect. Tissue Res.,* 9, 83, 1981.
25. **Inoue, H.,** Three-dimensional architecture of lumbar intervertebral discs, *Spine,* 6, 139, 1981.

26. **Coventry, M. B., Ghormley, R. K., and Kernohan, J. W.,** The intervertebral disc, its microscopic anatomy and pathology. II. Changes in the intervertebral disc concomitant with age, *J. Bone and Jt. Surg.,* 27, 233, 1945.

27. **Hansson, T. and Roos, B.,** The amount of bone mineral and Schmorl's nodes in lumbar vertebrae, *Spine,* 8, 266, 1983.

28. **Ball, J.,** New knowledge of intervertebral disc disease, *J. Clin. Pathol.,* 31, (Suppl., Royal College of Pathologists 12), 200, 1978.

29. **Gower, W. E. and Pedrini, V.,** Age-related variations in protein-polysaccharide from human nucleus pulposus, annulus fibrosus and costal cartilage, *J. Bone and Jt. Surg.,* 51A, 1154, 1969.

30. **Eyre, D. R.,** Biochemistry of the intervertebral disc, *Int. Rev. Connect. Tissue Res.,* 8, 227, 1979.

31. **Maroudas, A.,** Physical chemistry of articular cartilage and the intervertebral disc, in *The Joints and Synovial Fluid,* Vol. 2, Sokoloff, L., Ed., Academic Press, New York, 1980, chap. 6.

32. **Maroudas, A. and Urban, J. P. G.,** Swelling pressure of cartilagenous tissues, in *Studies in Joint Disease,* Vol. 1, Maroudas, A. and Holborrow, E. J., Eds., Pitman Medical, Tunbridge Wells, England, 1980, chap. 3.

33. **Bushell, G. R., Ghosh, P., Taylor, T. K. F., and Akeson, W. H.,** Proteoglycan chemistry of the intervertebral discs, *Clin. Orthop. Relat. Res.,* 129, 115, 1977.

34. **Hardingham, T. E. and Muir, H.,** The specific interaction of hyaluronic acid with cartilage proteoglycan, *Biochim. Biophys. Acta,* 279, 401, 1972.

35. **Muir, I. H. M.,** The chemistry of the ground substance in joint cartilage, in *The Joints and Synovial Fluid,* Vol. 2, Sokoloff, L., Ed., Academic Press, New York, 1980, chap. 2.

36. **Beard, H. K. and Stevens, R. L.** Biochemical changes in the intervertebral disc, in *The Lumbar Spine and Back Pain,* 2nd ed., Jayson, M. I. V., Ed., Pitman Medical, Tunbridge Wells, England, 1980, chap. 14.

37. **Bayliss, M. T.,** Proteoglycans: structure and molecular organisation in cartilage, in *Connective Tissue Matrix,* Hukins, D. W, L., Ed., Macmillan, London, 1984, chap. 3.

38. **Gelman, R. A. and Blackwell, J.,** Collagen — mucopolysaccharide interactions at acid pH, *Biochim. Biophys. Acta,* 342, 254, 1974.

39. **Hukins, D. W. L. and Aspden, R. M.,** Composition and properties of connective tissues, *Trends Biochem. Sci.,* 10, 260, 1985.

40. **Hukins, D. W. L.,** Tissue components, in *Connective Tissue Matrix,* Hukins, D. W. L., Ed., Macmillan, London, 1984, chap. 1.

41. **Lyons, G., Eisenstein, S. M., and Sweet, M. B. E.,** Biochemical changes in intervertebral disc degeration, *Biochim. Biophys. Acta,* 673, 443, 1981.

42. **Happey, F.,** A biophysical study of the human intervertebral disc, in *The Lumbar Spine and Back Pain,* 1st ed., Jayson, M. I. V., Ed., Sector Publishing, London, 1976, chap. 13.

43. **Happey, F.,** Studies of the structure of the human intervertebral disc in relation to its function and aging processes, in *The Joints and Synovial Fluid,* Vol. 2, Sokoloff, L., Ed., Academic Press, New York, 1980, chap. 3.

44. **Ghosh, P., Bushell, G. R., Taylor, T. F. K., and Akeson, W. H.,** Collagens, elastin and non-collagenous protein of the intervertebral disc, *Clin. Orthop. Relat. Res.,* 129, 124, 1977.

45. **Hirsch, C., Paulson, S., Sylvèn, B., and Snellman, O.,** Biophysical and physiological investigations on cartilage and other mesenchymal tissues: VI. Characteristics of human nuclei pulposi during aging, *Acta Orthop. Scand.,* 22, 175, 1952.

46. **Hallen, A.,** The collagen and ground substance of human intervertebral disc at different ages, *Acta Chem. Scand.,* 16, 705, 1962.

47. **Urban, J. P. G. and Maroudas, A.,** Measurement of fixed charge density in the intervertebral disc, *Biochim. Biophys. Acta,* 586, 116, 1979.

48. **Buckwalter, J. A., Maynard, J. A., and Cooper, R. R.,** Banded structures in human nucleus pulposus, *Clin. Orthop. Relat. Res.,* 139, 259, 1979.

49. **Hough, A. J., Mottram, L., and Sokoloff, L.,** The collagenous nature of amianthoid degeneration of human costal cartilage, *Am. J. Pathol.,* 73, 201, 1973.

50. **Hukins, D. W. L., Knight, D. P. and Woodhead-Galloway, J.,** Amianthoid change: orientation of normal collagen fibrils during aging, *Science,* 194, 622, 1979.

51. **Jenkins, J. P. R., Hickey, D. S., Zhu, X. P., Machin, M. and Isherwood, I.,** MR imaging of the intervertebral disc — a quantitative study, *Br. J. Radiol.,* 58, 705, 1985.

52. **Richardson, M. L., Genant, H. K., Helms, C. A., Gillespy, T., Heller, M., Jergesen, H. E., and Bovill, E. G.,** Magnetic resonance imaging of the musculoskeletal system, *Orthoped. Clin. N. Am.,* 16, 569, 1985.

53. **Modic, M. L., Pavlicek, W., Weinstein, M. A., Boumphrey, F., Ngo, F., Hardy, P., and Duchesneau, P. M.,** Magnetic resonance imaging of intervertebral disk disease, *Radiology,* 152, 103, 1984.

54. **Farrar, T. C. and Becker, E. D.,** *Pulse and Fourier Transform NMR: Introduction to Theory and Methods,* Academic Press, London, 1971.
55. **Mansfield, P. and Morris, P. G.,** *NMR Imaging in Biomedicine,* Academic Press, New York, 1982.
56. **Hickey, D. S., Checkley, D., Aspden, R. M., Naughton, A., Jenkins, J. P. R., and Isherwood, I.,** A method for the clinical measurement of relaxation times in magnetic resonance imaging, *Br. J. Radiol.,* 59, 565, 1986.
57. **McDonald, G. G. and Leigh, J. S.,** A new method for measuring longitudinal relaxation times, *J. Magn. Reson.,* 9, 358, 1973.
58. **Gathercole, L. J. and Keller, A.,** Light microscopic waveforms in collagenous tissues and their structural implications, *Structure of Fibrous Biopolymers,* Atkins, E. D. T. and Keller, A., Eds., Butterworths, London, 1975, 153.
59. **Stokes, I. and Greenapple, D. M.,** Measurement of surface deformation of soft tissue, *J. Biomech.,* 18, 1, 1985.
60. **Inoue, H.,** Three-dimensional observation of collagen framework of intervertebral discs in rats, dogs and humans, *Arch. Histologicum Japonicum,* 36, 39, 1973.
61. **Inoue, H. and Takeda, T.,** Three-dimensional observation of collagen framework of lumbar intervertebral discs, *Acta Orthop. Scand.,* 46, 949, 1975.
62. **Takeda, T.,** Three-dimensional observation of collagen framework of human lumbar discs, *J. Jpn. Orthop. Assoc.,* 49, 45, 1975.
63. **Hukins, D. W. L.,** Collagen orientation, in *Connective Tissue Matrix,* Hukins, D. W. L., Ed., Macmillan, London, 1984, chap. 8.
64. **Naylor, A., Happey, F., and Macrae, T.,** The collagenous changes in the intervertebral disc with age and their effects on its elasticity, an X-ray crystallographic study, *Br. Med. J.,* 2, 570, 1954.
65. **Horton, G. W.,** Further observations on the elastic mechanism of the intervertebral disc, *J. Bone and Jt. Surg.,* 40B, 552, 1958.
66. **Hickey, D. S. and Hukins, D. W. L.,** X-ray diffraction studies of the arrangment of collagenous fibers in human fetal intervertebral disc, *J. Anat.,* 131, 81, 1980.
67. **Hickey, D. S. and Hukins, D. W. L.,** Aging changes in the macromolecular organization of the intervertebral disc: an X-ray diffraction and electron microscopic study, *Spine,* 7, 234, 1982.
68. **Hickey, D. S. and Hukins, D. W. L.,** Effect of methods of preservation on the arrangement of collagen fibrils in connective tissue matrices: an X-ray diffraction study of annulus fibrosus, *Connect. Tissue Res.,* 6, 223, 1979.
69. **Hickey, D. S.,** Arrangement and structure of collagenous fibres in the annulus fibrosus of lumbar intervertebral discs: relationship to mechanical function, development and ageing, Ph.D. thesis, University of Manchester, Manchester, England, 1983.
70. **Klein, J. A. and Hukins, D. W. L.,** X-ray diffraction demonstrates reorientation of collagen fibres in the annulus fibrosus during compression of the intervertebral disc, *Biochim. Biophys. Acta,* 717, 61, 1982.
71. **Klein, J. A. and Hukins, D. W. L.,** Collagen fibre orientation in the annulus fibrosus of intervertebral disc during bending and torsion measured by X-ray diffraction, *Biochim. Biophys. Acta,* 719, 98, 1982.
72. **Hickey, D. S. and Hukins, D. W. L.,** Relation between the structure of the annulus fibrosus and the function and failure of the intervertebral disc, *Spine,* 5, 106, 1980.
73. **Aspden, R. M. and Hukins, D. W. L.,** Determination of the direction of preferred orientation and the orientation distribution function of collagen fibrils in connective tissues from high-angle X-ray diffraction patterns, *J. Appl. Crystallogr.* 12, 306, 1979.
74. **Berthet, C., Hulmes, D. J. S., Miller, A., and Timmins, P. A.,** Structure of collagen in cartilage of intervertebral disc, *Science,* 199, 547, 1978.
75. **Adams, P., Eyre, D. R. and Muir, H.,** Biochemical aspects of development and ageing of human lumbar intervertebral discs, *Rheumatol. Rehabil.* 16, 22, 1977.
76. **Herbert, C. M., Lindberg, K. A., Jayson, M. I. V., and Bailey, A. J.,** Changes in the collagen of human intervertebral discs during ageing and degenerative joint disease, *J. Mol. Med.* 1, 79, 1975.
77. **Eyre, D. R. and Muir, H.,** Types I and II collagens in intervertebral disc, *Biochem. J.* 157, 267, 1976.
78. **Eyre, D. R. and Muir, H.,** Quantitative analysis of types I and II collagens in intervertebral disc at various ages, *Biochim. Biophys. Acta,* 492, 29, 1977.
79. **Weiss, J. B.,** Collagens and collagenolytic enzymes, in *Connective Tissue Matrix,* Hukins, D. W. L., Ed., Macmillan, London, 1984, chap. 2.
80. **Jackson, D. S.,** Dermal scar, in *Collagen in Health and Disease,* Weiss, J. B., and Jayson, M. I. V., Eds., Churchill Livingstone, London, 1982, chap. 27.
81. **Farfan, H. F., Huberdeau, R. M., and Dubow, H. I.,** The influence of geometric features on the pattern of disc degeneration — a post mortem study, *J. Bone Jt. Surg.,* 54A, 492, 1972.
82. **Johnson, E. F., Chetty, K., Moore, I. M., Stewart, A., and Jones, W.,** The distribution and arrangement of elastic fibres in the intervertebral disc of the adult human, *J. Anat.* 135, 301, 1982.

83. **Buckwalter, J. A., Cooper, R. R., and Maynard, J. A.,** Elastic fibres in human intervertebral disc, *J. Bone Jt. Surg.,* 58A, 73, 1976.

84. **Hickey, D. S., and Hukins, D. W. L.,** Collagen fibril diameters and elastic fibres in the annulus fibrosus of human fetal intervertebral disc, *J. Anat.* 133, 351, 1981.

85. **Ross, R.,** The elastic fiber: a review, *J. Histochem. Cytochem.,* 21, 199, 1973.

86. **Hukins, D. W. L.,** Properties of spinal materials, in *The Lumbar Spine and Back Pain,* 3rd ed., Jayson, M. I. V., Ed., Pitman, Tunbridge Wells, England, 1987, chap. 6.

87. **Speer, D. P.,** Collagenous architecture of the growth plate and perichondral ossification groove, *J. Bone Jt. Surg.,* 64A, 399, 1982.

88. **Hukins, D. W. L., Aspden, R. M., and Yarker, Y. E.,** Fibre reinforcement and mechanical stability in articular cartilage, *Eng. Med.,* 13, 153, 1984.

89. **Myers, E. R., Armstrong, C. G. and Mow, V. C.,** Swelling pressure and collagen tension, in *Connective Tissue Matrix,* Hukins, D. W. L., Ed., Macmillan, London, 1984, chap. 6.

90. **Steven, F. S., and Thomas, H.,** Preparation of insoluble collagen from human cartilage, *Biochem. J.,* 135, 245, 1975.

91. **Maroudas, A., and Thomas, H.,** A simple physicochemical micro method for determining fixed anionic groups in connective tissue, *Biochim. Biophys. Acta,* 215, 214, 1970.

92. **Maroudas, A.,** Biophysical chemistry of cartilagenous tissues with special reference to solute and fluid transport, *Biorheology,* 12, 233, 1975.

93. **Hickey, D. S., Aspden, R. M., Hukins, D. W. L., Jenkins, J. P. R., and Isherwood, I.,** Analysis of magnetic resonance images from normal and degenerate lumbar intervertebral discs, *Spine,* 11, 702, 1986.

94. **Urban, J. P. G., Maroudas, A., Bayliss, M. T., and Dillon, J.,** Swelling pressures of proteoglycans at the concentrations found in cartilagenous tissues, *Biorheology,* 16, 447, 1979.

95. **Anderson, G. B., and Schultz, A. B.,** Effects of fluid injection on the mechanical properties of intervertebral discs, *J. Biomech.,* 12, 453, 1979.

96. **Tencer, A. F., and Ahmed, A. M.,** The role of secondary variables in the measurement of the mechanical properties of the lumbar intervertebral joint, *J. Biomech. Eng.,* 103, 129, 1981.

97. **Quandieu, P., Pellieux, L., Leinhard, F., and Valezy, B.,** Effects of the ablation of the nucleus pulposus on the vibrational behaviour of the lumbosacral hinge, *J. Biomech.,* 16, 777, 1983.

98. **Virgin, W. J.,** Experimental investigation into the physical properties of the intervertebral disk, *J. Bone Jt. Surg.,* 33B, 607, 1951.

99. **Ranu, H. S, and King, A. J.,** Correlation of intradiscal pressure with vertebral end plate pressure, in *Engineering Aspects of the Spine,* Institution of Mechanical Engineers, London, 1980, 37.

100. **Horst, P. and Brinckmann, P.,** Measurement of the distribution of axial stress on the end-plate of the vertebral body, *Spine,* 6, 217, 1981.

101. **Klein, J. A.,** Mechanics of the intervertebral disc: implications for the response of the lumbar spine to loading, Ph.D. thesis, University of Manchester, Manchester, England, 1982.

102. **Nachemson, A.,** Towards a better understanding of low back pain: a review of the mechanics of the lumbar disc, *Rheumatol. and Rehabil.,* 14, 129, 1975.

103. **Sonnerup, L.,** Semi-experimental stress analysis of the human intervertebral joint, *J. Soc. Exp. Stress Anal.,* 29, 142, 1972.

104. **Quinnell, R. C., Stockdale, H. R., and Willis, D. S.,** Observations of pressures within normal discs within lumbar spine, *Spine,* 8, 166, 1983.

105. **Nachemson, A. L., and Evans, J. H.,** Some mechanical properties of the third human interlaminar ligament (ligamentum flavum), *J. Biomech.,* 1, 211, 1968.

106. **Gordon, J. E.,** *Structures,* Penguin, Hamondsworth, Middlesex, England, 1978.

107. **Adams, M. A. and Hutton, W. C.,** Effect of posture on the fluid content of lumbar intervertebral discs, *Spine,* 8, 665, 1983.

108. **Agarwal, B. D. and Broutman, L. J.,** *Analysis and Performances of Fibre Composites,* Wiley, New York, 1980.

109. **Hukins, D. W. L.,** Biomechanical properties of collagen, in *Collagen in Health and Disease,* Weiss, J. B., and Jayson, M. I. V., Eds., Churchill Livingstone, London, 1982, chap. 4.

110. **Jeronimidis, G. and Vincent, J. F. V.,** Composite materials, in *Connective Tissue Matrix,* Hukins, D. W. L., Ed., Macmillan, London, 1984, chap. 7.

111. **Brown, T., Hansen, R. J., and Yorra, A. J.,** Some mechanical tests on the lumbo-sacral spine with particular reference to the intervertebral disc, *J. Bone J. Surg.,* 39A, 1135, 1957.

112. **Galante, J. O.,** Tensile properties of the human lumbar annulus fibrosus, *Acta Orthop. Scand.* Suppl. No. 100, 1967.

113. **Belytschko, T., Kulak, R., Schultz, A., and Galante, J.,** Finite element stress analysis of an intervertebral disc, *J. Biomech.,* 7, 277, 1974.

114. **Wu, H.-C. and Yao, R.-F.,** Mechanical behaviour of the human annulus fibrosus, *J. Biomech.* 9, 1, 1976.

115. **Harkness, R. D.,** Mechanical properties of collagenous tissues, in *Treatise on Collagen,* Vol. 2A, Gould, B. S., Ed., Academic Press, New York, 1968, chap. 6.
116. **Diamant, J., Keller, A., Baer, E., Litt, M., and Arridge, R. G. C.,** Collagen: ultrastructure and its relationship to mechanical properties as a function of ageing, *Proc. R. Soc.,* B180, 293, 1972.
117. **Elden, H. R.,** Physical properties of collagen fibres, *Int. Rev. Connect. Tissue Res.* 4, 283, 1968.
118. **Elliot, D. H.,** Structure and function of mammalian tendon, *Biol. Rev.,* 40, 392, 1965.
119. **Haut, R. C. and Little, R. W.,** A constitutional equation for collagen fibres, *J. Biomech.,* 5, 423, 1972.
120. **Kenedi, R. M., Gibson, T., Evans, J. H., and Barbenel, J. C.,** Tissue mechanics, *Phys. Med. Biol.* 20, 699, 1975.
121. **Rigby, B. J., Hirai, N., Spikes, J. D., and Eyring, H.,** The mechanical properties of rat tail tendon, *J. Gen. Physiol.* 43, 265, 1959.
122. **Torp, S., Arridge, R. G. C., Armeniades, C. D., and Baer, E.,** Structure-property relationships in tendon as a function of age, in *Structure of Fibrous Biopolymers,* Atkins, E. D. T. and Keller, A., Eds., Butterworths, London, 1975, 197.
123. **Vincent, J. F. V.,** *Structural Biomaterials,* Macmillan, London, 1982, 10.
124. **O'Brien, J. P.,** The role of fusion for chronic low back pain, *Orthop. Clin. N. Am.,* 14, 639, 1983.
125. **Hooley, C. J. and Cohen, R. E.,** A model for the creep behaviour of tendon, *Int. J. Biol. Macromol.,* 1, 123, 1979.
126. **Dlugosz, J., Gathercole, L. J., and Keller, A.,** Transmission electron microscope studies and their relation to polarising optical microscopy in the rat tail tendon, *Micron,* 9, 71, 1978.
127. **Minns, R. J., Soden, P. D., and Jackson, D. S.,** The role of the fibrous components and ground substance in the mechanical properties of biological tissues: a preliminary investigation, *J. Biomech.,* 6, 153, 1973.
128. **Cook, J. and Gordon, J. E.,** A mechanism for the control of crack propagation in all-brittle systems, *Proc. R. Soc.,* A282, 508, 1964.
129. **Klein, J. A., Hickey, D. S., and Hukins, D. W. L.,** Computer graphics illustration of the operation of the intervertebral disc, *Eng. Med.,* 11, 11, 1982.
130. **Pearcy, M. J. and Tibrewal, S. B.,** Intervertebral structures investigated *in vivo* using radiography, I. Lumbar intervertebral disc and ligament deformations in flexion and extension, *Clin. Orthop. Relat. Res.,* 191, 281, 1984.
131. **Pearcy, M. J., Portek, I., and Shepherd, J.,** Three-dimensional X-ray analysis of normal movement in the lumbar spine, *Spine,* 9, 294, 1984.
132. **Pearcy, M. J.,** Stereo-radiography of lumbar spinal motion, *Acta Orthop. Scand.,* Suppl. No. 212, 1985.
133. **Rolander, S. D.,** Motion of the lumbar spine with special reference to the stablising of posterior fusion. An experimental study on autopsy specimens, *Acta Orthop. Scand.,* Suppl. No. 90, 1966.
134. **Klein, J. A. and Hukins, D. W. L.,** Relocation of the bending axis during flexion-extension of lumbar intervertebral discs and its implications for prolapse, *Spine,* 8, 659, 1983.
135. **Adams, M. A. and Hutton, W. C.,** Prolapsed intervertebral disc: a hyperflexion injury, *Spine,* 7, 184, 1982.
136. **Higdon, A., Ohlsen, E. H., Stiles, W. B., Weese, J. A., and Riley, W. F.,** *Mechanics of Materials,* 3rd ed, Wiley, New York, 1976, 147.
137. **Broberg, K. B. and von Essen, H. O.,** Modeling of intervertebral discs, *Spine,* 5, 155, 1980.
138. **Klein, J. A., Hickey, D. S., and Hukins, D. W. L.,** Radial bulging of the annulus fibrosus during compression of the intervertebral disc, *J. Biomech.,* 16, 211, 1983.
139. **Reuber, A., Schultz, A., Denis, F., and Spencer, D.,** Bulging of lumbar intervertebral discs, *J. Biomech. Eng.,* 104, 187, 1982.
140. **Roaf, R.,** A study of the mechanics of spinal injuries, *J. Bone, Jt. Surg.,* 42B, 810, 1960.
141. **Tkaczuk, H.,** Tensile properties of human lumbar longitudinal ligaments, *Acta Orthop. Scand.,* Suppl. No. 115, 1968.
142. **Shah, J. S., Jayson, M. I. V., and Hampson, W. G. J.,** Mechanical implications of crimping in collagen fibres of human spinal ligaments, *Eng. Med.,* 8, 95, 1979.
143. **Jayson, M. I. V., Herbert, C. M., and Barks, J. S.,** Intervertebral discs: nuclear morphology and bursting pressure, *Ann. Rheum. Dis.* 32, 308, 1973.
144. **Schmorl, G. and Junghanns, H.,** *The Human Spine in Health and Disease,* 2nd ed, Beseman, E. F., Ed., Grune & Stratton, New York, 1971, 262.
145. **Vernon-Roberts, B., and Pirie, C. J.,** Healing trabecular microfractures, *Ann. Rheum. Dis.,* 32, 406, 1973.
146. **Sims-Williams, H., Jayson, M. I. V., and Baddely, H.,** Small spinal fractures in back pain patients, *Ann. Rheum. Dis.,* 37, 262, 1978.
147. **Batson, O. V.,** The vertebral venous system, *Am. J. Roentgenol.,* 78, 195, 1957.

Chapter 2

THE DEVELOPMENT OF THE HUMAN INTERVERTEBRAL DISC

James R. Taylor and Lance T. Twomey

TABLE OF CONTENTS

I. INTRODUCTION

There have been very few studies of growth and development of the human intervertebral disc in the past 20 to 30 years. The difficulty of collecting enough human material is the principal hindrance to such study. The following account of intervertebral disc development is based on an extensive review of the literature and on two doctoral studies,[1,2] the former, a histological and measurement study of prenatal and postnatal development and the latter, a measurement study with emphases on movement and age changes throughout the whole age range. Taylor's[1] study involved embedding and sectioning a graded series of 67 embryos, fetuses, infants, and children, with a cumulative total of 272 discs sectioned in a variety of planes and examined microscopically. Linear and area measurements were recorded, principally from midline sections. In addition, radiographic measurements were recorded from 29 cervical, 196 thoracic, and 321 radiographs. Twomey[2] sectioned, examined, and measured over 1000 lumbar intervertebral discs from more than 200 spines with an age range from 1 day to 97 years.

Twomey's measurements were made directly on fresh material;[2] Taylor's measurements were made on both sections and radiographs, with controls for contraction artifact (6 to 8%) and corrections for magnification error, respectively.[1]

A. General Description and Nomenclature:

In standard anatomical texts,[3,4] the intervertebral disc is described as consisting of a peripheral annulus fibrosus and a central nucleus pulposus. The intervertebral disc and, particularly, its nucleus undergo continuous change during development, maturation, and degeneration. The nucleus pulposus is notochordal in prenatal and infant life. It becomes fibrocartilaginous in adolescents and adults. The fibrous annulus, which is vascular in fetal and infant life, becomes almost avascular in adults. The fluid, mucoid "notochordal nucleus pulposus" of fetal and infant discs has clearly defined boundaries. However, in the mature disc, it is impossible to determine an exact boundary line between the fibrocartilaginous nucleus and the inner fibrocartilaginous annulus by histological means.

The description of the disc, simply as comprising an annulus fibrosus and a nucleus pulposus, is oversimplified, both in the immature and the mature disc for a number of reasons.[1]

1. Transitional Zones in the Developing Disc

In the prenatal disc, Peacock[5] describes a "transitional zone", Figure 1 a, of randomly oriented fibrocartilage lying between the annulus and the nucleus. This zone is often referred to as the "inner cell zone".[5,6] The inner cell zone disappears in the postnatal disc. Some authors describe an additional transitional zone (Figure 1 b), where the fibers of the annulus enter the peripheral parts of the adjacent cartilage plates.

2. The Continuity of the Annulus and Cartilage Plates

The lamellar structure described in the annulus fibrosus is not confined to the annulus, but also continues around, above, and below the nucleus, completely encapsulating it[1,7] (Figure 1). In the lamellar annulus, two parts can be distinguished: the fibrous outer lamellae which are continuous with the longitudinal ligaments of the vertebral column or inserted into the bone of the vertebral bodies, and the fibrocartilaginous inner layers, which are continuous with the cartilage plates, forming a complete "envelope" for the nucleus pulposus.

Historically, the cartilage plates capping the ends of the adjacent bony vertebral bodies were regarded as parts of the intervertebral disc,[8,9] but some authors and standard anatomical texts describe them as parts of the vertebral bodies.[3,6] Such controversy as to disc and vertebral boundaries is not surprising in view of their common origin from a single, con-

DIAGRAM of INTERVERTEBRAL DISC and
VERTEBRAL BODY of NEWBORN INFANT.

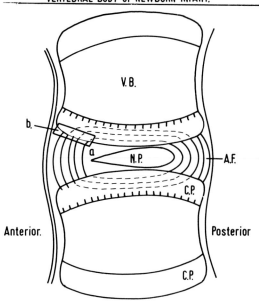

FIGURE 1. Diagrammatic median sagittal section of a
full-term fetal lumbar intervertebral disc, showing how the
cartilage plates (C.P.) and the annulus fibrosus (A.F.) form
a complete envelope for the nucleus pulposus (N.P.); V.B.
= vertebral body; a and b = "transitional zones".

tinuous mesenchymal vertebral column. Whatever the status of the cartilage plates, the
development of the annulus fibrosus and of the nucleus pulposus cannot be described adequately without reference to the concurrent development of the intimately related cartilage
plates. It is surprising that, in classical descriptions of the development of the intervertebral
disc,[5,6,10-13] scant attention is paid to the cartilage plates.

II. EARLY DEVELOPMENT

The first axial structures to appear in the embryo are the notochord, the neural tube, and
the dorsal aorta. The first vertebral column is formed by aggregation of mesenchyme around
the notochord. Descriptions of early development of the vertebral column are given by
Bardeen,[14] Wyburn,[15] Prader,[11] Sensenig,[16] Peacock,[5] Walmsley,[6] O'Rahilly and Meyer,[17]
and Verbout.[18] Bardeen[14] describes the stages of development of the vertebral column as:
(1) blastemal, (2) chondrogenous, and (3) osseogenous. Early development of the vertebral
column may be conveniently described using this classification:

A. Blastemal stage
1. Formation of the Mesenchymal Column
In embryos of 2 mm or more C.R.L. (crown to rump length) (3 weeks gestation) a
continuous mesenchymal column is formed around the cylindrical notochord. This is said
to be due to the active proliferation and medial migration of somitic mesoderm from the
ventromedial portions of the somites — termed sclerotomes.[19] The notochord becomes
separated from the gut tube and aorta ventrally and from the neural tube dorsally, as mesenchyme appears around it. The column appears first cranially and, at a later stage, caudally.[16]

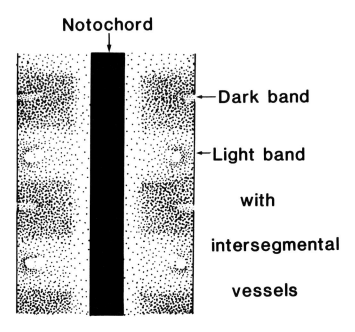

FIGURE 2.   Diagram of coronal section of 7-mm human embryo, showing segmentation of the perichordal blastemal vertebral column into successive light and dark bands. The dark band is the perichordal disc, whose central part retains a similar appearance to the "precartilage" of the light band which is the primordium of the vertebra. (From Taylor, J. and Twomey, L., *Modern Manual Therapy of the Vertebral Column*, Grieve, G., Ed., Churchill Livingstone, Edinburgh, 1986. With permission.)

Neural processes appear as condensations of the somitic mesenchyme at each side of the neural tube. These extend dorsally from the continuous column around the notochord. According to Verbout,[18] the loose axial mesenchyme, which develops first around the notochord, differs morphogenetically from the somitic mesenchyme and may not be initially derived from it. However, "commissural" communications are later established with the somitic mesoderm on each side. The continuous mesenchymal column thus formed around the notochord constitutes the anlagen of the vertebral bodies and intervertebral discs.

In embryos of about 4 mm C.R.L., "sclerotomic fissures" are traditionally described at midsegmental level. They are associated with Remak's[20] theory of resegmentation.[5,6,11,14-16] Intersegmental vessels also appear in "intersegmental fissures".[16] Recent work casts doubt on the existence of such fissures. "Sclerotomic fissures" are probably artifacts and "intersegmental fissures" are probably misinterpretations of the appearances in sections through the intersegmental vessels.[18,21] Some older authors also denied the existence of the sclerotomic fissure,[22,23] but its existence has become "enshrined in the literature", bringing unnecessary complexity to descriptions of early development. Baur,[21] Verbout,[18] and Taylor[24] contend that the blastemal column remains continuous, at least in its perichordal part, and that segmentation occurs only at a later stage, when the vertebrae and intervertebral discs differentiate in their definitive positions.

2. Segmentation

A banded pattern becomes evident in the mesenchymal vertebral column of embryos of about 5 mm C.R.L. (Figure 2). Light bands, at the level of the intersegmental vessels, alternate regularly with dark bands. The dark and light bands appear so because of a relatively greater nuclear density in the dark bands than in the light bands. *The dark bands are the forerunners of the intervertebral discs, including cartilage plates, and are known as the perichordal discs.* The light bands are the anlagen of the vertebral bodies. Dark and light bands are originally of equal height,[6] but the light bands grow in height more rapidly than the dark bands. The perichordal part of the dark band remains light or less dense throughout the column. The more rapid growth of the light bands may be related to their relation to the intersegmental vessels, which may play a role in the process of segmentation itself.[24,25]

B. Chondrogenous stage

In embryos of 10 to 12 mm C.R.L. (at about 6 weeks gestation), the onset of chondrification in the light bands is reported.[5,16,18] The differentiation of mesenchyme into embryonic hyaline cartilage takes place throughout the light bands at about the same time, and not from two centers of chondrification on the right and left of the notochord, as described (page 68) by Schmorl and Junghanns.[8] This differentiation is associated with the rapid increase in height of the light bands during the 6th week of gestation. The primitive vertebral bodies also change their shape, becoming convex at their cranial and caudal ends.

The perichordal disc in a 12.5-mm embryo shows a trilaminar arrangement; the middle lamina is darker, or more dense, with lighter strips cranially and caudally adjoining the primitive vertebrae.[15] At this stage, the outer mesenchymal cells of the perichordal disc begin to show a lamellar appearance, arranged with their long axes parallel to the craniocaudal axis of the embryo. In a 17-mm embryo (7 weeks gestation), Walmsley[6] reports that the notochord, still of relatively uniform diameter, shows localized aggregation of its cells at the intervertebral level, but the segmental dilatations of the notochord are first seen in embryos of about 20 mm C.R.L.[1,5,6]

In embryos of 20 to 40 mm C.R.L., the perichordal disc is a short cylinder, concave cranially and caudally. It has an outer dark lamellar zone of fibroblasts, the primitive annulus fibrosus, and light "inner cell zone" of embryonic cartilage bounding a fusiform or rhomboidal dilatation of the notochord (Figure 3). Notochordal cells gradually disappear from the cartilaginous vertebral body leaving only the "mucoid streak" connecting the "chordasegments".[5,10]

C. Osseogenous stage

In embryos of 40 to 50 mm C.R.L., the mucoid streak or notochordal track through the vertebra is interrupted by chondrocyte hypertrophy and the onset of ossification (Figure 4). The streak usually disappears gradually, as endochondral ossification progresses in the vertebral body, but traces of the notochordal track not infrequently persist in the cartilage plates into postnatal life.[9,26] The notochordal segment expands within the perichordal disc to form the notochordal nucleus pulposus.

D. Segmental Variations in the Notochord before the 20-mm Stage

1. Segmental flexures: transitory "chordaflexures" are described in man and other mammalian embryos as early as 6 mm and as late as 20 mm.[5,6,10,16,18,27] Prader[10] reviewed earlier descriptions of these chordaflexures. She found them in human embryos between 6 and 12 mm and agreed with Dursy[27] in attributing their existence to a relative excess of growth in length of the "chorda" compared with the vertebral column.
2. Dursy[27] described transitory spindle-shaped swellings of the notochord in the vertebral body anlagen of a 12-mm bovine embryo. Williams[28] stated that similar notochordal swellings were found in the precartilaginous vertebrae of many mammalian embryos.
3. Sensenig[16] claimed that in human embryos as early as 10 mm slight segmental differences in thoracic notochordal diameter could be detected, with the notochord up to 10% wider in the perichordal disc than in the vertebral body anlage.

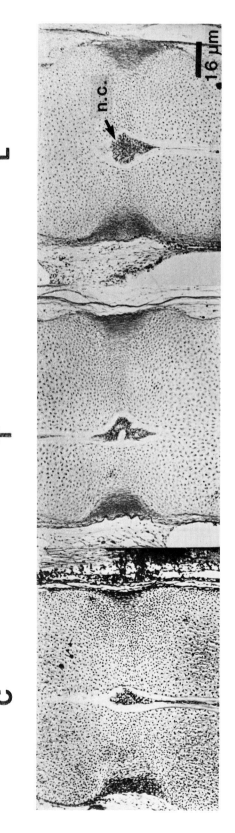

FIGURE 3.   Median sagittal sections of cervical (C), thoracic (T), and lumbar (L) regions of a vertebral column from a 30-mm human embryo (×60), showing the segmental swellings of the notochord in the perichordal discs; n.c. = notochordal segment.

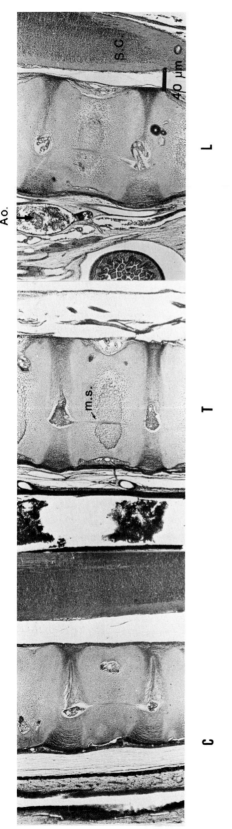

FIGURE 4. Median sagittal sections of discs and vertebrae from cervical (C), thoracic (T), and lumbar (L) regions of a 75-mm C.R.L. human fetus, showing the beginning of ossification in vertebral centra, expansion of notochordal segments in the primitive discs, and the "mucoid streak" passing through the developing primary ossification centers of the vertebrae (X25); m.s. = mucoid streak; Ao - aorta; and S.C. = spinal cord.

E. Notochordal Segmentation

Notochordal segmentation does not occur in all regions at the same time. In a 20 mm embryo, small fusiform enlargements are present in thoracic and lumbar disc anlagen, but the notochord is still cylindrical in the cervical region. By the 30-mm stage, fusiform enlargements are seen in all discs, though these are larger in lumbar and thoracic than in cervical discs (Figure 3). The foamy or vesicular appearance typical of notochordal tissue is already evident. This appearance is due to intercellular globules, but intracellular vacuoles are also seen.[1] At this stage, the perichordal zone of the disc has the appearance of embryonic hyaline cartilage.

In 13-, 18- and 22- week-old fetuses, the enlarged notochordal segments are stretched out as a "chorda reticulum" by the accumulation of a mucoid matrix between the cell strands. A mucoid streak remains in each cartilage model of a vertebral body. The notochordal tissue in infants and children retains essentially the same histological appearance as in fetuses[1] (Figure 5).

III. FURTHER DEVELOPMENT OF THE ANNULUS FIBROSUS

A. Differentiation and Growth

In 10- to 15-mm embryos, the elongated cells of the outer zone of the perichordal disc become oriented to give an outwardly convex curved lamellar pattern.[5,6,12] Collagen fibers first appear in this zone in embryos of 20 to 40 mm.[1,5,12] This outer lamellar zone constitutes the annulus fibrosus. As the annulus develops in the fetus, its outer part becomes almost entirely fibrous, with a concomitant decrease in its cellularity. The inner part, though lamellar, remains more cellular, becoming fibrocartilaginous,[1,5,6,12,29] The outer fibrous annulus is fused with the longitudinal ligaments of the vertebral column.[1,6] In the fetus, the fibers of the annulus are anchored to the cartilage plates on their caudal and cephalic aspects. The fibers of the outer third of the annulus simply insert into those areas of the cartilage plates where the ring apophysis will later appear (see V,B) Polarized light studies reveal the continuity of the curved lamellar pattern of the inner two thirds of the annulus fibrosus with the horizontal lamellar structure of the cartilage plates (Figures 1 and 6). Together, the annulus fibrosus and the cartilage plates encapsulate the nucleus pulposus.[1,7] But[30] defines the "perichordal disc" of the 2-month embryo as including three zones: (1) an outer fibrous zone, (2) an intermediate fibrocartilaginous zone, and (3) a hyaline cartilage "inner cell zone" around the notochord. The inner cell zone does not show any lamellar arrangement and is termed "precartilage" by Walmsley,[6] specialized embryonic cartilage by Peacock,[5] and hyaline cartilage by Prader[12] and But.[30] This zone becomes fibrocartilaginous in late fetal life, and it is said to contribute both to growth of the annulus fibrosus and the nucleus pulposus.[5,12] Hirsch and Schazowicz[31] state that growth of the annulus is both interstitial and appositional from the longitudinal ligaments of the vertebral column. Bohmig[9] and Donisch and Trapp[32] suggest that the annulus "grows interstitially from the cartilage plates", and relate this growth to the presence of vascular canals in the cartilage plates close to the annulus. This pronounced vascularity of fetal and infant cartilage plates is most evident near the inner, more cellular lamellae of the annulus, where these are in continuity with the lamellae of the cartilage plates.[1] This is also the region described as a "transitional zone" by Peacock[13] and where experiments in growing animals demonstrate more active $^{5}35$ uptake than in adjacent regions.[33] These various observations support the view that enlargement of the "envelope" to accommodate the growing nucleus takes place in this "transitional region" and in the inner annulus, by growth in length of the lamellae of both the annulus and the cartilage plates. Walmsley[6] states that growth of the anterior part of the annulus exceeds growth of its posterior part. Horton[34] believes that the annulus grows in thickness by increase in lamellar thickness rather than by increase in the number of its lamellae.

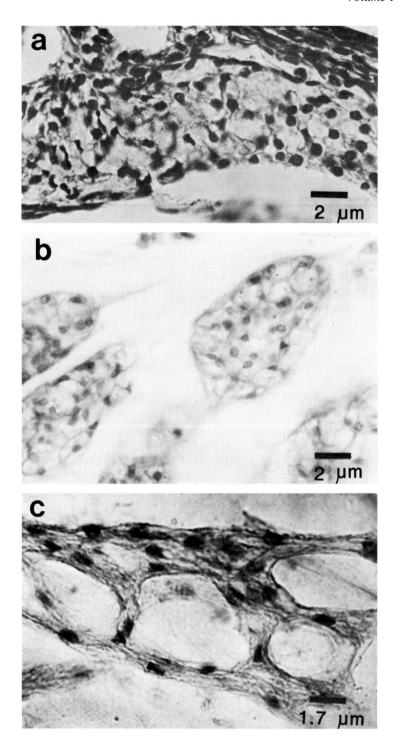

FIGURE 5. Notochordal tissue: (a) from the pharyngeal region rostral to the dens of C 2, in a 28-₋nm human embryo, 10-μm wax section, H.&E. (×500); (b) from a human nucleus pulposus of a full-term fetus, 150 μm celloidin section, stained haematoxylin and light green, (×480); (c) from the nucleus of a 4-month infant, 150 μm section, (×600). The changes from (a) to (c) relate to the accumulation of more mucoid matrix, rather than to any change in the cells.

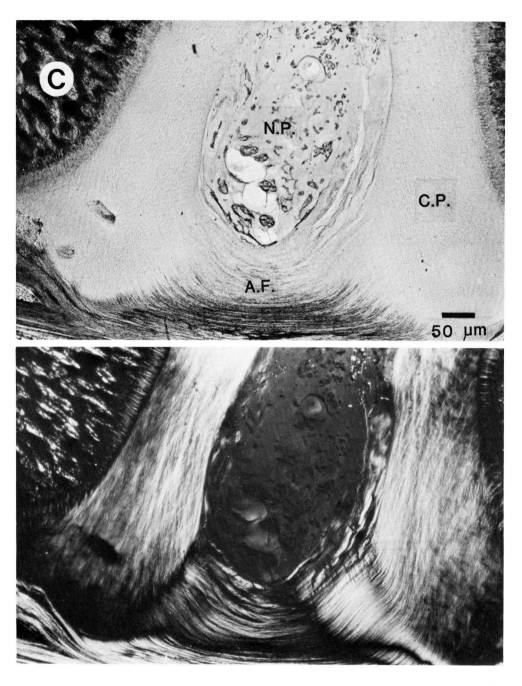

FIGURE 6.   150-μm median sagittal section of a full-term L4—5 disc showing the posterior annulus and nucleus. The same field is viewed by two different lighting techniques; above: normal transmitted light; below; polarized light. C = centrum; N.P. = nucleus pulposus; A.F. = annulus fibrosus; C.P. = cartilage plate. Note the continuity of the lamellar structure of annulus and cartilage plate; cf Figure 1.

B. Fiber Pattern

In a 40-mm embryo the fibers and cells of each lamella pass in a curved spiral sheet from one cartilaginous vertebra to the opposite vertebra. Since fibers in adjacent lamellae lie at different angles, a cruciate pattern of fibers is seen in vertical sections of the outer zone of the disc.[1,5,6] Uebermuth[35] believed that the outward convexity of the lamellae was due to

**VERTICAL
PLANE**

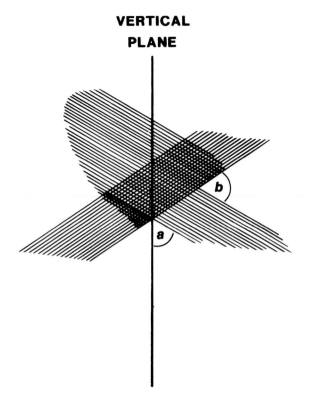

The angles "a" and "b" are both about 60° in lumbar discs

FIGURE 7.   The interstriation angles "a" and "b", represent the difference between fiber orientation in successive lamellae of the lumbar annulus fibrosus — see text.

the outward pressure of the notochordal aggregations, but this outward convexity is apparent before segmental dilatations of the notochord appear.[1,5,6,10] Walmsley[6] regards the pattern of the annulus as genetically determined.

The adult pattern is established in the annulus before birth, the inner cell zone being reduced and gradually disappearing, either by differentiating into lamellar fibrocartilage or by liquefaction and incorporation into the nucleus pulposus.[1,5,12] Walmsley[6] emphasizes the complexity of fiber pattern in the annulus by stating that it "almost defies description". However, in the lumbar intervertebral disc he describes 12 to 16 lamellae. Although lamellae do not form complete rings, there is a pattern of dovetailing and anastomosis between them[6]. From one cartilage plate the fibers of the inner two thirds of the annulus spiral round the nucleus pulposus into the opposite cartilage plate, but the fibers of the outer third pass out into the longitudinal ligaments or into the anterior surface of the adjacent vertebral body.[36] The "envelope" formed by annulus and cartilage plates resembles a flattened or elliptical sphere (Figure 1) which Franceschini[7] describes as a "parallelopiped". Franceschini[7] and Walmsley[6] state that the innermost lamellae of the mature annulus may be convex inwards towards the nucleus. It is possible that this configuration is an artifact due to contraction of the nucleus during dehydration and embedding.

At about 8 years, a ring apophysis forms in the periphery of each cartilaginous plate. Many outer fibers of the annulus gain attachment to this ring of new bone and, subsequently, with its fusion at 18 to 20 years to the vertebral body,[37] to the bony rim of the vertebra.

Rouviere[38] and Horton[34] studied the angle between fibers of adjacent lamellae of the annulus fibrosus (Figure 7). The angle "a" between the fibers and the vertical measures

50° in cervical and thoracic discs, increasing to 60° in lumbar discs. The greater angle in lower discs is said to reflect the greater weight borne by them.[38] These angles do not change from infancy to adult life. Horton[34] describes the "interstriation angle b" as about 57°, decreasing (in experiments on autopsy discs) with vertical compression of the intervertebral disc. Schmorl and Junghanns[8] describe "spanning fibers" binding adjacent lamellae together, but this has not been confirmed by other authors.

Walmsley[6] describes a change in the orientation of the fibrous structure of the posterior annulus, as seen in median sagittal sections of lumbar discs, after establishment of the secondary lumbar curvature. In the infant, the fibers pass in a gentle curve from the upper to the lower vertebra, but in the child of 11 years they are said to pass in a sharply curved or U-shaped course between the vertebrae.

IV. DEVELOPMENT OF THE NUCLEUS PULPOSUS

A. Role of the Notochord in the Origin of the Nucleus Pulposus

Luschka[39] gave the first detailed account of the formation of the nucleus pulposus from the intervertebral expansions of the notochord. Virchow[40] suggested a different origin, the nucleus arising "through a central growth of cartilage with softening of its ground substance". In 1858, Luschka,[41] while still maintaining that the intervertebral expansion of the notochord forms the original nucleus pulposus, accepted that it is later augmented by the liquefaction of fibrocartilaginous processes from the surrounding parts of the intervertebral disc. Kolliker[42,43] also described the origin of the nucleus pulposus from the notochord in man and other mammals. Robin[44] upheld the views of Luschka[41] and Kolliker[43] on the notochordal origin of the nucleus, though he is widely misquoted by Williams[28] and subsequent authors.[6,45] These authors take the contrary view, first advanced by Dursy[27] that the role of the notochord in human nucleus pulposus formation is minimal and confined to the early embryonic stages of development. Dursy[27] had wide experience of nonhuman, mammalian material, but had few human embryonic specimens at his disposal. Moreover, Dursy[27] confined his observations in man to the development of the cervical region of the vertebral column.

Four important studies, conducted between 1945 and 1953,[5,6,10,16] though often lacking regional precision or comparison in their descriptions of development, were based on observations of extensive series of human embryos. These agreed that the notochord plays an essential role in the origin of the nucleus pulposus, and that it continues to do so in the development of the nucleus at least during the first half of prenatal life. Three further studies, using histochemical and histological measurement methods, have shown that *the notochordal cells also continue to multiply and remain active in postnatal life, at least in infancy.*[1,46,47] These will be described later.

As stated earlier, notochordal dilatations at the level of the perichordal disc appear at the 20-mm stage of human embryonic development and increase progressively in size. Recognizable notochordal cells disappear from the intravertebral course of the notochord leaving the notochordal sheath — a clear homogenous cell-free strand — as a "mucoid streak" through the center of the primitive cartilaginous vertebral body. Kolliker,[43] Williams,[28] Keyes and Compere,[45] Prader,[10] Sensenig,[16] and Peacock[5] attribute the segmental changes of the notochord to passive displacement of the notochordal cells, from rapidly growing cartilaginous vertebral bodies to looser, more slowly growing adjacent perichordal discs. Walmsley[6] believes that active multiplication of notochordal cells in the discs and concurrent death of cells in the vertebral bodies account for the segmental changes. He cites a 17-mm embryo where the notochord is still of uniform diameter, but a greater cell density is seen at intervertebral levels compared with vertebral levels. Taylor[1] also notes a greater nuclear density in the disc portions than in the vertebral parts of a cylindrical cervical notochord in

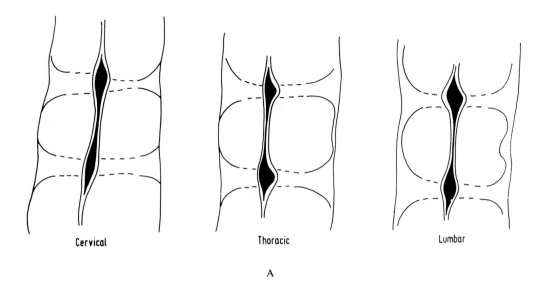

Cervical   Thoracic   Lumbar

A

FIGURE 8. (A to E) Tracings of median sagittal section outlines, showing vertebral centra and disc outlines in the cervical, thoracic, and lumbar regions of the developing vertebral column, at different stages. Changes in the shape of the notochordal segments (black), associated with their growth, can be traced through five stages (A to E) — not to scale. Within the vertebral body outlines, the white areas represent cartilage and the stippled areas represent bone. A, 30-mm C.R.L., 8 weeks; B, 75-mm C.R.L., 13 weeks; C, 115-mm C.R.L., 17 weeks; D, 295 C.R.L., 34 weeks; E, 14-month infant.

a 20-mm human embryo. Some doubt remains as to whether the differential "growth pressures" of a more rapidly growing vertebral anlage passively displace notochordal tissue into the perichordal discs, or whether the notochordal tissue actively segments by a differential growth pattern at disc and vertebral levels, respectively.

The notochordal dilatations in the perichordal discs are usually fusiform or rhomboidal in shape (Figures 4 and 5). Bohmig[9] describes a variety of shapes of "chordasegment" as seen in an 86-mm embryo, particularly, rhomboid, mushroom-shaped, and fusiform but also a "V-form", usually found in the cervical region. Peacock[5] was unable to find such well-defined forms. Peacock,[5] Prader,[10] and Taylor[1] describe the horizontal expansion of the notochordal segments, predominantly in a posterior direction, in embryos and fetuses. Figure 8 illustrates the expansion of the notochordal tissue in the discs at five stages from the 30-mm embryo to the 14-month infant.

Notochordal segmentation heralds a change in the activity of the notochordal cells, as extracellular matrix begins to appear around the notochordal cells. Robin[44] first gave a clear description of how "the central cavity of the intervertebral disc is produced by expansion of the notochordal segments with multiplication of the notochordal cells" and of the appearance of a gelatinous matrix which separates the cell mass into small clumps. Different authors note the first appearance of extracellular substance in embryos at various stages between 20 and 55 mm C.R.L.[1,5,6,10,30,48] At the same time, a change in the notochordal cells is described with the appearance of vacuoles or vesicles in their cytoplasm. Virchow[40] described chordoma cells as "physaliferous" (or "bubble-bearing"), though he mistook the origin of the chordoma and referred to it as a tumour of cartilage. Robin[44] described the appearance of "sarcoid droplets" in the notochordal cells from 3 months of intrauterine life (about 100 mm C.R.L.) onwards. Prader[10], Bradford and Spurling,[48] Peacock,[5] and But[30] also describe the appearance of intracellular vesicles in the notochordal cells of embryos of from 21 to 70 mm onwards. Thereafter, increasing quantities of "mucoid matrix" of similar appearance to the substance in the intracellular vacuoles[1,6] appear around the notochordal

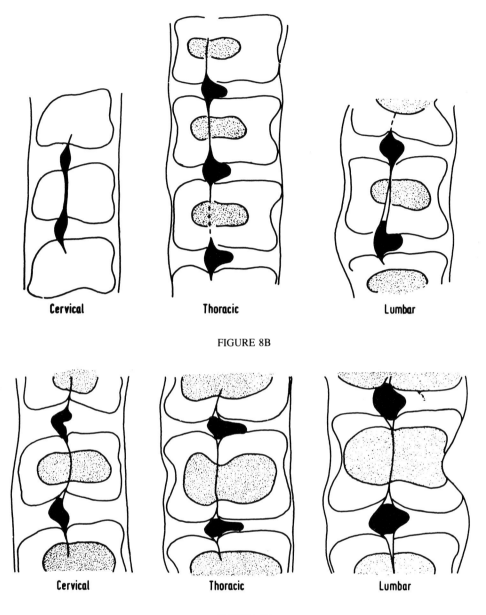

Cervical   Thoracic   Lumbar

FIGURE 8B

Cervical   Thoracic   Lumbar

FIGURE 8C

cells. The accumulation of matrix splits up the originally compact mass of notochordal cells into cellular clumps and strands which form a loose network known as a "chorda reticulum".[1,5] The ealier view that notochordal cells form a syncytium[6,28] has been shown to be false by electron microscopy (Figure 9). Cell membranes are complete at all stages of notochordal cell development.[49-51]

Ultrastructural studies[51] and Figure 9 show that the "physaliferous" appearance of the chorda reticulum is, in the main, due to accumulation of matrix between cells which are joined by multiple cell processes around these intercellular vesicles. The notochordal cells are large with large ovoid nuclei. The cytoplasm contains a Golgi apparatus, a plentiful rough endoplasmic reticulum which surrounds the few mitochondria, and a number of spherical vesicles. There are also a number of lysosomes; occasionally, centrioles are seen. Fibrillar material and glycogen are plentiful in some cells (Figure 9).

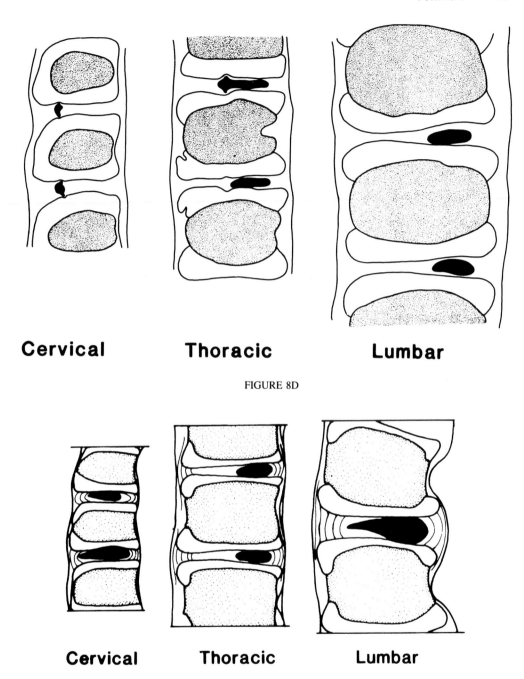

Cervical **Thoracic** **Lumbar**

FIGURE 8D

Cervical **Thoracic** **Lumbar**

FIGURE 8E

B. Survival of Notochordal Cells

The appearance of vesicles in the notochordal cells has been mistakenly described as a sign of degeneration,[9,45] referring to the increase of matrix as "mucoid degeneration" of notochordal cells. This view was widely disseminated.[10,30,48] However, as early as 1868, Robin[44] performed in vitro experiments on fresh notochordal cells and described the accumulation and disappearance of droplets in these cells as a reversible process. More recently, Fell[52] observed the vesicular appearance associated with endocytosis and exocytosis in a variety of connective tissue cells in culture.

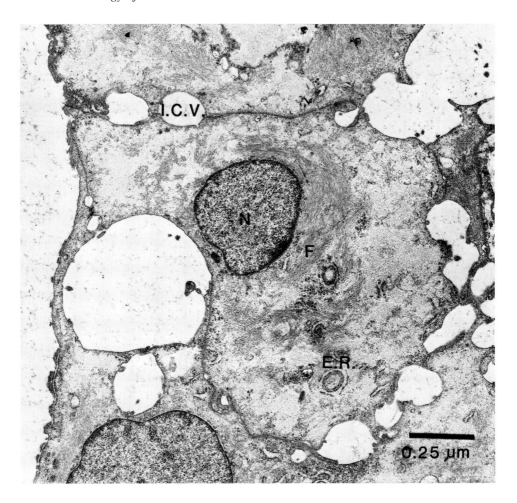

FIGURE 9.   Electron micrograph of notochordal tissue from a human fetus, fixed by immersion in glutaraldehyde within 1 hour of death. Note the large cell and nuclear size, perinuclear fibrillar material, spherical vesicles surrounded by ribosomes and intercellular accumulations of matrix. N. = nucleus; F. = fibrillar material; I.C.V. = intercellular vesicles; E.R. = ribosomes around vesicle.

There is wide variation in estimates of the period during which notochordal cells continue to survive, multiply, or show other activity. Many authors have wrongly restricted noto-chordal cell multiplication and activity to the prenatal period. Prader[10] observed mitoses only in notochordal cells of her earliest group of embryos (3 to 5 mm). She described "involutional changes" (pyknotic nuclei and acidophilic cytoplasm) from 70 mm onwards. While "clearly recognizable notochordal cells" were described in full-term fetuses, all the cells were said to "show degenerative appearances". Prader[10] associated the "degeneration" of the vesicular notochordal cells with the accumulation of mucoid matrix. Bradford and Spurling[48] went further and claimed that the notochordal cells were reduced in number by 157 mm. They even stated that "they are inconspicuous" in the "full-term" nucleus pul-posus. They may have been misled by appearances in cervical discs, in which notochordal development is retarded and unpredictable compared to lumbar discs (Figure 8d). Peacock[5] claimed that notochordal cells were fewer in number by 210 mm, though he described the full-term nucleus pulposus as predominantly notochordal.

Other workers attribute more prolonged activity to the cells. Keyes and Compere[45] em-phasize the rapid growth of notochordal tissue in fetuses up to 157 mm C.R.L., maintaining that the notochord is the chief source of the nucleus pulposus up to full term. Walmsley[6] describes an increase "in size and number" of notochordal cells during the first 6 months of intrauterine life and a full-term nucleus pulposus consisting mainly of mucoid material containing "scattered notochordal cells". Malinski[46] states that the chorda reticulum in full term fetuses is "widespread". On the basis of his histochemical studies, he considers that notochordal cells remain active in the production of glycosaminoglycans until the 5th or 8th year of postnatal life. From histochemical investigations on fetal and infant intervertebral discs, Wolfe, et al.[47] conclude also that *notochordal cells actively contribute to the matrix in the postnatal period,* probably by the production of glycosaminoglycans, since they contain the necessary enzyme systems. Using autoradiography, Amprino[53] and Souter and Taylor[33] show that notochordal cells in immature small mammals incorporate ^{35}S sulfate, and conclude that the cells produce glycosaminoglycans.

In a series of measurement studies, Taylor[1] *confirmed that notochordal cells remain active postnatally.* He demonstrated continuing increase in the volume of the notochordal tissue of the lumbar nucleus pulposus, both prenatally and postnatally. There is a 30-fold increase in the volume of the notochordal nucleus in the human fetus from 18 weeks to 40 weeks, principally due to an 18-fold increase in the number of notochordal cells. This is followed by a 10-fold increase in the volume of notochordal tissue from birth to 3 years. The postnatal increase in volume is largely due to the increase in mucoid matrix. However, nuclear counts show a further increase in notochordal cell numbers after birth in the 1st year of life. Then the number of notochordal cells remains at about the same level from 1 to 3 years in lumbar nuclei pulposi. There is further evidence that these cells remain active in infancy and early childhood, as they produce alcianophilic material in the surrounding matrix. The alcian blue staining is most dense in the rim of matrix surrounding the cells.[1] In many cases in the author's series, notochordal cells retain essentially the same appearance from embryonic life until early childhood (Figure 5). Healthy cell clumps and cells showing necrotic changes are present in the same notochordal nucleus of some 2-year-old discs. The notochordal cells appear to die off and disappear fairly quickly in the period from 3 to 5 years, with no notochordal tissue being found by light microscopy in 7- and 10-year specimens, though much necrotic cell debris is seen.[1,54] They are replaced by a different population of cells similar to fibroblasts and chondrocytes.[54]

Most modern authors agree that notochordal cells disappear from the human disc during infancy and childhood. Meachim and Cornah[54] found that most notochordal cells disappeared by 4 years; Taylor[1] did not find any cells which could be clearly identified as notochordal in the nucleus pulposi of children over the age of 5 years, though there were many necrotic or disintegrating cells; Malinski[46] did not observe them after the age of 8 years; and Peacock[5] and Walmsley[6] could not detect any notochordal cells in discs in children of more than 10 years of age.

Schwabe,[55] on the other hand, describes persistence of notochordal tissue in sacral-disc remnants of adults ranging from 22 years to 45 years, attributing their persistence in this situation to the "absence of mechanical attrition". Trout et al.,[51] in an electron microscopic study, also describe notochordal cells persisting in adult lumbar nuclei pulposi. Their micrographs of fetal notochordal cells are good, but their published illustration of adult "notochordal cells" is unconvincing. In a recent survey of the histology of end-plate lesions (Schmorl's nodes) in the cartilage plates and vertebral end-plates of 19 lumbar spines from subjects between 5 and 35 years of age, we have observed typical notochordal cell clumps in a Schmorl's node in a 17-year-old male. Chordomas are of notochordal origin, and the occurrence of these rare tumors presupposes the survival of notochordal cells in some individuals, usually near the cranial or sacral ends of the original notochordal track.[56] They are locally invasive, produce necrotic changes in the tissues they infiltrate, and may show some variation in their histological pattern, e.g., being described as "stellate", "physaliferous", or "chondroid".[56-58]

C. Changes at the Periphery of the Notochord

In embryos of about 20 mm C.R.L., a clear homogenous notochordal sheath is described surrounding the original diamond-shaped notochordal dilatation[5,10,42] (see Figure 8a). This sheath initially separates the notochordal cells from the embryonic hyaline cartilage cells of the surrounding perichordal disc. As early as the 35-mm stage[6] the sheath may break down, leading to a "blending and interaction" between notochordal cells and the cells of the "inner-cell zone" or perichordal zone. Walmsley[6] describes active invasion of the inner-cell zone by the notochordal cells in a 72-mm embryo and postulates that degenerative changes observed in the cells of the inner zone are a direct result of this invasion. He suggests, as did Luschka,[41] that by its degeneration and liquefaction, the inner-cell zone adds to the volume of the expanding nucleus pulposus. Keyes and Compere,[45] Prader,[10] Peacock,[5] and But[30] also agree that interaction between notochordal cells and the cells of the surrounding inner-cell zone plays an essential part in the growth and expansion of the nucleus pulposus. But[30] maintains that the soft central mass cannot properly be called a "nucleus pulposus" until this interaction has taken place.

The rapid increase in notochordal nucleus pulposus volume in fetuses from 29 to 40 weeks is accompanied by incorporation and apparent liquefaction of tissue from the inner-cell zone.[1] This involves infiltration of the inner-cell zone and inner annulus by notochordal tissue and loosening of the connective tissue strands at the periphery of the notochordal nucleus (Figures 10 and 11). These connective tissue elements around the boundary of the notochordal nucleus frequently show a hyaline, necrotic appearance (Figure 12). At this stage, the inner-cell zone no longer consists of hyaline cartilage, but its numerous closely packed cells have elongated nuclei like fibroblasts and its plentiful matrix contains some randomly oriented collagen bundles. The main mass of the notochordal nucleus lies posterior of the center of the disc, and the inner-cell zone tissue lies mostly anterior to the notochordal tissue in thoracic and lumbar discs. In cervical discs, where the notochordal tissue expansion is relatively delayed, "inner-cell zone" tissue occupies most of the center of the disc.[1]

The first appearance of fine fibrous elements in the matrix of the nucleus pulposus was described by Walmsley[6] in a 94-mm embryo and by Keyes and Compere[45] in a 157-mm specimen. Prader[12] and Taylor[1] also reported "flaking off" of collagen bundles into the nucleus pulposus in full-term fetuses, but these appeared to be "liquefied" or "digested" in some way by the notochordal tissue. The increase of visible collagen in the nucleus pulposus was most marked in postnatal rather than prenatal life.[1,5]

D. Postnatal Changes in the Nucleus Pulposus

The newborn lumbar nucleus pulposus is relatively large, with clearly demarcated margins bounded by a "perichordal" zone of fibrocartilage. Its matrix is an apparently homogeneous mucoid substance, containing scattered clumps and strands of notochordal cells. The innermost part of the surrounding fibrocartilage, the main mass of which lies anterior to the notochordal nucleus, appears to be undergoing liquefaction. Similar but less obvious changes are occurring at the faces of the cartilage plates. The 5-month-old nucleus pulposus has a similar appearance.[1,5] Luschka[41] stated that during childhood, villous processes of fibrocartilage project into the notochordal nucleus. Such villi are illustrated in Figure 12. In full-term and infant discs, there is further evidence of invasion of the inner cell zone by notochordal cells, with some mixing of the notochordal cell clumps and the "cartilage cells" (Figures 11 and 12). The inner-cell zone tissue at the boundary of the nucleus often has a necrotic hyaline appearance with indistinct cell boundaries. Strands of the inner cell zone tissue or "ghosts" of lamellae of the inner annulus are seen within the notochordal nucleus pulposus of infants and 2-year-old children (Figure 12). These are partly necrotic and disintegrating.[1] At 1 year, fine collagen is appearing in the matrix of the nucleus.[59] In early childhood, despite continuing increase in the volume of notochordal tissue, there is gradual

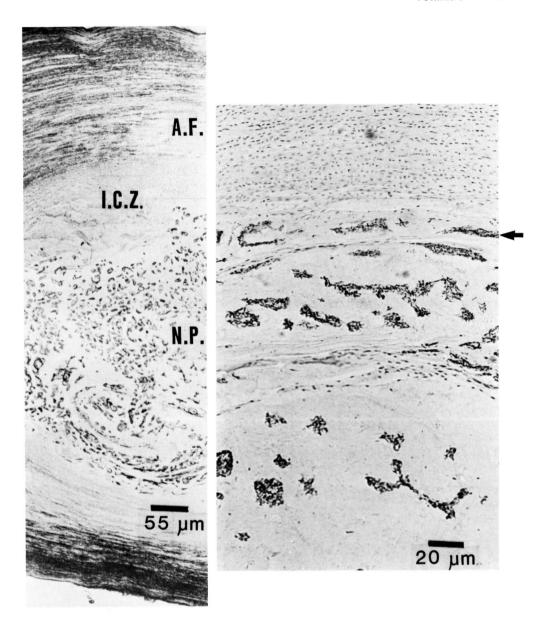

FIGURE 10.   Horizontal 50 μm sections of low viscosity nitrocellulose embedded lumbar discs, from a 30-week fetus, showing "invasion" of the inner cell zone by notochordal cell clumps (arrow); A.F. = annulus; I.C.Z. = inner cell zone; N.P. = nucleus pulposus.

change in the character of the tissue. Some cells remain active, and probably multiply, while others show nuclear pyknosis and loss of cytoplasmic staining. By 4 years, an irregular network of collagen is seen in the matrix and only a few isolated clumps of notochordal cells persist, many of which are degenerate.[1]

Measurements of the anteroposterior dimensions of the annulus and nucleus in midsagittal sections of lumbar discs show that, during the phase of rapid nucleus pulposus growth in infancy, the nucleus grows at the expense of the annulus (Figure 13). Similar data from vertical measurements in the same sections suggest that the cartilage plates are also eroded at their inner margins during the same period.[1] Growth in thickness of the annulus and cartilage plates resumes at the end of this phase, i.e., at about 3 years (Figure 13).

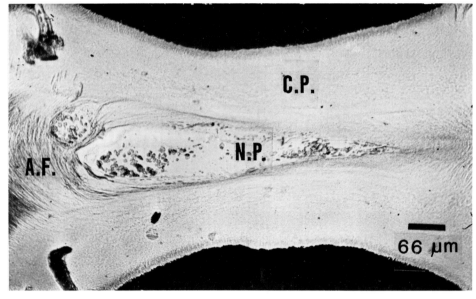

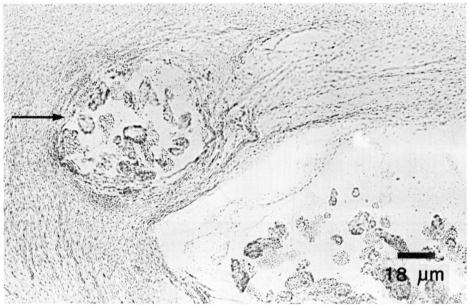

FIGURE 11.   Median sagittal 150-μm section of a full-term fetal L4-5 disc showing "invasion" of the inner part of anterior anulus by notochordal tissue; above: (×15) (A.F. = annulus, N.P. = nucleus, C.P. = cartilage plate); below: the invading notochordal tissue is shown by the arrow (×55).

The outlines in Figures 8 and 14 illustrate the typical shape, extent, and position of the notochordal nucleus pulposus at different stages from fetal life to childhood. Figures 8 and 14 compare median sagittal outlines of notochordal segments in cervical, thoracic, and lumbar discs in embryos, fetuses, infants, and children. At all stages of infancy and childhood, the nucleus pulposus occupies a large part of the area of a lumbar disc as seen in median sagittal section, but as age increases, the boundary between the nucleus pulposus and the surrounding fibrocartilage becomes blurred, while the collagen fiber content of the nucleus increases.[13] The progressive increase in its collagen content and the gradual change in its cell content from large groups of notochordal cells in clumps or strands to relatively few cells resembling

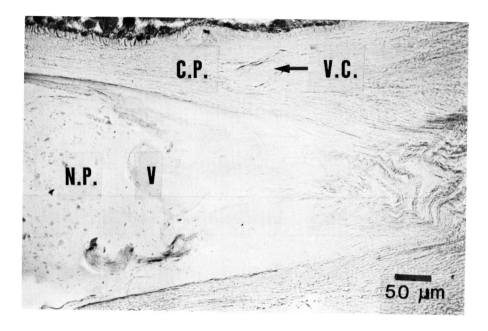

A

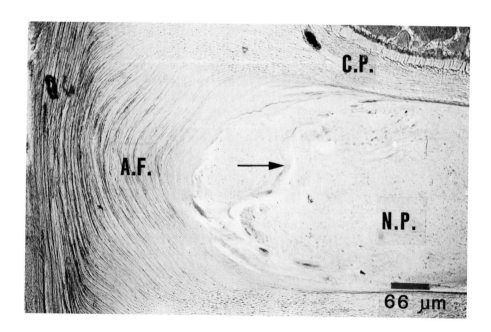

B

FIGURE 12.   Median sagittal 150-μm section of a 14-month infant L4-5 disc, showing: (A) above (×20): a "villus" (V) of inner cell zone tissue, with hyaline necrotic appearance, projecting into the posterior part of the notochordal nucleus. Note the former vascular canal (V.C.), now without a vessel and plugged by connective tissue; C.P. = cartilage plate; N.P. = nucleus pulposus. (B) Below (×15): the "ghost" of a lamella of the anterior annulus (arrowed), now being incorporated into the expanding nucleus; A.F. = annulus; N.P. = nucleus; C.P. = cartilage plate.

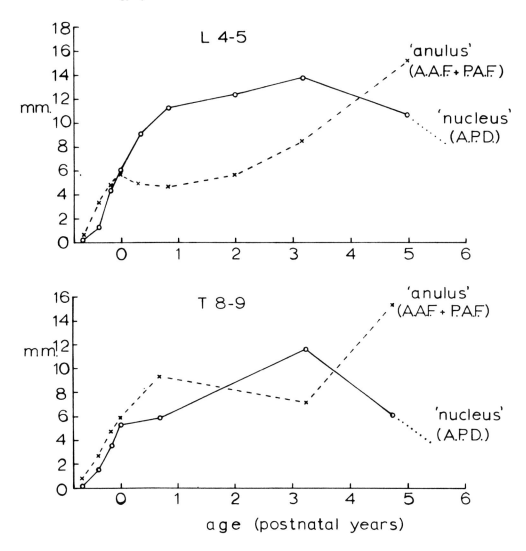

FIGURE 13.   Graph comparing the anteroposterior median sagittal dimensions of the "annulus" and the noto-chordal nucleus pulposus ("annulus" is the sum of anterior annulus, posterior annulus, and inner cell zone). L4—5 dimensions were measured in 36 discs and T 8-9 dimensions in 26 discs. Comparison of six full-term lumbar discs with seven infant lumbar discs (mean age 5 months) shows a decrease in "annulus" from 5.8 mm to 4.5 mm; using a Student *t*-test the probability that this decrease is significant is $p < 0.01$.

chondrocytes, occurring singly or in small groups, so alter the appearance of the nucleus pulposus during childhood (3 to 8 years) that the nucleus of an adolescent or of a young adult appears fibrocartilaginous.[1,5,6,59] The relative size of the lumbar notochordal nucleus pulposus, compared to the disc as a whole, peaks in the age range 1 to 3 years when it constitutes 75% of the anteroposterior extent of the lumbar disc in median sections, 30% of the area of the disc in horizontal sections, and 10% of the volume of the disc — see Table 1 and Figures 15 and 16.[1] There is considerable regional variation in development of the notochordal segments.[60] The nucleus pulposus is never as large in thoracic discs as in lumbar discs, and the cervical notochordal nucleus varies much more in its extent, being extensive in some infants and quite limited in others (Figures 8 d and e). After about 5 years, a "notochordal nucleus pulposus" can no longer be defined. Its mucoid matrix persists, but it is largely masked by the increasing collagen content.[13]

Corresponding with its histological changes during maturation, the water content of the

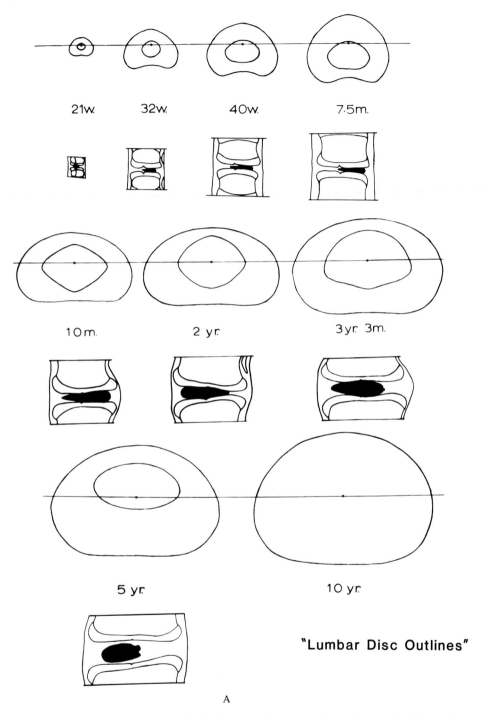

21w.   32w.   40w.   7·5m.

10m.   2 yr.   3 yr. 3m.

5 yr.   10 yr.

"Lumbar Disc Outlines"

A

FIGURE 14. (A) shows L4—5; (B) shows T8—9; diagrammatic reconstructions of intervertebral disc and notochordal nucleus pulposus outlines (× 2.4); ages are shown with horizontal outlines above and median sagittal
outlines below. In the sagittal section outlines, notochordal tissue is shown black and anterior is to the left. The
"points" at the "center" of each horizontal outline represent the position of the "notochordal defects" in each
pair of cartilage plates. These "defects" are visible as small triagular depressions in the cartilage plates on the
median sagittal outlines (see figures 19 and 22); this permits assessment of the extent of anterior and posterior
growth from these "points". Note the "change in posture" between the 10-month and 2-year stages in 14(A),
the absence of notochordal tissue in the 10-year lumbar disc, and the indeterminate anterior boundary of the
notochordal nucleus in the 6-year thoracic disc.

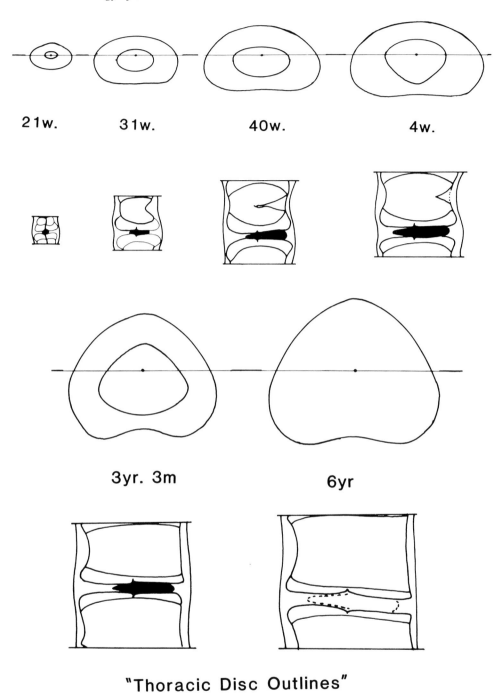

21w.   31w.   40w.   4w.

3yr. 3m   6yr

"Thoracic Disc Outlines"

FIGURE 14B.

nucleus decreases with age, from 88% in the newborn to 76% in the 3rd decade of life.[61] The most rapid reduction in water content takes place during the growth period, with relatively little further change during adult life. The young adult nucleus still contains much mucoid substance around an irregular fibrocartilaginous network.[13] Nachemson[62] maintains that, despite its dramatic change in appearance during postnatal development and maturation, the

Table 1
MIDSAGITTAL PROPORTIONS OF THREE PARTS OF LUMBAR DISCS

Age group	% of Disc Proper due to NCNP X̄ S. D.		% of disc proper due to A.F. X̄ S. D.		% of disc proper due to ICZ. X̄ S. D.	
Fetuses (5)	7.1 ± 2.2		75.0 ± 5.5		17.5 ± 4.2	
Newborn (3)	6.7 ± 0.3		69.7 ± 5.9		23.3 ± 4.2	
Infants and children (4)	10.4 ± 2.1		67.3 ± 4.1		22.7 ± 5.1	

Note: NCNP = notochordal nucleus pulposus; A.F. = annulus fibrosus; ICZ = inner cell zone (which becomes fibrocartilage — see text); X̄ = mean; SD = standard deviation. Using Student's *t*-test, the postnatal increase in the % of the disc proper due to the notochordal nucleus is statistically significant at the $p < 0.05$ level.

nucleus pulposus of the normal adult still behaves as a fluid, redistributing axial compression forces equally in all directions to the cartilage plates and annulus fibrosus. That the nucleus pulposus is under pressure in the absence of any external load is shown by the fact that it bulges out from the cut surface on section of the disc, the internal pressure in vivo exceeding the external load by 50%.[62]

Almost two thirds of the adult population are said to show radiological signs of disc degeneration.[63] According to Stevens,[64] the basis of this is that the loss of water content and decreasing turgor of the nucleus lead to horizontal "flat-tire" bulging of the annulus and stripping of the periosteum from the vertebral body margins with the formation of osteophytes. This is contradicted by the recent observations of Twomey and Taylor[65] that the average mid-disc height of aged intervertebral discs is increased compared to young adults, though the peripheral height may be marginally reduced and small osteophytes may be common. The conflict would appear to arise from the fact that clinical interpretations of age changes in discs have been based on biased populations with chronic degenerative back problems. Wrong conclusions on disc thickness may have been drawn from radiological images where marginal osteophytes with some marginal narrowing of the disc space may mask well preserved central disc thickness. Post-mortem examination of an unselected population shows that 70% of elderly lumbar discs are not thin or "degenerate" as judged by Rolander's classification.[65]

E. The Position of the Notochordal Nucleus Pulposus within the Disc
1. In the Prenatal Disc

In embryos, the notochord lies anterior to the center of the vertebral column[1,5,6,30,45] — see Figures 4 and 8. In the discs, posterior expansion takes place from the original anterior position. By its enlargement, as seen in the median plane, the nucleus pulposus comes to occupy about half the anteroposterior extent of thoracic and lumbar discs in 30- to 40-week fetuses, with the main mass of the nucleus posterior to the center of the disc.[1] Prader[10] attributes this predominantly posterior expansion to a lesser tissue pressure in the posterior parts of the kyphotic fetal vertebral column. This interpretation is supported by the later observation of the change in position of the lumbar nucleus, when lordosis is established in early childhood (see below).[1]

"Notochordal flexures", quite distinct from those described in the unsegmented notochord, are described in older embyos where the mucoid streak is still visible (up to 150 mm). These are seen in the later cartilaginous and early ossification stages of vertebral development (about 35 to 150 mm) and are said to be due to the fixed position of the mucoid

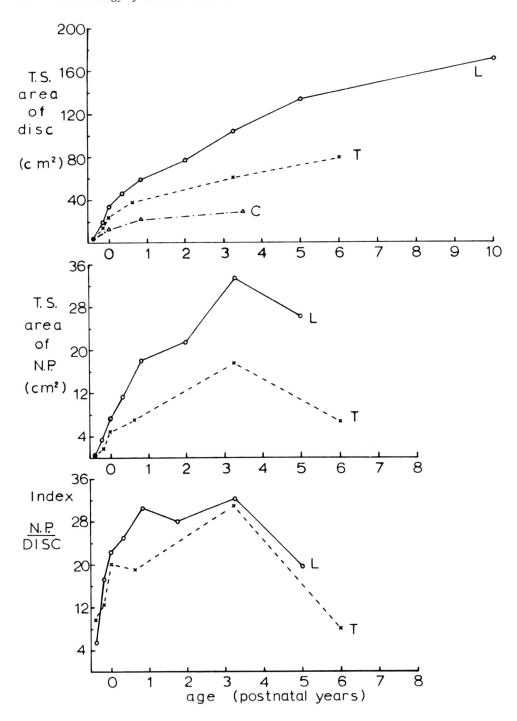

FIGURE 15.   Transverse sectional areas of the disc and the nucleus (N.P.) for L4—5 and T8—9, with the nucleus-to-disc ratio; areas were measured by planimentry of projected sections of 9 lumbar, 6 thoracic, and 4 cervical discs. Notochordal nucleus pulposus area was not consistently measurable in cervical discs.

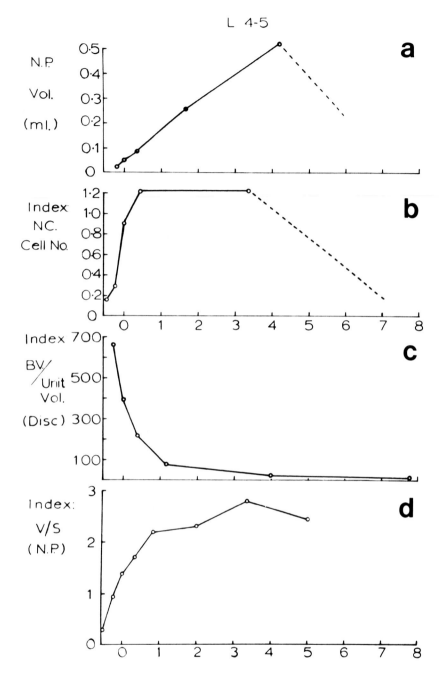

FIGURE 16. (a) Volume of the lumbar notochordal nucleus (N.P.) with age, based on plan-imetry of consecutive sections;[1] (b) estimate of notochordal cell (N.C.) numbers with age, based on nuclear counts;[1] (c) vascularity of the lumbar disc is based on counting the vascular canals (B.V.) in the cartilage plates; this is then related to the volume of the "disc proper" (i.e., annulus plus nucleus, excluding cartilage plates); (d) index of volume to surface area ratio for the nucleus (V/S), indicates the relation of available absorptive area to the mass requiring nutrition.

streak in the ossifying vertebral body, while the notochordal segment in the disc is able to shift its position.[1] Such flexures would appear to indicate different growth patterns in discs compared to vertebral bodies, e.g., appositional growth of bone and interstitial growth in discs. Most chordaflexures in embryos of mammals other than man show a ventral convexity in the vertebral bodies.[10,18,27] In human fetuses, flexures with a dorsal convexity in the vertebral bodies and a ventral convexity in the discs are described.[1,9,10,27]

2. Position of the Nucleus in the Postnatal Disc

Bohmig[9] and But[30] maintain that the position of the nucleus is influenced by the curvature of the vertebral column, being posterior in kyphotic regions and anterior in lordotic regions. This was confirmed by Taylor[66] in studies of the changing position of the lumbar notochordal nucleus pulposus during infancy and early childhood (Figure 14a). The newborn notochordal nucleus pulposus is wedge-shaped in median sagittal section, large and rounded towards the posterior annulus, and tapering forwards into the "inner cell zone". On assumption of the erect posture, with the establishment of lumbar lordosis in the 2nd year of life, there is a shift in both the position and shape of the lumbar nucleus from a "posterior wedge" to a mirror image "anterior wedge". In the thoracic spine, where the primary curve is maintained, the nucleus retains its posterior position (Figure 14b). In older children, the lumbar nucleus pulposus is centrally situated.

V. THE CARTILAGE PLATES

Some authorities do not include the cartilage plates in descriptions of the intervertebral disc[5,6,12,13] while others do.[8,9,36,59,67] These tissues are parts of the original cartilage model of the vertebra, which remain unossified as "cartilaginous epiphyses", capping the cephalic and caudal surfaces of each centrum. They are also essential parts of the envelope which encloses the nucleus pulposus, with a lamellar structure in continuity with the annulus fibrosus.[1,7]

A. Origin and Role in the Growth of the Vertebral Column

At an early stage of development (12.5 mm), the mesenchymal tissue of the dark band between the developing cartilaginous vertebral bodies — the perichordal disc — is described as consisting of three parts[15]: a middle component or plate, the anlage of the "intervertebral disc proper", and cranial and caudal components or plates, which chondrify from the vertebral bodies and become the primordia of the cartilage plates.[1,5,15]

Once ossification has begun in the vertebral bodies, the cartilage plates fit over the cephalic and caudal surfaces of the bony vertebral body "as an overhanging lid fits a jampot".[8] The cartilage plates in fetuses, infants, and children (Figure 17) may be regarded as including: (1) the growth zone with its palisade arrangement of cartilage cells in columns vertical to the advancing ossification front of the vertebral body, and (2) a layer of hyaline cartilage with flattened cells oriented horizontally, adjacent to the intervertebral disc. Each "cartilage layer" has the fibers of the annulus fibrosus anchored in it peripherally, as seen by normal light microscopy. With the annulus, the cartilage layers bound and enclose the nucleus pulposus centrally.[1,6,7,13,67]

Small blood vessels which penetrate the cartilage plates from the periphery from the 75-mm stage onwards provide nutrition for the cartilage plates and the adjacent intervertebral disc during growth[1,5,32] and persist into the 2nd decade of life.[9,35] These are associated during childhood and adolescence with radially running grooves at the junction of the cartilage plates and bony vertebral body.[24,68] The cartilage plate is described as loosely cemented to the underlying bone by a calcareous layer, presumably calcified cartilage.[8] In the growing individual, it is clearly distinguishable in ordinary light microscopy from the annulus and

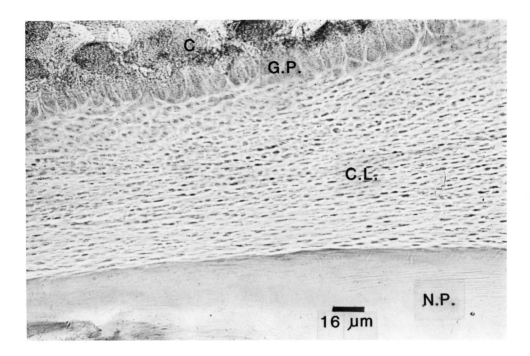

FIGURE 17. A 150-μm sagittal section of the upper cartilage plate of the L4—5 disc of a 14-month infant (× 60), showing the "cartilage layer" (C.L.) adjacent to the nucleus (N.P.); the growth plate (G.P.) is adjacent to the centrum (C) above.

nucleus,[5,6] though Peacock describes the junction of annulus and cartilage plate as a transitional zone. The polarized light studies of Franceschini[7] and Taylor[1] show the continuity of the lamellar structure of the annulus fibrosus into the horizontally oriented "cartilage layer" (Figures 1 and 6). The "cartilage layer" is said to contribute to the "interstitial growth" of the annulus, a growth possibly induced by the vascular canals in the cartilage.[32] During the rapid growth of the nucleus pulposus in the fetus and infant, the "cartilage layer" appears to be eroded by the expanding nucleus.[1,5,6] It is said to be thicker during the first years of life than at later stages,[8,32] but measurement studies[1] show a diminution in the thickness of lumbar cartilage plates during the first 2 postnatal years when the lumbar nucleus is expanding rapidly (Figure 15).

B. Formation of the Ring Apophysis

Before adolescence, foci of calcification appear in the peripheral parts of the "cartilage layer" which ossify to form a bony ring,[9] described as an apophysis (Figure 18), since it makes no independent contribution to vertebral growth.[69] Hanson[70] reviewed the 19th century literature on the "vertebral epiphyses" which were said to appear during adolescence. In a radiological study, Hanson[70] found that their earliest appearance was in a girl of 6 years. The foci of calcification usually appear at about 8 years in girls and 9 years in boys. Ossification follows immediately and proceeds to fusion with the vertebral body from 18 to 20 years.[37] The major, central part of the "cartilage layer" does not ossify. It separates the vertebral spongiosa from the nucleus pulposus and permits nutrition of the avascular nucleus from the vascular spongiosa.[71]

C. Defects in the Cartilage Plate

Bohmig[9] described a funnel-shaped defect or identation into each "cartilage layer" at the junction of the nucleus pulposus with the situation of the former notochordal track through

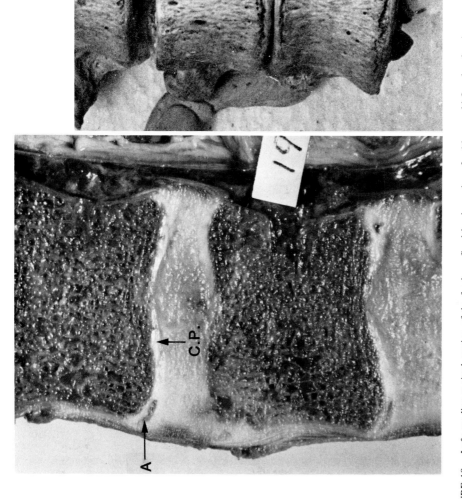

FIGURE 18.   Left: median sagittal section of the fresh, unfixed lumbar spine of a 16-year-old female, showing an unfused ring apophysis (A) in the periphery of a cartilage plate (C.P.). Ring apophyses are seen at the anterior margin of the upper cartilage plate in both discs and at the posterior margin of the upper cartilage plate in the lower disc. Right: fusing ring apophyses (A) in vertebrae from a young adult male: small holes for vascular canals are visible, both in the anterior vertebral body surface and between the centrum and apophyseal rings.

the cartilage plate. This funnel-shaped defect, also described by Taylor[1,24,26] in median sagittal sections of developing discs, is continuous at its apex with a translucent, cell-free area of matrix in the cartilage plate along the line of the former notochordal track (Figure 19). These features are described from fetal life onwards, persisting up to 20 or 25 years. They constitute central weak points in the cartilage plates through which herniations from the nucleus into the vertebral spongiosa frequently occur[9,24] (see Figure 20). Such herniations, known as Schmorl's nodes, are found in 38% of adult vertebral columns on median sagittal sectioning of the columns.[2,9,24] In addition to the central weakness in each cartilage plate, attributable to the notochordal track, there are "peripheral" weaknesses in the cartilage plate related to attrition of vascular canals. These may also be related to disc herniations in later life[24] (see Figures 21 and 22).

VI. NUTRITION OF THE INTERVERTEBRAL DISCS

Nutrition of the intervertebral disc during growth and development may be derived from two sources: (1) from vertebral blood vessels ramifying close to the annulus and nucleus in the cartilage plates (Figure 22), and (2) by blood vessels entering the periphery of the annulus fibrosus (Figure 23).

A. Vertebral Sources

A consideration of the vertebral blood supply is germane to the question of nutrition of the intervertebral disc.

An anastomotic network is formed in the vertebral canal on the dorsal aspect of the vertebral bodies from arteries entering the intervertebral foramina. A large branch from this network enters the center of the dorsal surface of each vertebral body.[1,72,73] This "primary" or nutrient artery[1,72] branches out to all parts of the vertebral body, particularly to the cranial and caudal metaphyses.

A series of smaller blood vessels ramify within the periosteum of the anterior and lateral surfaces of the "waist" of the vertebra. Branches from this plexus termed "secondary blood vessels"[72] arch radially around the caudal and cephalic surfaces of the centrum *into the cartilage plates* (like epiphyseal vessels). The cartilage plate vessels give off side branches in the direction of the annulus and nucleus (Figure 22). These usually end in capillary plexuses or "glomeruli" near the junction of the cartilage plate and "disc proper".[1,9,32,72,73] Some cartilage plate vessels form anastomotic arcades through the metaphysis with vessels in the centrum.[1] A third group of vessels appearing to emerge from the centrum, to end blindly in the cartilage plate, are probably former cartilage plate vessels which have become enclosed by the advancing ossification front.[1,24] Bohmig[9] describes vessels passing close to all parts of the annulus and nucleus, but Donisch and Trapp[32] state that the vessels are mainly confined to the peripheral (circumferential) part of the cartilage plate and end close to the annulus fibrosus. The vascular canals from the anterior periosteum of the centrum, arching around the bone-cartilage plate junction, are responsible for the "toothed appearance" of the immature caudal and cephalic vertebral end-surfaces.[1,24,68] With the advance of the ossification front, these vessels may disappear or become included in the bony centrum.[1,32] Taylor[1] performed "vascular counts" on the vascular canals in 10 fetal infants' and childrens' intervertebral discs and related the progressive reduction in disc vascularity with growth to the attrition and replacement of notochordal cells in the nucleus pulposus (Figures 16 and 24).

Experiments in immature rabbits, tracing the diffusion of fluorochrome into the intervertebral discs of animals sacrificed at given intervals after intravenous injection, have shown that the blood vessels of the cartilage plate play an important role in the nutrition of the developing disc, since diffusion takes place from the cartilage plate to the disc.[74] However,

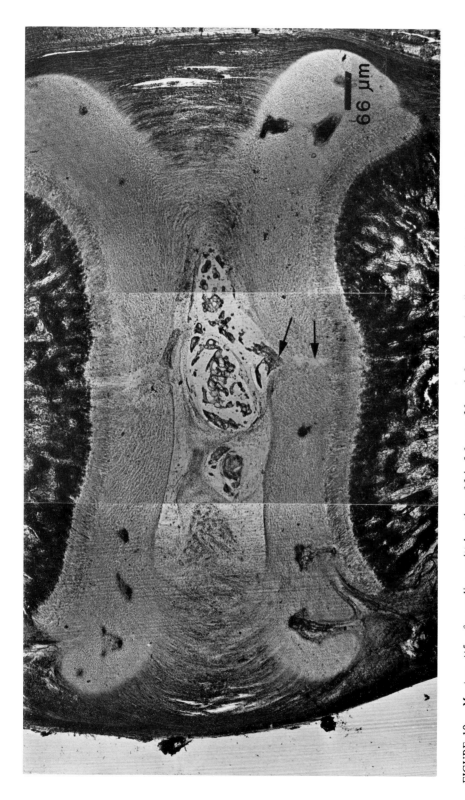

FIGURE 19.   Montage, ×5, of a median sagittal section of L4—5 from a 36-week fetus, showing "notochordal defects" (arrows) in the cartilage plates; a funnel-shaped depression extends from the notochordal nucleus into the cartilage plate and is continous at its apex, with a clear cell-free linear translucency extending towards the centrum; these "defects" follow the "line" of the former notochordal track; they persist into adolescence.[1]   (From Taylor, J. and Twomey, L., *Modern Manual Therapy of the Vertebral Column*, Grieve, G., Ed., Churchill Livingstone, Edinburgh, 1986. With permission.)

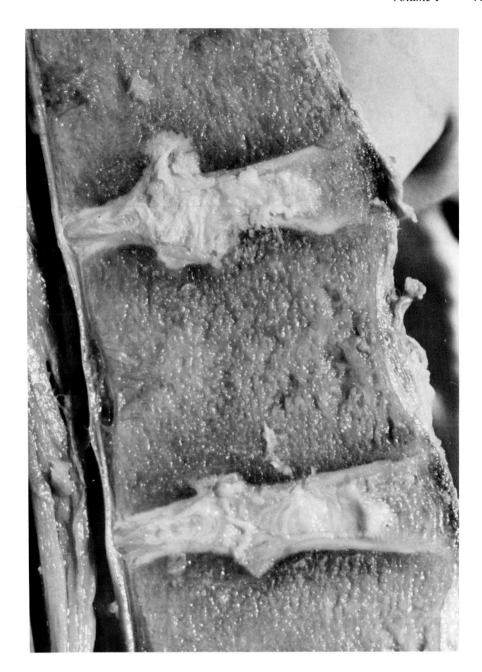

FIGURE 20. Midline section of young adult lumbar vertebrae and discs; multiple, aligned Schmorl's nodes (prolapses of disc material into the vertebral spongiosa) are in the line of the former notochordal track.[1,2]

the blood vessels of the human cartilage plate gradually disappear during growth and finally disappear by about 25 years.[1,9,24,35] In the adult, relatively few blood vessels from the spongiosa perforate the calcified cartilage layer binding the cartilage plate to the bony vertebra.[75] In childhood and adolescence, the sites of the original blood vessels are occupied by plugs of soft fibrocartilage[1,9,55] (see Figure 12a). Deformations or "outpouchings" of the nuclei pulposi of children are described opposite the sites of these "cartilage degeneration zones". These weak points in the cartilage plates predispose to herniations forming Schmorl's nodes.[1,8,9,24,55]

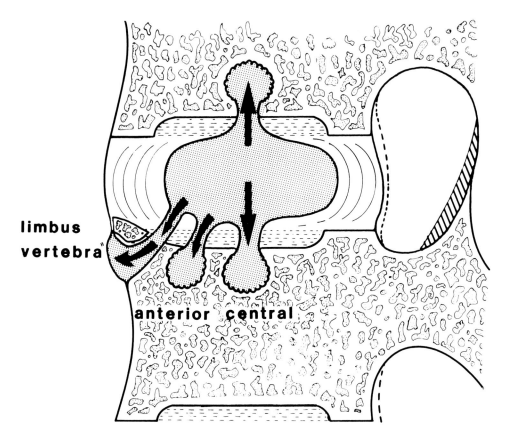

limbus vertebra

anterior central

FIGURE 21.   Varieties of Schmorl's nodes: central nodes are related to "notochordal defects" in the cartilage plates; anterior nodes are probably related to weaknesses left by attrition of former vascular canals; a "limbus vertebra" is a disc prolapse between the centrum and the ring apophysis. (From Taylor, J. and Twomey, L., *Modern Manual Therapy of the Vertebral Column,* Grieve, G., Ed., Churchill Livingstone, Edinburgh, 1986. With permission.)

B. Blood vessels in the Annulus Fibrosus

Small blood vessels in the annulus fibrosus were first described by Luschka.[41] Numerous small vessels are found in the outer annulus of fetuses, infants, and children, particularly in the posterior annulus.[1,5] The largest vessels in the fetus are found dorsolaterally.[72] Taylor[1] describes their appearance in a 75-mm embryo. Prader[12] and Somogyi[72] considered that they were entirely separate from the blood vessels of the vertebral body, entering the outer surface of the annulus radially. However, Taylor[1] showed that they establish loop-like links with the marrow vessels in fetuses and infants. Mineiro[73] describes many small blood vessels in the outer annulus fibrosus anastomozing with vessels in the longitudinal ligaments. Only the outer third or half of the annulus is vascular in fetuses and infants (Figure 23) and a few small blood vessels may persist in this peripheral part of the annulus in adults[1,6,30,72] Although Bohmig[9] described small blood vessels in the prenatal nucleus pulposus, his illustration of them suggests that he was describing an artifact, and it is generally stressed that the nucleus is always devoid of blood vessels.[1,5,6,45] The growing nucleus can therefore only be nourished by diffusion from the surrounding tissues. The number of blood vessels in the annulus and the number of vascular canals in the cartilage plates, both of which increase in the fetus up to full term, remain approximately static through infancy and decrease progressively during childhood. At the same time, the mass of the intervertebral disc is increasing rapidly, e.g., a $\times 12$ increase in nucleus pulposus volume from birth to 3 years.

a)

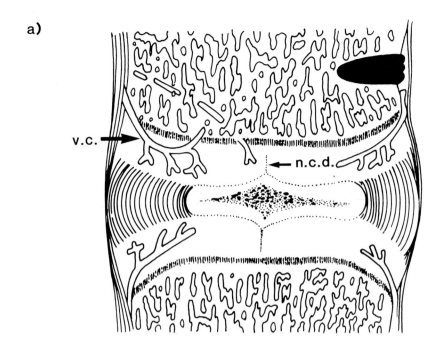

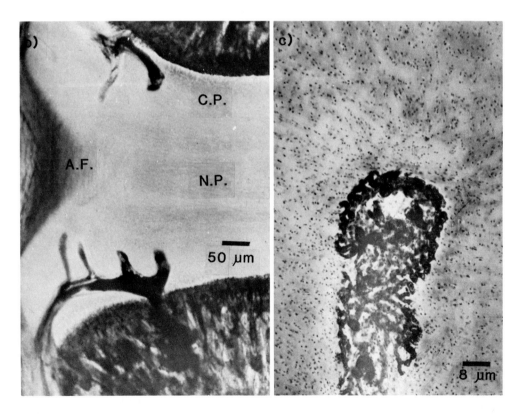

FIGURE 22.   (a) diagram of a median sagittal section of a lumbar disc, showing vascular canals (v.c.) and "notochordal defects" (n.c.d.) in cartilage plates (anterior is to the left); branches of the vascular canals end near the boundary with the "disc proper" (annulus and nucleus); (b) vascular canals loop from the anterior vertebral periosteum to the marrow of the centrum, with side branches towards the "disc proper", in a sagittal section of a 34-week fetal L4—5 disc (×20); A.F. = annulus; N.P. = nucleus; C.P. = cartilage plate; (c) each vascular canal ends with a capillary tuft or "glomerulus", as seen in this 150-μm section of a cartilage plate (×120).

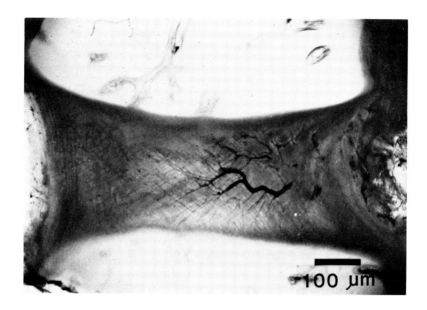

FIGURE 23.   Branching small blood vessels in the annulus of an L3—4 disc from a 30-week fetus, at 2-mm depth from the surface of the annulus, ×12; the outer third of the annulus is extremely vascular in fetuses and infants.

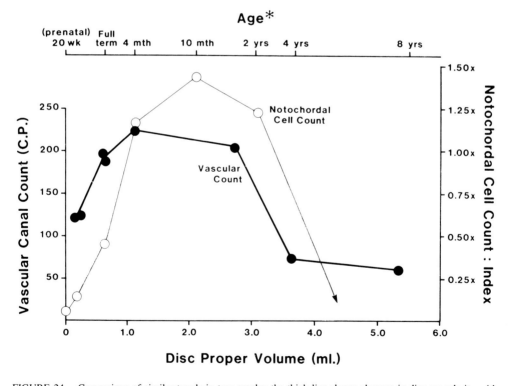

FIGURE 24.   Comparison of similar trends in two graphs; the thick line shows changes in disc vascularity with age; the thin line shows changes in notochordal cell counts with age.[1] The vertical axes represent vascular canal counts in the cartilage plates and notochordal cell counts; the horizontal axes represent age (not to scale), and volume of the disc proper (annulus plus nucleus); as disc volume increases, after infancy, vascularity and notochordal cell counts decrease in parallel. (From Taylor, J. and Twomey, L., *Modern Manual Therapy of the Vertebral Column,* Grieve, G., Ed., Churchill Livingstone, Edinburgh, 1986. With permission.)

As nuclear volume increases, there is a decrease in its surface area to volume ratio (Figure 16). All these changes make the nutritional status of the notochordal tissue progressively more unfavorable.[1] This coincides, in the period after 3 years, with the disappearance of notochordal cells from the nucleus, to be replaced by cells resembling chondrocytes and fibroblasts — cells renowned for their ability to survive in less vascular situations. It seems likely that the change in vascularity is responsible for the change in cell population (Figure 24). Trout et al.[51] dispute the claims of histologists that notochordal cells disappear from the nucleus during childhood and cite the paucity of mitochondria and presence of plentiful glycogen granules in notochordal cells as evidence that they may be equipped to survive in anaerobic conditions. However, the electron microscopic study of Trout et al.[51] does not provide acceptable evidence of survival of notochordal cells in adults. In the authors' experience, notochordal cells have some electron microscopic features in common with chondrocytes, but as a tissue, notochordal tissue has a histological appearance quite different from cartilage. While it is possible that an occasional notochordal cell may persist, masked by the massive increase in collagen content, in the nucleus pulposus of adults, repeated histological examinations by many workers have been unable to demonstrate them,[1,5,6,54] except possibly in the sacrum.[55] Both the cellular and tissue characteristics of the adult nucleus are most unlike those of the notochordal nucleus of infancy and early childhood.[54]

VII. THE EFFECTS OF ERECT POSTURE ON DISC AND VERTEBRAL GROWTH

Growth of vertebrae and intervertebral discs in childhood involves not only increase in size but also changes in shape. These changes in shape appear to be influenced by the mechanical effects of weightbearing in the erect posture.[66] They include: (1) change of the pattern of vertical growth of vertebral centra and intervertebral discs (including cartilage plates) such that the centra change from convex vertebral end-plates to concave end-plates and the disc becomes biconvex rather than biconcave (Figures 1 and 18); (2) an increase in the anteroposterior growth rate of vertebral bodies and discs, relative to lateral and vertical growth rates, so that indices of AP diameter/transverse diameter and the vertebral index of AP diameter/height, both increase (Figure 25).

Fetal and infant centra are rounded and convex towards the discs. Two factors contribute to the appearance of concavities in the lumbar vertebral end-plates. These are the rapid increase in the volume of the notochordal nucleus pulposus and the change in its position, consequent upon assumption and establishment of the erect posture at the beginning of the 2nd postnatal year. The increase in nucleus pulposus volume has already been described. When the secondary lumbar curve is established in the 2nd year of life, the main mass of the notochordal nucleus moves from a predominantly posterior to a predominantly anterior or central position (Figure 14a). With weightbearing in the erect posture, there is a considerable increase in pressure transmitted to the fluid nucleus, which redistributes this vertical pressure in all directions exerting outward force on the envelope formed by the annulus and cartilage plates. As a consequence, there is compressive loading of the centers of the vertebral end-plates and tension exerted on the vertebral rims by the traction of the outer annulus (Figure 26). The observation that a concavity begins to appear in the lumbar vertebral end plates from the age of 3 years onwards[66] opposite the maximum bulge of the large nucleus pulposus, may relate either to the pressure exerted by the compressed nucleus on this central area, or to the tension exerted on the vertebral rims, or in part to both mechanical influences. Comparison of ambulant and nonambulant groups confirms that the normal growth in thickness of lumbar intervertebral discs and the appearance of the concavities in lumbar vertebral end-plates are conditional upon weightbearing in the erect posture (Figures 27 and 28).

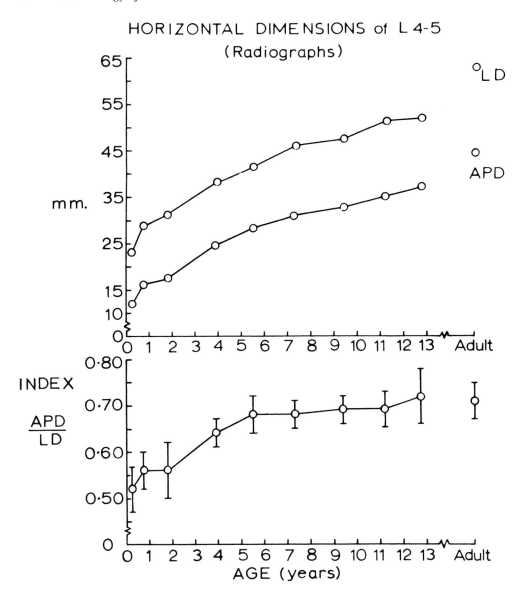

FIGURE 25. Comparison of growth in transverse (LD) and anteroposterior dimensions (APD) from corrected radiographic measurements; anteroposterior growth is greater than transverse growth from 2 to 6 years. Similar data are obtained from the post-mortem material, where increments in anteroposterior dimensions exceed increments in transverse dimensions from 2 to 7 years. This alters the shape of the disc (Figure 14).

There is also an acceleration of anteroposterior growth of the anterior elements of the lumbar column, relative to their vertical and transverse growth. This is most evident from 2 to 3 years, but the trend persists until 6 or 7 years.[2,66] This changes vertebral shape from high square lumbar vertebral centra to rectangular outlines on lateral X-ray, with the longer dimension in the horizontal plane. One may speculate that this change in direction of growth (Figure 29), which is demonstrably dependent on assumption of the erect posture,[66] represents an adaptation to the muscle forces required for balance in the sagittal plane. This redirection of growth may be the response of the forces of vertebral and disc growth to the combined mechanical influences of weightbearing in the erect posture and the associated postural muscle activity (Figure 28).

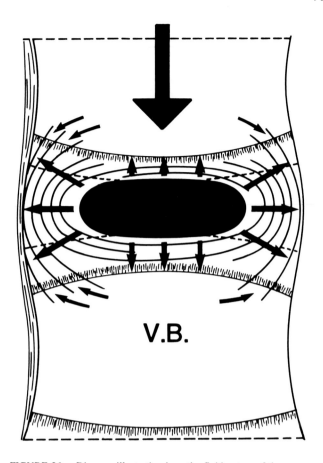

FIGURE 26.   Diagram illustrating how the fluid nature of the young nucleus ''redirects axial loads'' to its surrounding envelope; the continuity of the lamellar structures of both annulus and cartilage plate is an essential part of this mechanism. (From Taylor, J. and Twomey, L., *Modern Manual Therapy of the Vertebral Column*, Grieve, G., Ed., Churchill Livingstone, Edinburgh, 1986. With permission.)

VIII. SEXUAL DIMORPHISM IN SPINAL STRUCTURE AND FUNCTION

From about 6 or 7 years, anteroposterior growth rate of the anterior elements of the vertebral column slows down. This coincides with the time of closure of the neurocentral growth plates. From about 8 years onwards through adolescence, there are sex differences in the growth pattern of vertebrae and intervertebral discs.[76] Transverse growth of both vertebrae and discs is greater in males than in females, while vertical growth (in vertebral height) is greater in females than in males (Figure 29). This results in wider more squat vertebrae in males than in females, who have a more slender vertebral column.

This difference may also be related to sex differences in muscle development in early adolescence. Lordosis also becomes more pronounced in the lumbar spine of females than in males during the adolescent period. The ranges of lumbar spinal movement also become greater, on average, in females than in males during the same period.[77] The sex differences in vertebral shape, lumbar vertebral column posture, and lumbar spinal movement appear at puberty and disappear after the menopause, suggesting that hormonal factors may be responsible for producing and maintaining the differences. Muscle effects may be mediated by male hormones producing indirect effects on bone growth, the discs simply adapting in shape to the vertebral bodies bounding them. Greater female lordosis may be a reflection

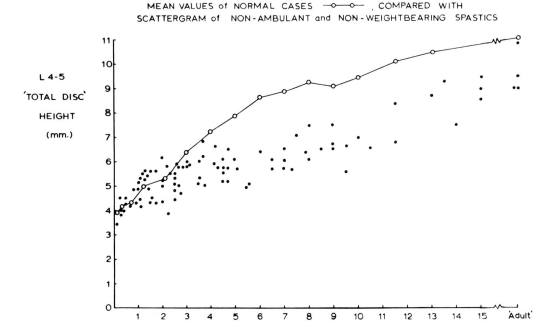

FIGURE 27.   A comparison of "total disc" heights (radiolucent disc space) in ambulent and nonambulant children.[1,66] The measurements in 362 normal ambulant children and adults are represented by mean values for 16 age groups; the values for nonambulant children with cerebral palsy are plotted individually. Nonambulant in this context means using a wheel-chair and nonweightbearing means confined to bed. (From Taylor, J., *J. Anat.*, 120, 49, 1975. With permission.)

Tracings from Radiogaphs (L.)

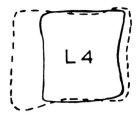

———— spastic non-ambulant female (14 yrs.)

- - - -   normal female (15 yrs.)

FIGURE 28.   Tracings of L 4 vertebral outlines from lateral radiographs, comparing the vertebral shape typical of ambulant and nonambulant children. (From Taylor, J., *J. Anat.*, 120, 49, 1975. With permission.)

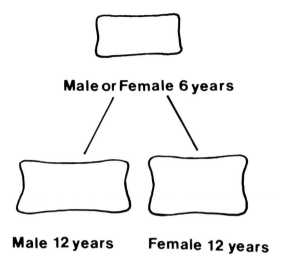

Male or Female 6 years

Male 12 years   **Female 12 years**

FIGURE 29.   Sexual dimorphism in vertebral shape: tracings
of outlines from radiographs illustrate the typical sexual dim-
porphism which develops between 6 and 12 years and is maintained into adult life. There are corresponding sex differences
in the horizontal dimensions of thoracic and lumbar intervertebral discs. Associated with these changes in shape, movement
ranges become greater in females than in males (see text).

of relaxin activity on connective tissues. However, the more slender the vertebral column,
the greater the expected range of movement, other factors being equal.

IX. REGIONAL VARIATION IN DEVELOPMENT OF INTERVERTEBRAL DISCS

New features do not appear in all regions of the vertebral column simultaneously, and
the sequence of development is not the same in the anterior elements (vertebral bodies and
discs) as in the posterior elements.[78] Regional variations in the development of the nucleus
pulposus were reported in the age range from 6 weeks of intrauterine life (20-mm embryo)
until 3 years of age.[1,60] The original notochordal segments appear in thoracic and lumbar
regions first and slightly later in cervical discs. By the 30-mm stage, fusiform enlargements
are visible in all three presacral regions, largest in lumbar discs and smallest in cervical
discs (Figure 8). Thoracic chordasegments assume a rhomboid form and lumbar segments
an asymmetrical elliptical or "mushroom" shape.[9] By the 75-mm stage, the thoracic and
lumbar chordasegments are expanding posteriorly in the perichordal discs while the cervical
chordasegments are little changed from the 30-mm stage, but with slight ventral convexities
of the notochordal track at disc levels. The cervical segments retain the same appearance
in a 115-mm fetus, though all the notochordal material is now in the perichordal discs. In
thoracic and lumbar discs, posterior expansion of the chordasegments has taken place.
Thoracic discs contain a flattened ellipse of notochordal tissue; and lumbar discs, by virtue
of their greater height, have a more globular or rounded chordasegment. The mucoid streak
is visible in all regions in this 115-mm fetus. At the 295-mm stage, again the cervical
segment has scarcely enlarged, and it retains its primitive anterior position within the perichordal disc, while the posterior expansion of the notochordal nucleus within the other discs
continues. The chordasegments are discontinuous with no mucoid streak visible. By full
term, the lumbar notochordal nucleus occupies half of the anteroposterior extent of the disc,

the thoracic nucleus one third of the AP extent of the disc, but the cervical nucleus is quite variable in its extent.

This prenatal increase in size of the chordasegments in thoracic and lumbar discs is largely due to an increase in the number of notochordal cells; since the lumbar notochordal segment is initially larger, it is not surprising that the full-term lumbar nucleus is largest. However, it is strange that the cervical nuclear growth is so delayed in comparison to the other regions and that in some cases it does not expand at all. Indeed, no notochordal tissue can be found in some full-term cervical discs, while a large notochordal nucleus is present in cervical discs of other individuals. In postnatal discs, lumbar notochordal nuclei pulposi continue to grow most rapidly in volume, principally by accumulation of mucoid matrix, but also with some increase in cell numbers in infancy. By one year, the lumbar nucleus occupies 75% of the A.P. extent of the disc, the thoracic nucleus 33%, and the cervical nuclei remain variable in their extent. In the 2nd year, the lumbar nucleus moves to a central and anterior position and changes shape in conformity with the change in disc shape when the lumbar column becomes lordotic. The thoracic nucleus remains posterior in position and is generally of much smaller volume. The cervical discs (from C 2—3, to C 6—7) differ from thoracic and lumbar discs in that cervical discs do not extend to the lateral margins of the vertebral bodies they join together. In this lateral area, during childhood, uncinate processes grow from the vertebral body below each disc to make contact, by about 8 years, with the lower lateral margins of the vertebral body above each disc. These processes form adventitious joints with bursa-like synovial cavities, termed uncovertebral joints, at the lateral margins of typical cervical intervertebral discs. These joints were originally described by Luschka.[41]

The differences in size and position of thoracic and lumbar nuclei probably relate to the development of differences in shape of thoracic and lumbar centra in childhood when pronounced concavities appear at the center of lumbar vertebral end-plates, while only shallow concavities appear posteriorly in thoracic vertebral end-plates. Persistence of the notochordal track occurs in some infants, most commonly in thoracic and lumbar regions. It is postulated that the "Cupid's bow" appearance of some lower lumbar vertebrae on radiographs[79] relates to late persistence of the notochordal track and its effect on ossification.

REFERENCES

1. **Taylor, J. R.,** Growth and Development of the Human Intervertebral Disc, Ph.D. thesis, University of Edinburgh, Edinburgh, 1973.
2. **Twomey, L. T.,** Age Changes in the Human Lumbar Vertebral Column, Ph.D. thesis, University of Western Australia, Nedlands, W.A., 1981.
3. **Williams, P. L. and Warwick, R.,** *Gray's Anatomy,* 36th Ed., Churchill Livingstone, Edinburgh, 1980, 444.
4. **Romanes, G. J. R.,** *Cunningham's Anatomy,* 12th ed., Oxford University Press, London, 1981, 244.
5. **Peacock, A.,** Observations on the prenatal development of the intervertebral disc in man, *J. Anat.,* 85, 260, 1951.
6. **Walmsley, R.,** The development and growth of the intervertebral disc, *Edinburgh Med. J.,* 60, 341, 1953.
7. **Franceschini, M.,** Richerche sull'architettura dei dischi intervertebrale, *Atti Accad. Sci. Med. Ferrara,* 26, 1, 1947.
8. **Schmorl, G. and Junghanns, H.,** *The Human Spine in Health and Disease,* 2nd Am. Ed., Grune & Stratton, New York, 1971.
9. **Bohmig, R.,** Die Blutgefassversorgung der Wirberbandscheiben das Verhalten des intervertebralen Chordasegments, *Arch. Klin. Chir.,* 158, 374, 1930.
10. **Prader, A.,** Beitrag sur Kenntnis der Entwicklung der Chorda dorsalis beim Menschen, *Rev. Suisse Zool.,* 52, 598, 1945.
11. **Prader, A.,** Die Fruhembryonale Entwicklung der menschlichen Zwischenwirbelscheibe, *Acta Anat.,* 3, 68, 1947.

12. **Prader, A.,** Die Entwicklung der Zwischenwirbelsheibe beim menschlichen Keimling, *Acta Anat.,* 3, 115, 1947.
13. **Peacock, A.,** Observations on the postnatal structure of the intervertebral disc in man, *J. Anat.,* 86, 162, 1952.
14. **Bardeen, C. R.,** Development of thoracic vertebrae in man, *Am. J. Anat.,* 4, 163, 1905.
15. **Wyburn, G. M.,** Observations on the development of the human vertebral column, *J. Anat.,* 78, 94, 1944.
16. **Sensenig, E. C.,** The early development of the human vertebral column, in *Contributions to Embryology,* Carnegie Inst., Washington, D.C., 33, 1949, 23.
17. **O'Rahilly, R. and Meyer, D. B.,** The timing and sequence of events in the development of the human vertebral column during the embryonic period proper, *Anat. Embryol.,* 157, 167, 1979.
18. **Verbout, A. J.,** *The Development of the Vertebral Column,* Springer-Verlag, Berlin, 1985.
19. **Goodsir, J.** (1857); cited in Walmsley, R., Development and growth of the human intervertebral disc, *Edinburgh Med. J.,* 60, 341, 1953.
20. **Remak, R.** (1855); cited in Walmsley, R., Development and growth of the human intervertebral disc, *Edinburgh Med. J.,* 60, 341, 1953.
21. **Baur, R.,** Zum Problem der Neugliederung der Wirbelsaule, *Acta Anat.,* 72, 321, 1969.
22. **Froriep, R.,** (1886); cited in Walmsley, R., Development and growth of the human intervertebral disc, *Edinburgh Med. J.,* 60, 341, 1953.
23. **Gadow, H. and Abbott, E. C.,** (1895); cited in Walmsley, R., Development and growth of the human intervertebral disc, *Edinburgh Med. J.,* 60, 341, 1953.
24. **Taylor, J. R. and Twomey, L. T.,** The role of the notochord and blood vessels in vertebral column development and in the aetiology of Schmorl's nodes, in *Modern Manual Therapy, Vol. 1 The Vertebral Column,* Grieve, G., Ed., Churchill Livingstone, Edinburgh, 1986, chap. 1.
25. **Tanaka, T. and Ulthoff, H. K.,** The pathogenesis of congenital malformations, *Acta Orthop. Scand.,* 52, 413, 1981.
26. **Taylor, J. R.,** Persistence of the notochordal canal in vertebrae, *J. Anat.,* 111, 211, 1972.
27. **Dursy, E.,** *Zur Entwicklungsgeschichte des Kopfes des Menschen und der Hoheren Wirbeltiere,* Laupp, Tübingen, FRG, 1869.
28. **Williams, L.,** The later development of the notochord in mammals, *Am. J. Anat.,* 8, 251, 1908.
29. **Dahmen, G.,** Studies on the maturation of human connective tissue, *Z. Orthop.,* 100, 359, 1965.
30. **But, N. I.,** Development of the intervertebral disc in human embryogenesis (Russian) *Arkiv Anatomii Gistologii i Embriologii (Moscva)* 36, 30, 1959 (British National Lending Library Translation RTS 6907).
31. **Hirsch, C. and Schazowicz, F.,** Studies on structural changes in the lumbar anulus fibrosus, *Acta Orthop. Scand.,* 22, 184, 1953.
32. **Donisch, E. W. and Trapp, W.,** The carilage endplates of the human vertebral column, *Anat. Rec.,* 169, 705, 1971.
33. **Souter, W. A. and Taylor, T. K. F.,** Sulphated acid mucopolysaccharide metabolism in the rabbit intervertebral disc, *J. Bone Jt. Surg.,* 52B, 371.
34. **Horton, W. G.,** Further observations on the elastic mechanism of the intervertebral disc, *J. Bone Jt. Surg.,* 40B, 552, 1958.
35. **Uebermuth, H.,** Über die Altersveranderungen der menslichen Zwischenwirbelsheibe und ihre Beziehung zu den chronischen Gelenkleiden der Wirbelsaule, Berlin Sachs, *Geschichte Akad. Wissenschafte* (Leipzig), 81, 111, 1929.
36. **Beadle, O. A.,** *The Intervertebral Discs,* M.R.C. Special report, Series No. 161, Her Majesty's Stationary Office, 1931.
37. **Dale-Stewart, T. D., and Kerley, E. R.,** *Essentials of Forensic Anthropology,* Charles C Thomas, Springfield, Ill., 1979, 136.
38. **Rouviere, H.,** Sur le texture des disques intervertebraux, *C. R. Soc. Biol.,* 85, 156, 1921.
39. **Luschka, H. von,** cited in Walmsley R., Development and growth of the human intervertebral disc, *Edinburgh Med. J.,* 60, 341, 1953.
40. **Virchow, R.,** *Untersuchungen uber die Entwicklung des Schadelgrundes,* Reimer, Berlin, 1857.
41. **Luschka, H. von,** *Die Halbgelenke des Menschlichen Korpers,* Reimer, Berlin, 1858.
42. **Kolliker, A.,** *Entwicklungsgeschichte des Menschen und der Hoheren Wirbelthiere,* Engelman, Liepzig, 1861.
43. **Kolliker, A.,** *Entwicklungsgeschichte des Menschen und der Hoheren Wirbelthiere,* Zweite Auflage, Engelman, Leipzig, 1879.
44. **Robin, C.,** *Memoire sur l'Evolution de la Notochord,* Bailliere, Paris, 1868.
45. **Keyes, D. C. and Compere, E. L.,** The normal and pathological physiology of the nucleus pulposus of the intervertebral disc, *J. Bone Jt. Surg.,* 14, 897, 1932.
46. **Malinski, J.,** Histochemical demonstration of carbohydrates in human intervertebral discs during postnatal development, *Acta Histochem.,* 5, 120, 1958.

47. **Wolfe, H. J., Putschar, W. G. J., and Vickery, A. L.,** Role of the notochord in human intervertebral discs. I. Fetus and infant, *Clin. Orthop.,* 39, 205, 1965.

48. **Bradford, F. K. and Spurling, R. G.,** *The Intervertebral Disc,* 2nd ed., Thomas, Baltimore, 1945.

49. **Leeson, T. S. and Leeson, C. R.,** Observations on the histochemistry and fine structure of the notochord in rabbit embryos, *J. Anat.,* 92, 278, 1958.

50. **Jurand, A.,** The development of the notochord in chick embryos, *J. Exp. Morphol.,* 10, 602, 1962.

51. **Trout, J. J., Buckwalter, J. A., Moore, K. C., and Landas, S. K.,** Ultrastructure of the human intervertebral disc: notochordal cells, *Tissue Cell,* 14, 359, 1982.

52. **Fell, H. B.,** Role of biological membranes in some skeletal reactions, *Ann. Rheum. Dis.,* 28, 213, 1969.

53. **Amprino, R.,** Autoradiographic research on S35 sulphate metabolism in cartilage and bone differentiation and growth, *Acta Anat.,* 24, 121, 1955.

54. **Meachim, G. and Cornah, M. S.,** The fine structure of the juvenile nucleus pulposus, *J. Anat.,* 107, 337, 1970.

55. **Schwabe, R.,** Untersuchungen uber die Ruckbildung der Bandscheiben im menschlichen Kreuzbein, *Virchow's Arch.,* 287, 651, 1933.

56. **Friedman, I., Harrison, D. F. N., and Bird, E. S.,** Fine structure of chordoma with particular reference to the physaliferous cell, *J. Clin. Pathol.,* 15, 116, 1962.

57. **Harvey, W. F. and Dawson, E. K.,** Chordoma, *Edinburgh M. J.,* 48, 713, 1941.

58. **Heaton, J. M. and Turner, D. R.,** Reflections on notochordal differentiation arising from a study of chordomas, *Histopathology,* 9, 543, 1985.

59. **Amprino, R. and Bairati, A.,** Studi sulle transformazioni delle cartilagini dell'uomo nell'accrescimento e nella senescenza. III. Cartilagini fibrose, *Z. Zellforsch. Mikrosk. Anat.,* 21, 448, 1934.

60. **Taylor, J. R.,** Regional variation in the development and position of the notochordal segments of the human nucleus pulposus, *J. Anat.,* 110, 131, 1971.

61. **Puschell, J.,** Der Wassergehalt normaler und degenerierter Zwischenwirbelscheiben, *Beitrag Pathol. Anat.,* 84, 123, 1930.

62. **Nachemson, A. and Elfstrom, G.,** Intravital dynamic measurements in lumbar discs, *Scand. J. Rehabil. Med.* (Suppl. 1), 1, 1960.

63. **Lawrence, J. S.,** Disc degeneration: its frequency and relationship to symptoms, *Ann. Rheum. Dis.,* 28, 121.

64. **Stevens, J.,** Low back pain, Med. Clin. North Am., 52, 55, 1968.

65. **Twomey, L. and Taylor, J.,** Age changes in lumbar intervertebral discs, *Acta Orthop. Scand.,* 56, 496, 1985.

66. **Taylor, J. R.,** Growth of human intervertebral discs and vertebral bodies, *J. Anat.,* 120, 49, 1975.

67. **Harris, R. I. and MacNab, I.,** Structural changes in the lumbar intervertebral discs, *J. Bone Jt. Surg.,* 36B, 304, 1954.

68. **Theiler, K.,** Die Enstehung der Randleistenzahne der Wirbelkorper, *Z. Anat. Entwicklungsgesch.,* 124, 533, 1965.

69. **Bick, E. M. and Copel, J. W.,** Longitudinal growth of human vertebrae, *J. Bone Jt. Surg.,* 32A, 803, 1950.

70. **Hanson, R.,** Development of vertebrae as seen on skiagrams from late foetal life to age of fourteen, *Acta Radiol.,* 5, 112, 1926.

71. **Wiley, A. M. and Trueta, J.,** The vascular anatomy of the spine, in relation to pyogenic vertebral osteomyelitis, *J. Bone Jt. Surg.,* 41B, 796, 1959.

72. **Somogyi, B.,** Blood supply of the fetal spine, *Acta Morphol. Acad. Sci. Hung.,* 12, 261, 1964.

73. **Mineiro, J. D.,** Coluna Vertebral Humana: alguns aspectos de sua estrutura e vascularizacao, M. D. Thesis, Faculty of Medicine, Lisbon, 1965.

74. **Brodin, H.,** Paths of nutrition in articular cartilage and intervertebral discs, *Acta Orthop. Scand.,* 24, 177, 1955.

75. **Maroudas, A., Nachemson, A., Stockwell, R. A., and Urban, J.,** Factors involved in the nutrition of the adult human lumbar intervertebral disc, *J. Anat.,* 120, 113, 1975.

76. **Taylor, J. R. and Twomey, L. T.,** Sexual dimorphism in human vertebral body shape, *J. Anat.,* 138, 281, 1984.

77. **Taylor, J. R. and Twomey, L. T.,** Sagittal and horizontal plane movement of the human lumbar vertebral column in cadavers and in the living, *Rheumat. Rehab.,* 19, 223, 1980.

78. **Taylor, J. R.,** Scoliosis and growth, *Acta Orthop. Scand.,* 54, 596, 1983.

79. **Dietz, G. W. and Christensen E. E.,** Normal Cupid's bow contour of the lower lumbar vertebrae, *Radiology,* 121, 577, 1976.

Chapter 3

COMPARATIVE ANATOMY AND DEVELOPMENT OF THE MAMMALIAN DISC

Wallace F. Butler

TABLE OF CONTENTS

I. INTRODUCTION

Mammalian discs are similar in basic plan in all species. Thus, they all consist of a tough fibrous capsule called the annulus fibrosus, which encloses a soft nucleus pulposus.

Although the discs develop in a similar manner in the embryo,[1-11] changes occur, either in the late fetus or postnatally, that result in detailed differences between species.

This chapter will discuss the newborn disc and the changes which occur with aging.

II. THE NEWBORN DISC

Intervertebral discs (Figures 1 and 2) are interposed between two adjacent vertebral bodies in each of the cervical (C), thoracic (T), lumbar (L), and caudal or coccygeal (Co) regions. They are absent from between the skull and the first cervical vertebra (C1), from between C1 and C2, and from between the fused vertebrae forming the sacrum (S). The number of vertebrae, and therefore the number of discs, varies between species and may occasionally vary within species.

The cartilaginous model of the fetal vertebra is partly ossified by birth, though the differentiation of epiphyses at the cranial and caudal ends of the centrum (Figures 1a and 2b) occurs at different times. Thus, no epiphyses are present in the newborn cat[12] and dog,[13] but they will have developed within a month of postnatal life. In the horse, however, they develop before birth.[14]

A. The Annulus Fibrosus

The annulus of all species so far examined has a common structure (Figures 1 and 2).[15,16] Although terminology varies with author, we can recognize an outer annulus composed of well-defined lamellae of dense white fibrous tissue whose constituent collagen fibers are from 180 to 700 nm in diameter in the rat.[15] The outer annulus merges with an inner annulus which is formed from fibrocartilage.

The fibers of the lamellae of the outer annulus run obliquely between the vertebral bodies (centra) rather than directly, the fibers of adjacent lamellae lying at an angle of about 120° to each other.[12] The most peripheral lamellae are slightly arched in their course and their fibers enter the vertebra at the level of the future epiphyseal plate.[12] The deeper lamellae of the outer annulus are more arched in their course,[12] particularly dorsally.[12] The reason for this may be related to the shape of the disc, which reflects the shape of the vertebral surfaces (Figures 1 and 2). The fibers of the inner annulus are even more arched and completely encircle the nucleus pulposus in many species.[11,12,16] The cells of the annulus vary with their position. In the outer annulus they resemble fibrocytes,[12] but at the junction with the cartilaginous end of the vertebra they appear chondrocytic. The cells of the inner annulus (Figure 4) are also chondrocytic,[12,16] but, at the sharp border with the nucleus pulposus that is seen in the newborn of many species,[9,12,19] some of the cells appear necrotic. The fibers associated with these innermost cells appear to break down and to aid in the formation of the clear gel (Figures 2a, c, and e) at the periphery of the nucleus pulposus in these species. In other species[18,19] there is not such sharp demarcation of the annulus from the nucleus pulposus. There is, instead, a gradual disorientation of the fibers of the annulus centrally.

Elasticity of the disc has been considered by many investigators to be due solely to the lamellar arrangement. However, elastic fibers have been found in the fetal ox,[20] the 7-day-old cat,[20] and the adult dog[21] where they are randomly oriented within the lamellae and radially oriented between them.

B. The Nucleus Pulposus

In all species the nucleus pulposus (Figures 1 and 2) starts in fetal life as a gelatinous

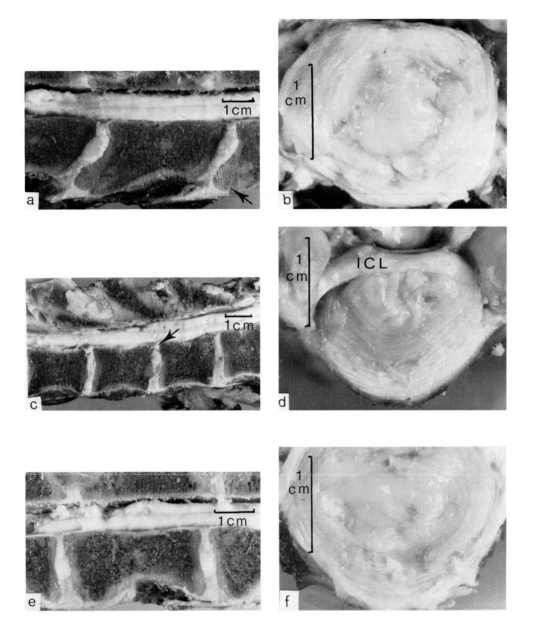

FIGURE 1. Discs of adult sheep. In all sections, the annulus merges gradually into the softer, but fibrous, nucleus pulposus. In the cervical region (a and b) the discs are obliquely oriented but in the thoracic (c and d) and lumbar (e and f) regions they are more vertical. An intercapital ligament (ICL in d, arrow in c) joins many pairs of ribs across the disc, replacing much of the dorsal annulus in the thoracic region. A remnant of the epiphyseal plate of cartilage can be seen arrowed in a. *Note*: cranial is to the right in (a) and (c), and to the left in (e); dorsal is at the top in all pictures.

mass in the center of the developing disc. During this stage, it consists of notochordal cells surrounded by, and sometimes divided up by, a gel. The gel, sometimes called the notochordal sheath,[3,7,11,22,23] is formed from highly hydrated proteoglycans in which collagen fibers are embedded.

At birth, the nucleus pulposus is of similar structure in the cat,[12] dog,[19] mink,[24] pig,[11,14] mouse and rat,[11,25,26] and the rabbit.[27-30] In these animals, the nucleus (Figure 2) of the newborn appears as a cloudy mass of notochordal cells embedded in a clear gel. With the

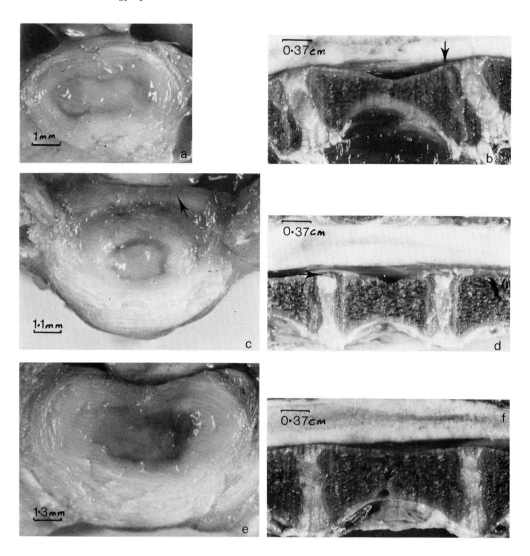

FIGURE 2.   Discs of adult cat and dog. **Transverse sections:** a, cervical; c, thoracic; e, lumbar cat discs. An intercapital ligament (arrow) is present dorsally (top of picture c). The nucleus pulposus is gelatinous and contains notochordal cells as a cloudy central region. The inner annulus is amorphous and merges with the lamellae of the outer annulus. **Sagittal sections:** b, cervical; d, thoracic; and f, lumbar dog discs. The cervical discs are obliquely arranged and remnants of the epiphyseal plate are shown by the arrow. An intercapital ligament is present in the thoracic region (arrow) ventral to the dorsal longitudinal ligament. *Note:* cranial is to the left.

light microscope, viable vacuolated cells (Figure 10) are seen embedded in a basophilic matrix. These cells are surrounded by a peripheral basophilic cell-free region that contains fine collagen fibers[31] which merge with the encircling fibers of the inner annulus. This would indicate that the nucleus pulposus may be enlarging at the expense of the inner annulus, where the cells are dying and the fibers disintegrating.[31]

In contrast, the nucleus pulposus of the newborn foal contains no notochordal cells, and in other species (e.g., the calf[16]), it may only contain a few isolated groups of these cells. Such a nucleus pulposus (Figure 1) is putty-like at birth and merges with the inner annulus. While there is not experimental evidence to support the idea, it seems likely that most or all of the notochordal cells have died or have changed into other cell types. At the same time, the inner annulus has proliferated inwards to replace them. The idea that viable noto-chordal cells can prevent invasion by the annulus was suggested more than 30 years ago,[9] and, in the fetal pig, there is evidence that living notochordal cells encroach upon the inner annulus, which is reduced in proportion.[11]

C. Ligaments Associated with the Disc

A dentate dorsal longitudinal ligament is attached to the vertebral bodies throughout the vertebral column. Dorsal to each disc, it widens to form a broad attachment to the annulus or, in the thoracic region, to the intercapital ligament.

A finer ventral logitudinal ligament is attached to the vertebrae and discs and is well developed from the midthoracic region caudally. The head of each rib is attached to adjacent vertebrae and to the intervening disc by a radiate ligament. In addition, there is an intercapital ligament (conjugal ligament) which joins the heads of paired ribs across the dorsal surface of many discs (Figures 1 and 2). This ligament is found in most mammals,[12,19,24,32,33] but not in all primates and marsupials.[32] In the ox and carnivores, the ligament joins across discs T1—10 or 11,[12,19,33-36] and in the horse (with 18 thoracic vertebrae), it joins across discs T2—15.[36] In all species, it replaces part of the outer annulus and is not additional to the annulus[12,17] (Figures 1 and 2). Williams[11] suggests that it may have been converted into a ligament by changes in the dorsal annulus.

A synovial membrane, an extension of the costovertebral joint capsule, separates the intercapital ligament from the dorsal annulus, but not usually from the dorsal longitudinal ligament.[32,35] Species differences exist in the detailed arrangement of the synovial membrane, and the rabbit may have none, since the fibers of the ligament are incorporated into the disc.[32] Furthermore, a recent report suggests that the synovial membrane completely surrounds the ligament in the cat.[34] However, no evidence for this could be found by others,[12] who noticed, instead, that the intercapital ligament is attached to the dorsal longitudinal ligament by loose connective tissue.

D. Innervation of the Disc

While most investigators[17,25,37-41] have been unable to find any nerve fibers within the discs of man, monkey, rat, cat, and dog, they have been able to find them in the surrounding connective tissue between the dorsal longitudinal ligament and the disc and in the ligament itself. Others have found occasional nerve fibers in the outer layers of the annulus.[42,43] (See also Chapter 5.)

In primates, these nerves originate from the sinuvertebral (meningeal) nerves[39,40] and contain both somatic and autonomic fibers. However, their origin in other species is not clear. While sinuvertebral nerves were suggested to be present in the dog,[17] none were subsequently found in either the cat or dog.[41,42]

E. Vascular Supply of the Disc

In the newborn cat,[44] branches from the developing vertebral epiphyseal arteries supply the periphery of the disc. Later on, the supply becomes more profuse laterally and ventrally until, in the adult (Figure 3), the metaphyseal and epiphyseal vessels become continuous. Branches from these vessels reach to within 10 μm of the disc[45] by passing through the very attenuated cartilaginous vertebral end-plate, particularly in the central region.

A similar arrangement exists in the dog,[17,46,47] where terminal branches give rise to a densely woven network beneath the thin cartilage end-plate, particularly in the region of the nucleus pulposus.[48] It is here that fine vessels cause pitting of the surface of the vertebral end-plate.

Vascularization of the outer lamella of the rabbit disc may, or may not, occur.[30,53] It does not occur in the ox disc or in the human disc,[49-51] though those vessels found beneath the vertebral end-plate are most important nutritionally.[47,51,52] Venules leave the vertebral epiphyses of the dog[46] to join the longitudinal vertebral venous sinuses that run dorsal to the vertebrae.

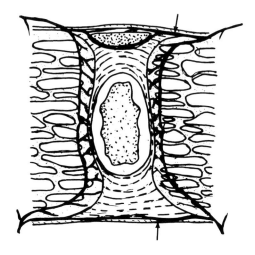

FIGURE 3.   Arterial supply to the cat disc. Two dorsal and two ventral arteries supply the epiphyseal region and each gives a branch to the disc surface. Branches (arrows) from these penetrate the more superficial lamellae of the annulus, particularly ventrally and laterally. The epiphyseal vessels give rise to branches which penetrate the bone to abut on the disc centrally.

III. THE ADULT DISC

A. The Size of the Adult Disc

1. Disc Size as a Whole

Growth of the disc is very rapid at first, the dorsoventral depth of the cat disc increasing threefold between birth and 6 months of age (Figures 4 and 5). There then appears to be a further slow increase throughout life. However, this could be due to an increase in the depth of the ruptured discs which were present in the sample examined, (Figures 12 and 13) since the number of ruptured discs increases with age[54] and their depth is greater than that of intact discs (Figure 6).

Craniocaudal thickness is difficult to measure in most mammals, because of the irregular shape of the end of each vertebra (Figures 1, 2, and 13 a, b, and c). In spite of this, attempts have been made to measure it, and the results show that the proportional thickness varies with species. For example, discs occupy between 12% and 18% of the spinal length in the cat,[17,34] 17% in the dog,[17] and 11% in the horse.[17] Regions of the vertebral column also vary. While the cervical discs are usually thickest[17,55] in absolute measurement, they may only occupy 7% of the vertebral column length in the sheep, 14% in the cat, and 12% in the dog. Thoracic discs are usually thinnest[17,55] but, because the vertebrae are short, they occupy 10% of the column length in the dog, 12% in the sheep, and 15% in the cat. Lumbar discs are proportionally shorter, occupying 4% of the column in the sheep, 6% in the cat, and 9% in the dog.[55]

It is difficult to relate these measurements to vertebral mobility, though the cervical region is most mobile in the dog where the discs are proportionally thickest.[17,56] The mobility of the rest of the spine does not, however, correlate with the figures, and other factors must play a part.[56] The mechanics of the vertebral column is discussed in Chapter 10.

2. Annulus Size

An examination of the depth of the dorsal annulus[55] in a sample of ten discs from each of six cats between birth and three years of age (i.e., before large ruptures are present) confirms that growth occurs mainly in the first 6 months of life (Figure 7) and shows that

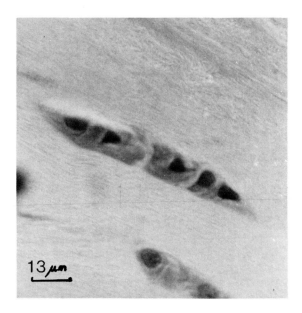

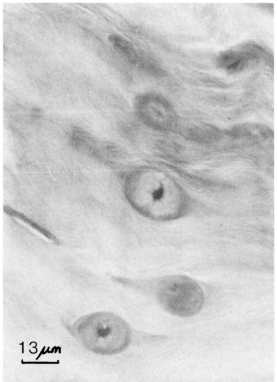

FIGURE 4. Cat inner annulus cells. Upper picture, (T7—8) stained with H & E, shows cells surrounded by basophilic pericellular material in a 10-week-old cat. Lower picture, (L7—S1) stained by PAS, shows pericellular material which is more extensive in a 2-year-old cat. (T = thoracic, L = lumbar, and S = sacral.)

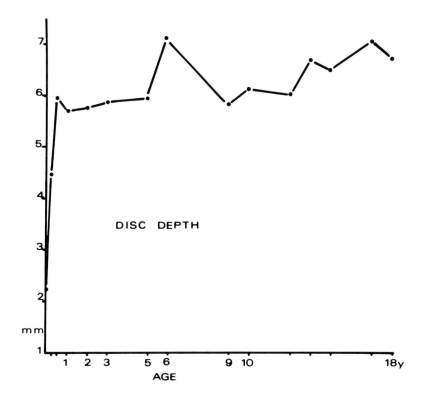

FIGURE 5. Age changes in the dorsoventral depth of cat discs. The mean dorsoventral depth of a sample of 10 discs from 15 cats between birth and 18 years of age is shown. The figures include both ruptured and nonruptured discs. There is a sharp rise between birth and 6 months and a gradual rise thereafter. Correlation between disc depth and age from 6 months is statistically significant ($r = 0.66$, $\upsilon = 12$).

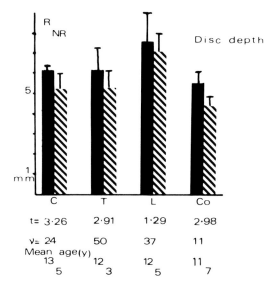

FIGURE 6. Dorsoventral depth of cat discs. The histogram shows that ruptured discs (R) are deeper than normal discs (NR). The differences are statistically significant in all but the lumbar region (L). C = cervical, T = thoracic, L = lumbar, Co = coccygeal or caudal, t = Student's *t*-test, and υ = degrees of freedom.

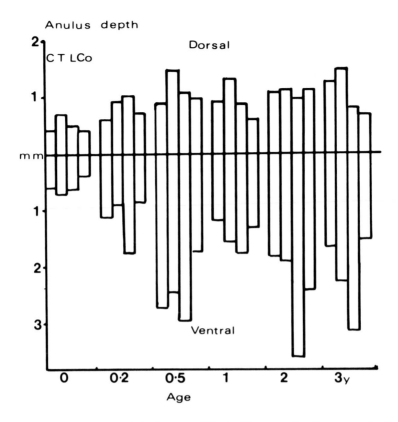

FIGURE 7. Age changes in the dorsoventral depth of the cat annulus. The mean regional depths of the dorsal and ventral parts of the annulus are shown for animals between birth and 3 years. Beyond this age the loss of notochordal cells and consequent reduction in size of the nucleus pulposus (Figure 8) makes measurement of the annulus meaningless. The symmetry of the newborn annulus changes quickly with a great increase in the ventral part by 6 months. Greatest asymmetry is seen in the lumbar region. C = cervical (mean of 2 discs); T = thoracic (mean of 4 discs); L = lumbar (mean of 3 discs); and Co = coccygeal (one disc).

the dorsal annulus is thickest in the thoracic region. The ventral annulus, however, grows much more than the dorsal annulus in the juvenile period (Figure 7) and, while individuals vary, there is clearly much greater growth in the lumbar region.

The ratio of the thickness of ventral to dorsal annulus in the cat is least in the thoracic region (1.3:1), intermediate in the cervical region (1.8:1), and greatest in the lumbar region (3.2.:1). These figures are a measure of the excentricity of the nucleus pulposus and suggest that, in the absence of other factors, ruptures of the annulus with protrusion of the nucleus pulposus might be greatest dorsally, particularly in the lumbar region. Dorsal protrusions are more numerous than ventral ones in the cat,[57] but the highest incidence is found in the cervical rather than in the lumbar region. Other factors are also clearly at work. The relative thickness of the dorsal and ventral annulus in the dog is quite different from that of the cat; the ratios being 2.3:1 for the cervical region, 2.8:1 for the thoracic, and 2.0:1 for the lumbar.[17] However, the very high incidence of dorsal protusions in the lumbar region of this species[58] also shows that other factors are important.

It has often been suggested that normal spinal curvatures are responsible for the excentricity of the nucleus pulposus but, as Scott et al.[4] have pointed out, this is not true for the rabbit,[27] nor is it true for other quadrupedal mammals. The absolute thickness of the annulus (Figure 7) might have an effect upon the incidence of protrusions in a particular region and, in fact,

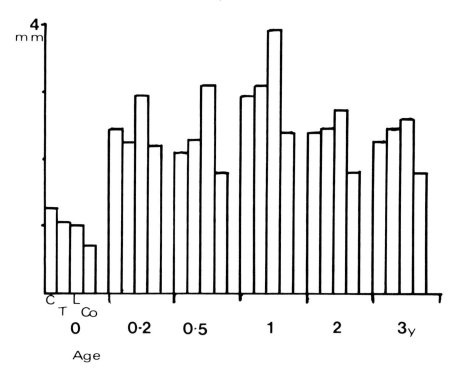

FIGURE 8.   Age changes in the dorsoventral depth of the cat nucleus pulposus. The mean depth is shown for animals between birth and 3 years. Beyond this age, loss of material from the nucleus pulposus makes measurement meaningless. (See Figure 14.) C = cervical (mean of 2 discs); T = thoracic (mean of 4 discs); L = lumbar (mean of 3 discs); and Co = coccygeal (one disc).

dorsal protrusions in the cat are minimal in the thoracic region and maximal in the cervical region.[59] However, since the incidence of dorsal ruptures of the annulus,[54] as distinct from protrusions at the surface, is high in the thoracic region, other factors must be operating to prevent material from reaching or being seen at the surface. One of these factors is the presence of the intercapital ligament, which can direct the protruded material towards the rib head where notochordal cells can be found in histological sections.[54]

3. Nucleus Pulposus Size

The gelatinous nucleus pulposus of the cat increases greatly in depth in the first 10 weeks of life (Figure 8). Little further change occurs unless material is lost through ruptures of the annulus. Except at birth, the lumbar region has the deepest nucleus pulposus (Figure 8).

Increase in size of the nucleus pulposus is clearly at the expense of the inner annulus, which degenerates and adds material to the nucleus. Indeed, at the beginning of this century, Williams[11] observed that, as pig embryos grew from 24 mm to 250 mm CR length, the notochordal mass not only increased in absolute size but also occupied a greater proportion of the disc; during this period, it increased from 20% to 58%. At the same time, the inner annulus decreased from a proportion of 41% to 8%, the outer annulus remaining unchanged at about 33%. The same sort of changes occur in human embryonic discs.[49,60]

B. The Morphology of the Adult Disc

1. The Normal Outer Annulus

The lamellae of the outer annulus increase in thickness and become less cellular as the animal matures.[45,61] The outermost cells remain as fibrocytes except at the junction with the vertebra, where they change into chondrocytes.[16,20,45] The inner cells become surrounded by basophilic matrix that increases in thickness towards the center of the disc. In those species with a gelatinous nucleus pulposus, this pericellular matrix also increases with age to reach a peak in the young adult: e.g., 2 years in the pig, 3 years in the cat, and 4 years in the dog.[16,45] In species without a gelatinous nucleus pulposus (e.g., horse and ruminants[16]), this change occurs much earlier in life. Electron microscopy shows that the basophilic matrix contains granules and fibrils[15] (Figure 9) that are beaded or banded.[20]

Collagen fibrils increase in diameter with age. In the newborn cat, they are 40 to 50 nm in diameter[20] and increase up to 83 nm in the young adult.[62] In the newborn, the fibrils that enter the cartilaginous vertebra split into finer ones, 8 to 10 nm in diameter.[20] Collagen fibrils are aggregated into larger fibers, with a diameter of between 180 nm and 2900 nm in the rat.[15] In the adult, they pass through the cartilage end-plate of the vertebra (e.g., in horse, ruminants, pig, and dog) or directly into the vertebra where it is absent.[16,27]

2. The Normal Inner Annulus

Microscopic studies reveal that the lamellar arrangement becomes increasingly obscured towards the disc center. At the same time, the macroscopic semitranslucency of the outer annulus (perhaps a function of the regular arrangement of these fibers) changes gradually to the opaque whiteness of the inner annulus.

In species that have few or no notochord cells,[16] the inner annulus merges imperceptibly with the nucleus pulposus and the consistency changes from firmness to puttiness[18] (Figure 10). In species in which the nucleus pulposus contains mainly or only notochordal cells,[16] there is an abrupt change from the opaque inner annulus to the clear gel which surrounds the notochordal mass (Figure 2), a state that may be retained throughout life in some discs.[16,63]

Light microscopy shows that the collagen of the inner annulus becomes increasingly disorientated towards the nucleus pulposus, and that it stains increasingly with basophilic and metachromatic dyes.[16,17,27,28,63,64] Basophilia increases with age in the cat disc until about three quarters of the annulus is so stained by the end of the 1st year of life;[45] staining intensity continues to increase until the 3rd year. This staining is probably due to the presence of glycosaminoglycans whose concentration decreases peripherally and increases with age.[64,65] The largest proportion of the glycosaminoglycans consists of chondroitin sulfate with smaller amounts of keratan sulfate and hyaluronate, though the proportion of keratan sulfate increases with age.[29,65-71] The cells of the inner annulus show degenerative changes with increasing age[16,45] and towards the disc center (Figures 4 and 9). There is an accumulation of basophilic material around them, and many become necrotic in the cat and dog[16,17,45] or show chondroid change, particularly in chondrodystrophoid breeds.[16,67]

The fine structure of the inner annulus shows that the inner annulus cells of the 2-month-old cat[72] are either fibrocytes or chondrocytes, though some cells are degenerating. They contain intracytoplasmic filaments, microtubules, and occasional centrioles, as well as the usual organelles. The plasma membrane contains numerous micropinocytotic vesicles. In older animals, cellular organelles decrease and degenerate cells increase in number. At the same time, "bays" in the cell surface (Figure 9b) increase and become continuous with the dilated endoplasmic reticulum in degenerate cells (Figure 9c). Many cells are surrounded by granular densities (Figure 9b). These may be derived from the intracellular granular bodies[72] and may represent the pericellular granules[73] of light microscopy (Figure 9a). The fibrils that surround the cells sometimes show beading and banding in the cat[72] as in other species.[20,74] They are associated with material that is amorphous or finely granular in routine electron microscopic sections, but which stains densely with Alcian Blue[62] (Figure 9d). Alcian Blue also stains a sheath around the collagen fibrils, a feature which indicates that glycosaminoglycans are associated closely with them.

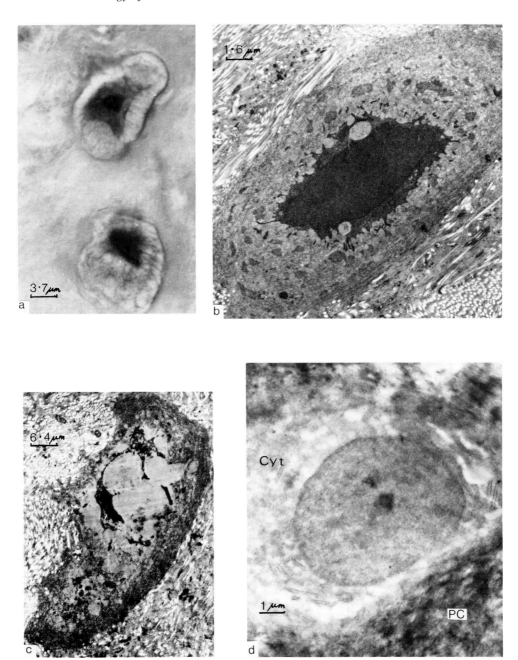

FIGURE 9.   Inner annulus cells. (a.) Adult horse, stained Alcian Blue in 0.3 *M* MgCl$_2$ at pH 5.6; light microscope section. The cells are similar to those of the cat (Figure 4); pericellular material contains fibrils and granules and is embedded in disorientated collagen fibers. (b.) Cat, 10 months, uranyl acetate, lead citrate stained. This electron micrograph shows granular masses in the pericellular material; amorphous areas at the cell surface may be derived from intracellular vacuoles; (c.) Same animals as (b). Degenerate cytoplasm lies in a mass of amorphous substance, which in turn is surrounded by the usual fibrillogranular material. (d.) Cat, 6 months, stained Alcian Blue in 0.3 *M* MgCl$_2$ at pH 5.6. This thick electron microscope section shows that the pericellular material (PC) is densely stained and is likely to contain large amounts of proteoglycan. In the cytoplasm (Cyt) there is some evidence of staining of the endoplasmic reticulum. (From Butler, W. F. and Heap, P. F., *Histochem. J.*, 14, 113, 1982. With permission.)

3. The Normal Nucleus Pulposus

In some species, the notochordal cells have either been completely lost by birth (e.g., the horse) or only a few cells remain at birth to be lost within the 1st year of life (e.g., the ox and sheep[1,16]). Much of the reduction in notochordal cell numbers is due to cell death, though some may be transformed into chondrocytes[16] (Figure 10e). In these species the nucleus pulposus is formed largely or completely by tissue that has proliferated from the inner annulus. Macroscopically, it usually appears as a soft putty-like mass, though in about 3% of horse discs it may be "gelatinous".[75] Microscopically, the tissue is seen to be formed, like the inner annulus, from a basophilic meshwork of collagen fibers in which chondrocytes, and in some species, the occasional notochordal cell are embedded. The cells[16] are similar to those of the inner annulus and are surrounded by granulofibrillar material (Figure 9a). Alcian Blue staining shows that both collagen and the pericellular material contains a high concentration of glycosaminoglycan.[19,73] This type of nucleus pulposus is also found in the adult antelope and gorilla[55] and in the young monkey.[76] Detailed description of the human disc occurs elsewhere in this volume (Chapter 2), but it should be noted that most of the cells of the human nucleus pulposus are chondrocytes, even in the late fetus,[8,77,78] though isolated notochordal cells have been detected as late as 67 years of age.[79]

Many other species have a nucleus pulposus that is quite different from that just described. In these, naked-eye examination reveals the nucleus pulposus to be clearly demarcated from the surrounding tissue (Figure 2) and to consist of a transparent gel in which a central cloudy mass is embedded. Such species include rodents,[11,17,25,26,82] lagomorphs,[27,28] and artiodactyls.[16] In the cat, the nucleus pulposus retains this clear separation throughout life in discs that have not undergone pathological change.[63] In other species, changes occur earlier and result in a fibrous type of nucleus pulposus, either in the juvenile period or in early or mid adulthood. Thus, rabbit notochordal cells are infrequent after 6 weeks of age and have mostly disappeared by 11 months[27] or later in life.[28,83] In young rabbits, they are found in groups rather than in a solid mass.[83]

The dog is a special case since there is a difference between normal breeds and those showing chondrodystrophy, or between strains within a breed.[17,80] In all breeds, the nucleus pulposus has a similar form in early life. In normal breeds,[17] a gelatinous nucleus pulposus occurs in about 75% of discs at 4 years of age, but in less than 19% beyond 7 years. Chondrodystrophic breeds, however, usually lose their gelatinous nucleus pulposus in the 1st year.

The age changes that can be seen with the light microscope have been described in detail for the dog and cat. In the dog,[17] and particularly in chondrodystrophoid breeds, the notochordal mass becomes lobulated, with some cells undergoing necrosis in the first 9 months of life. In normal dogs, degeneration of the cells continues until the remnants are found as groups within a collagenous network in animals over 7 years of age. As these changes proceed, the inner annulus proliferates to replace the degenerating notochordal area. In chondrodystrophoid breeds the changes are accelerated, with early death of notochordal cells and replacement by proliferating chondroid tissue from the inner annulus. In the cat,[31,63] the changes progress much more slowly so that, in nonruptured discs, the final result is some degeneration of the notochordal cells, particularly in the center of the mass (Figure 10c). Occasionally there is grouping of the cells with metamorphosis of them into chondrocytes (Figure 10e). In a disc with an intact annulus, there is no invasion of the nucleus pulposus by proliferating inner annulus cells, as has been described for the dog. This interesting difference leads one to agree with Walmsley,[10] that the presence of notochordal cells inhibits proliferation of the inner annulus. Indeed, since in embryonic pigs[11] and growing cats (Figure 8) the nucleus pulposus enlarges at the expense of the annulus, it is tempting to suggest that viable notochordal cells can destroy the inner annulus. Once their influence is removed, whether before or after birth, the annulus is free to invade the disc center, resulting in the variation in morphology seen in different species.

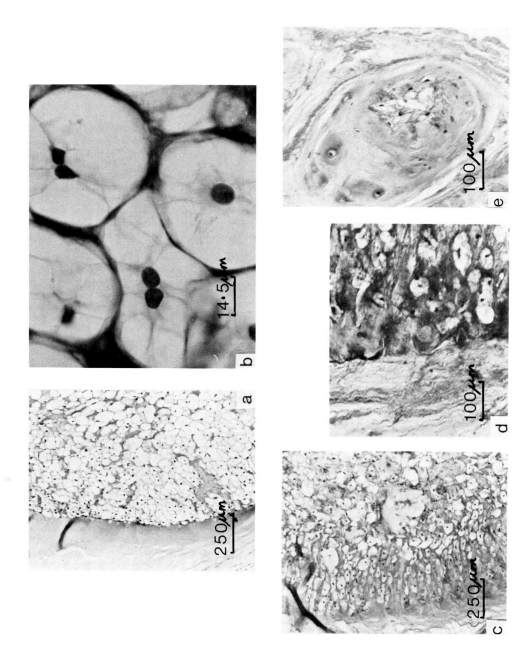

FIGURE 10.. Cat nucleus pulposus. a. Disc C2—3 from 6-month old cat, stained H & E. The nucleus pulposus consists of a mass of highly vacuolated notochordal cells, partly separated by amorphous basophilic matrix; basophilic matrix also separates the cells from the inner annulus (bottom left). (From Butler, W. F. and Smith, R. N., *Res. Vet. Sci.*, 8, 151, 1967. With permission.) b. High power light microscope picture of the cells stained with H & E; the intercellular material is basophilic; the vacuolated cells contain a network of cytoplasm and may be binucleate. c. Disc T4—5 from 3-year-old cat, stained H & E. The notochordal cells are degenerating in the central area (right of picture); the surrounding matrix is more densely stained than in (a) and is fibrillar. (From Butler, W. F. and Smith, R. N., *Res. Vet. Sci.*, 8, 151, 1967. With permission.) d. Disc L7—S1 from 18-year-old cat, stained H & E. Notochordal cells are still present in some discs at this age but are reduced in number; the matrix is fibrillar and acidophilically stained (dark fibers on left) (From Butler, W. F. and Smith, R. N., *Res. Vet. Sci.*, 151, 1967. With permission. e. As in (d). Some parts of the nucleus pulposus show islands of shrunken notochordal cells (center) as well as chondrocytes (upper left). (From Butler, W. F. and Smith, R. N., *Res. Vet. Sci.*, 151, 1967. With permission.)

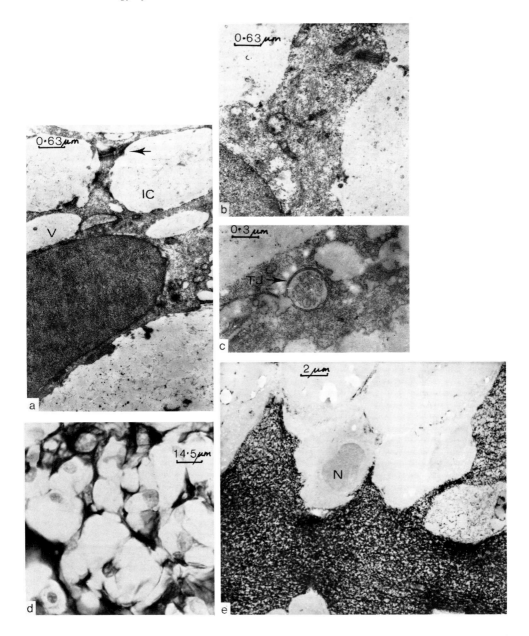

FIGURE 11.   Cat notochordal cells. a. Electron micrograph showing intracellular vacuoles (V), intercellular space (IC) and desmosome (arrow top); uranyl acetate and lead citrate. b. Similar to (a), showing possible centrioles (top right) and intracytoplasmic filaments. c. Similar to (a), showing a tight junction (arrow, center). d. Light micrograph of cells stained with Alcian Blue at pH 3.0 (Figure 10b); the pericellular material is densely stained and the cytoplasm and nuclei are pale. e. Electron micrograph of cells stained with Alcian Blue in 0.3 M MgCl$_2$ at pH 5.6; the intercellular material is densely stained and appears to form a filamentous network. (From Butler, W. F. and Heap, P. F., *Histochem. J.*, 11, 137, 1979. With permission.)

Electron microscopy of the cat disc (Figure 11) reveals that the notochordal cells vary in form, but usually contain large vacuoles separated by wisps of cytoplasm in which a few organelles are found. The vacuoles may be derived from dilated endoplasmic reticula.[3] Some glycogen is present in the cells of young animals,[84] but a striking feature is the presence of many filaments which converge upon desmosomes that join the cells to each other (Figure 10a). None of these filaments penetrate the cell membrane in the cat, although penetrating filaments have been seen in embryonic mouse cells.[3] Tight junctions also join the cells to each other (Figure 10c).[84] They have been seen in mouse embryos,[3] where they were thought to be possibly developing desmosomes. Micropinocytotic vesicles are numerous in the cells of the young cat,[84] as well as in mouse embryonic cells.[3] Electron microscopic examination[3,5,84] of the notochordal cells has dispelled the idea that they are syncytial, though it is impossible to distinguish separate cells with the light microscope (Figure 10).

In the intercellular space, the matrix contains collagen fibrils[84] as well as glycosaminoglycans[85] that, perhaps due to processing, appear as a network (Figure 10d and e) in Alcian Blue-stained sections or as granules or filaments in other preparations.[83,86] The cells are also bordered by remnants of a basement lamina that is common to embryonic notochord.[3]

4. Disc Degeneration

Detailed descriptions of the degenerative changes which discs undergo have been given for a few species, but most reports have concentrated on the dog and the cat. Macroscopic examination has led to the use of the terms prolapse (or protrusion), where internal tissue has either distorted the outer surface of the annulus or has burst through it. Disc degeneration is used to describe situations where the internal structure shows pathological change(s) with or without prolapse.

In a classical work on the discs of the dog, Hansen[17] has shown that prolapse can be recognized from the age of about 3 years, but that breeds differ in the age of onset and the proportion of discs involved. In chondrodystrophoid breeds, prolapses may be found as early as 3 years of age, when 17% of dogs are affected, and increase to 75% after 7 years of age. In normal breeds, however, they are first seen at 4 years, with 6% affected, and increase much more slowly, 24% being affected in animals over 7 years of age. It is clear from these data that the abnormality in cartilage development is associated with precocious disc degeneration in certain breeds of dog.

Hansen[17] classified the prolapses into two types. Type I occurs chiefly in chondrodystrophoid breeds and can be seen macroscopically in sectioned discs. It starts in the inner annulus where the ruptured lamellae radiate circularly around the disc, until the outer lamella is pierced. The rupture is often situated adjacent to the vertebral body. Type II protrusions occur chiefly in normal breeds and older animals and do not involve damage to the outer lamellae; often they can be seen only in serial microscopic sections. Thus, these protrusions are considered to arise as a senile phenomenon.

Degeneration, which can only be seen in sectioned discs, involves disorganization of the lamellar structure, ruptures (either internal or penetrating), sometimes calcification of the disc center, and a brown discoloration that is often, if not always, due to hemorrhage. This bleeding may arise from the vessels in the annulus. The rarity of protrusions through the vertebral end-plate[17,71] suggests that this is not a primary source of the blood. Degeneration of the annulus is considered by Hansen[17,71] always to follow degeneration of the central part of the disc.

There appear to be no sex differences in the incidence of disc prolapse in the dog, but there are regional differences along the vertebral column, most occurring in the lumbar region, fewer in the cervical region, and very few in the thoracic region.[58] This lack of dorsal protrusion in the region T1—10 is explained by Hansen[17] and by Hoerlein[88] as being due to the presence of the intercapital ligament dorsal to these discs. King,[87] however, pointed out that because the ligament is thinnest at T2—3 and T9—10 and thickest in the center of the series, there should be a gradient of incidence with a minimum at T6—7. This does not occur, so that other factors must operate. Dorsal prolapses are more common than ventral or lateral ones, perhaps because of the dorsal excentricity of the nucleus pulposus.

In contrast to the dog, which suffers clinically from disc disease,[17,88,89] the cat rarely does

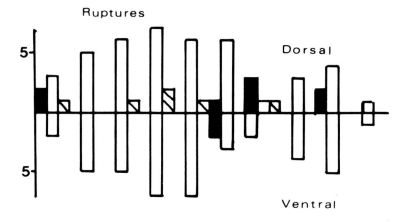

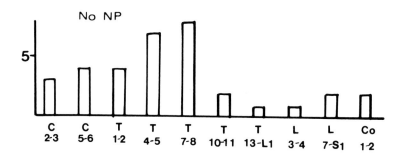

FIGURE 12. Incidence of ruptures and absence of nucleus pulposus in cat discs. The upper histogram shows the distribution of ruptures in serial microscope sections in a sample of 10 discs from each of 15 cats between birth and 18 years of age. Black bars represent ruptures of the internal annulus only, hatched bars represent ruptures of external annulus only, and white bars represent ruptures of the whole annulus. The lower histogram (No NP) represents the numbers of discs whose notochordal cells have been completely replaced by annulus fibrosus (Figure 14). C = cervical; T = thoracic; L = lumbar; S = sacral; and Co = coccygeal or caudal.

so.[90] Yet, pathological changes are very common in discs of the cat and result in extensive damage in later stages.[54] Detailed studies of the macroscopic changes that occur in cat discs have been made.[57,59,91-94] In random series using adult cats,[59,91] as many as 5% of the discs showed protrusions which ranged from small bulges to perforation of the outer lamellae. While some discs had an exceptionally high or low incidence, the regional distribution along the (Figure 12) vertebral column was similar to that of the nonchondrodystrophoid dog in that protrusions were rarest in the region T1—11. However, in contrast to the nonchondrodystrophoid dogs, protrusions were commonest in the cervical region of the cat spine (Figure 12). Dorsal protrusions were evident at about 6 years of age, and, since they increased until all discs were affected by about 15 years, the changes may be considered as a senile phenomenon like those of nonchondrodystrophoid dogs. The cervical region is affected earlier than the others. The incidence of ventral protrusions[57] also increases with age, but, in contrast to the dorsal situation, most occur in the lumbar region. The thicker ventral annulus in this region may be responsible for the smaller number of ventral protrusions.[57]

Macroscopic examination of transversely sectioned discs for degeneration, as distinct from protrusion, has shown that at least one third of the discs are affected and that the greatest incidence is seen in the region T1—10. The absence of dorsal protrusions in the thoracic region is not due to the mere presence of the intercapital ligament as is often suggested, but exists because extruded nucleus pulposus from discs showing degeneration (which includes ruptures) is directed to the costovertebral articulation by way of the synovial space beneath the ligament. This conclusion is supported by light microscopic observations.[54]

Examination of serial sections with the light microscope[54] shows that most disc ruptures start from about 5 years and increase with age, though small internal ruptures may be seen as early as 6 months. Early changes that are seen with the light microscope involve ruptures in the annulus with an intact nucleus pulposus (Figure 13 a and b). The ruptured fibers allow normal nucleus pulposus to escape into the annulus and, as the rupture enlarges, the notochordal tissue escapes to the outside. This allows the inner annulus to collapse inwards (Figure 13c) and the annulus cells to proliferate as chondrocytes, rather than to degenerate at the interface as in normal discs. The influence of notochordal cells on the inner annulus has already been discussed (see Section II, B). No proliferation of tissue of the vertebral surface at the level of the nucleus pulposus occurs, however, so that sagittally sectioned discs show an H-shaped slit (Figure 13c and d). The central brittle fibrocartilage (Figure 13d) then begins to break up and, at this time, the blood vessels in the vertebral surface become blocked by the proliferation of cartilage within these channels (Figure 13e). Bone-to-bone contact is made, the bone surface becomes eroded, and granulation tissue proliferates within the marrow spaces (Figure 13f) in an attempt at healing. Figure 14 summarizes these events which summarize the changes seen macroscopically and are described as very advanced degeneration, partial destruction, total destruction, and ankylosis.[95]

The changes just described are undoubtedly very similar, if not identical, to those called by Hansen[71] "osteochondrosis vertebrae." A high incidence of this condition has been found in the lumbosacral disc of cattle as well as in discs of camels and young pigs, and it is worth noting that this author[71] considers that the condition is secondary to a disc lesion. In pigs with erysipelas, osteochondrosis vertebrae is extensive in the vertebral column.[71]

Other changes occur in association with the disc changes just described. For instance, the intercapital ligament is often damaged and shows increased vascularity.[24,54] Avulsion of bone fragments also occurs from the outer edge of the vertebral body with hemorrhage[18,24,54] and vertebral osteophytes are formed.[54,99]

The latter condition, which has many synonyms,[99] is an important sequel to rupture of the ventral, but probably not the dorsal, annulus.[97] Experimental ventral incision of the discs of rabbits (a species with viable notochordal cells) has shown that, not only does loss of the nucleus pulposus and disc degeneration inevitably follow, but that osteophytes are produced with eventual ankylosis of the vertebrae (Figure 14). This condition is found particularly in the region T10—S1 of the dog vertebral column, where it is associated with disc degeneration. In a detailed study of the condition in the dog, Morgan[98] found that it increased with age, that incidence is high in the region T11—S1, and that it is rare dorsally. He also agreed that changes in the annulus play a major role in development of the condition both naturally and after experimental lesions and suggested that strain of the ventral longitudinal ligament was not of importance in the etiology of the condition in the dog.

In contrast to the dog, the condition in cats occurs most commonly in the thoracic region.[99] It is here also that most disc degeneration occurs (Figure 12).[54] Many other species are affected by vertebral osteophytes,[100-102] which are related to disc disease, at least in some animals. In the bull, but not in the cow, it is common at the lumbosacral disc so that a sex difference exists in this species.[100]

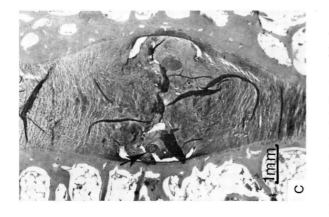

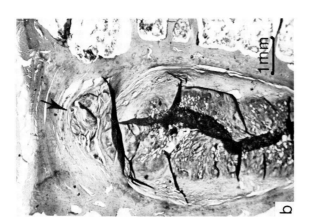

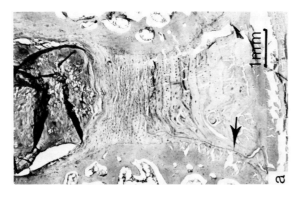

FIGURE 13. Ruptures of the cat disc. a. Rupture of outer annulus (arrow); the nucleus pulposus is intact; H & E stained. b. Rupture of the inner annulus with extrusion of notochordal cells and matrix (arrow); as in (a) there is no inward bulging of the inner annulus in this early change; H & E stained. c. Loss of most of the nucleus pulposus due to rupture (not in this section); remnants of the notochord (arrow) are present in the center, which is encroached upon by the inwardly bulging inner annulus; H & E stained. (From Butler, W. F., *Res. Vet. Sci.,* 9, 130, 1968. With permission.) d. Later stage. The inwardly bulged annulus has proliferated as fibrocartilage, but no proliferation has occurred at the vertebral surface at the junction with the nucleus pulposus (center); H & E stained. (From Butler, W. F., *Res. Vet. Sci.,* 9, 130, 1968. With permission.) e. The central vertebral surface of a disc similar to (d). Blood vessels have become blocked by proliferating cartilage from the vertebral surface; Toluidine Blue stained. f. Late stage of disc degeneration. The disc appears as a space which is closed peripherally by granulation tissue (lower left) and craniocaudally by the vertebrae that have been eroded, with the marrow spaces filled by granulation tissue (center left).

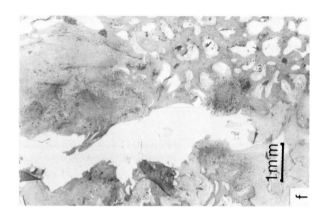

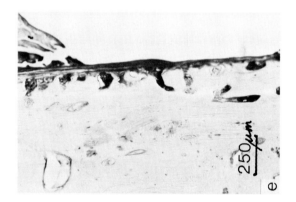

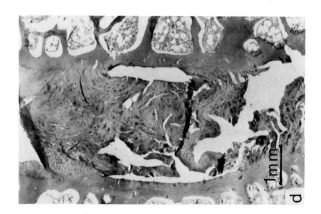

FIGURE 13 (continued)

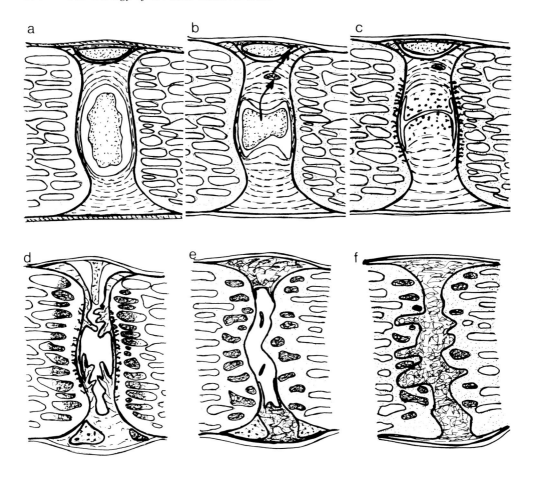

FIGURE 14.   The sequence of changes in ruptured cat discs. a. A normal thoracic disc in sagittal section. b. A dorsal rupture has allowed notochordal cells to be extruded and to enter the synovial sheath of the intercapital ligament (arrows); the inner annulus bulges inwards. c. Inner annulus cells proliferate and become chondrocytes instead of degenerating; an H-shaped slit is left in the area of the nucleus pulposus; blood vessels in the nearby bone become blocked with proliferating cartilage. d. Later, the more brittle central mass of fibrocartilage breaks up, allowing the vertebral faces to approach each other, and the intercapital ligament is compressed; new bone is forming in the ventral annulus (osteophytes). e. An attempt at healing with granulation tissue takes place peripherally; the bone surfaces are eroded and granulation tissue also proliferates in the marrow spaces; the osteophytes are fusing with the vertebral bodies. f. Finally, erosion of the vertebrae is extensive and the disc is replaced by granulation tissue.

IV. CONCLUSIONS

Although the structure of the intervertebral disc is basically similar in all mammals, it is clear from the description given above that there are important differences in morphology between and within species. One of the major differences is that the notochordal cells have a life span that may be purely embryonic, may extend into the juvenile period, or may last throughout life. Their presence clearly has an effect on the function of the annulus, which appears to be prevented from encroaching upon the disc center as long as a viable mass of notochordal cells is present. When these are lost, either by their degeneration or metamorphosis, or by their extrusion through ruptures, the inner annulus can proliferate to form a nucleus pulposus of quite a different texture and perhaps functional ability.

The sequence of changes that result in complete destruction of the disc is similar in many species, though serial sections are needed to confirm that this occurs in others. The incidence of the changes also indicates that it is usually a senile phenomenon, that there are no sex differences, but that species differ in the susceptibility of different regions of the vertebral column. These may be the result of many different influences, not the least of which are those of a functional nature and which are discussed elsewhere in this volume.

REFERENCES

1. **Carlier, E. W.,** The fate of the notochord and development of the intervertebral disc in the sheep, *J. Anat. Phys.,* 24, 573, 1890.
2. **Haldiman, J. T. and Gier, H. T.,** Bovine notochord origin and development, *Zentralbl. Veterinaermed. C.,* 10, 1, 1981.
3. **Jurand, A.,** Some aspects of the development of the notochord in mouse embryos, *J. Embryol. Exp. Morphol.,* 32, 1, 1974.
4. **Lauscher, C. K. and Carlson, E. C.,** The development of proline-containing extracellular connective tissue fibrils by chick notochord epithelium in vitro, *Anat. Rec.,* 182, 151, 1975.
5. **Leeson, T. S. and Leeson, C. R.,** Observations on the histochemistry and fine structure of the notochord in rabbit embryos, *J. Anat.,* 92, 278, 1958.
6. **Paavola, L. G., Wilson, D. B. and Center, E. M.,** Histochemistry of the developing notochord, perichordal sheath and vertebrae in Danforth's short tail (Sd) and normal C57BL/6 mice, *J. Embryol. Exp. Morphol.,* 55, 227, 1980.
7. **Sensenig, E. C.,** The origin of the vertebral column in the deermouse, *Peromyscus maniculatus sufiris, Anat. Rec.,* 86, 126, 1943.
8. **Trout, J. J., Buckwalter, J. A. and Moore, K. C.,** Ultrastructure of the human intervertebral disc. II. Cells of the nucleus pulposus, *Anat. Rec.,* 204, 307, 1982.
9. **Walmsley, R.,** Development and growth of the intervertebral disc, *Edinburgh Med. J.,* 60, 341, 1953.
10. **Walmsley, R.,** Anatomy and development, in *Modern Trends in Diseases of the Vertebral Column,* Nassim, J. R. and Burrows, H. J., Eds., Butterworth & Co., London, 1959, chap. 1.
11. **Williams, E. W.,** The latter development of the notochord in mammals, *Am. J. Anat.,* 8, 251, 1908.
12. **Butler, W. F. and Smith, R. N.,** The anulus fibrosus of the intervertebral disc of the newborn cat, *Res. Vet. Sci.,* 4, 454, 1963.
13. **Hare, W. D.,** Zur Ossification und Vereinigung der Wirbelepiphysen beim Hund, *Wien Tierarztl. Monatschr.,* 4, 48, 1961.
14. **Smith, R. N.,** personal communication, 1985.
15. **Postacchini, F., Bellocci, M. and Massobrio, M.,** Morphologic changes in annulus fibrosus during aging; an ultrastructural study in rats, *Spine,* 9, 596, 1984.
16. **Pousty, I.,** Microscopic studies on the intervertebral disc of domestic animals, Ph.D thesis, University of Bristol, Bristol, England, 1975.
17. **Hansen, H. J.,** A pathologic-anatomical study on disc degeneration in dog, *Acta Orthop. Scand.,* Suppl. 11, 1952.
18. **Hansen, H. J.,** Studies of the pathology of the lumbosacral disc in female cattle, *Acta Orthop. Scand.,* 25, 161, 1956.
19. **Butler, W. F. and Pousty, I.,** Staining of glycosaminoglycans in intervertebral disc cells, *Res. Vet. Sci.,* 23, 351, 1977.
20. **Knese, K. H.,** Kristallisation und Auflosung von Kollagenfibrille während der Histogenese der Zwischenwirbelscheibe, *Acta Anat. (Basel),* 100, 328, 1978.
21. **Johnson, E. F., Caldwell, R. W., Berryman, H. E., Miller, A. and Kothapada, C.,** Elastic fibres in the annulus fibrosus of the dog intervertebral disc, *Acta Anat.,* 118, 238, 1984.
22. **O'Rahilly, R., Miller, F. and Meyer, D. B.,** The human vertebral column at the end of the embryonic period proper. I. The column as a whole, *J. Anat.,* 131, 565, 1980.
23. **Trout, J. J., Buckwalter, J. A., Moore, K. C., and Landas, S. K.,** Ultrastructure of the human intervertebral disc. I. Changes in the notochordal cells with age, *Tissue-Cell,* 14, 359, 1982.
24. **Abe, M.,** A study on the intervertebral disc of the mink, *Jpn. J. Vet. Res.,* 8, 213, 1960.
25. **Kumar, S. and Davis, P. R.,** Lumbar innervation and intra-abdominal pressure, *J. Anat.,* 114, 47, 1973.
26. **Berry, R. J.,** Genetically controlled degeneration of the nucleus pulposus in the mouse, *J. Bone Jt. Surg.,* 43B, 387, 1961.
27. **Scott, N. A., Harris, P. F. and Bagnall, K. M.,** A morphological and histological study of the postnatal development of the intervertebral discs in the lumbar spine of the rabbit, *J. Anat.,* 130, 75, 1980.

28. **Souter, W. A. and Taylor, T. K. F.,** Sulphated acid mucopolysaccharide metabolism in the rabbit intervertebral disc, *J. Bone Jt. Surg.,* 52B, 371, 1970.

29. **Lipson, S. J. and Muir, H.,** Vertebral osteophyte formation in experimental intervertebral disc degeneration. Morphological and proteolycan changes over time, *Arthritis Rheum.,* 23, 319, 1980.

30. **Smith, J. W. and Walmsley, R.,** Experimental incision of the intervertebral disc, *J. Bone Jt. Surg.,* 33B, 612, 1951.

31. **Butler, W. F. and Smith, R. N.,** The nucleus pulposus of the intervertebral disc of the newborn cat, *Res. Vet. Sci.,* 5, 71, 1964.

32. **Cleland, D.,** On a peculiar ligament connecting opposite ribs in certain vertebrata, *Proc. R. Soc. Edinburgh,* 4, 101, 1858.

33. **King, A. S. and Smith, R. N.,** A comparison of the anatomy of the intervertebral disc in dog and man, *Br. Vet. J.,* 3, 135, 1955.

34. **Lohse, C. L. and Baba, Y. M.,** Comparitive anatomy of intervertebral discs and related structures in the cat and jaguar, *Zentralbl. Veterinaermed. C.,* 11, 334, 1982.

35. **Evans, H. E. and Christensen, G. C.,** *Miller's Anatomy of the Dog,* 2nd ed., W. B. Saunders & Co., Philadelphia, 1979, 239.

36. **Mayer, P.,** Ueber ein neuentdicktes Band, Jochband der Rippen (ligamentum costarum conjugale), *Arch. Anat. Phys. und Wiss. Med.,* 273, 1834.

37. **Kunzel, E.,** Beitrag zum fuktionellen Anatomie der Zwischerwirbelscheibe des Hundes mit Berucksichtigung der Discopathien, *Berl. Muench. Tieraerztl. Wochenschr.,* 83, 101, 1960.

38. **Pedersen, H. E., Blunck, C. F. J. and Gardner, E.,** The anatomy of the lumbosacral posterior rami and meningeal branches of spinal nerves, *J. Bone Jt. Surg.,* 38A, 377, 1956.

39. **Stillwell, D. R.,** The nerve supply of the vertebral column and its associated structures in the monkey, *Anat. Rec.,* 125, 139, 1956.

40. **Wiberg, G.,** Back pain in relation to the nerve supply of the intervertebral disc, *Acta Orthop. Scand.,* 29, 211, 1948.

41. **Bogduk, N.,** The lumbosacral dorsal rami of the cat, *J. Anat.,* 122, 653, 1976.

42. **Forsythe, W. B. and Ghoshal, N. G.,** Innervation of the canine thoracolumbar vertebral column, *Anat. Rec.,* 208, 57, 1984.

43. **Malinsky, J.,** Ontogenetic development of nerve terminations in the intervertebral discs of man, *Acta Anat.,* 38, 96, 1959.

44. **Lee, D. G.,** The arterial supply of the intervertebral disk of the domestic cat *(Felis domestica)* from fetal life to old age, *Am. J. Vet. Res.,* 23, 1072, 1962.

45. **Butler, W. F. and Smith, R. N.,** Age changes in the anulus fibrosus of the non-ruptured intervertebral disc of the cat, *Res. Vet. Sci.,* 6, 280, 1965.

46. **Crock, H. V.,** The arterial supply and venous drainage of the vertebral column of the dog, *J. Anat.,* 94, 88, 1960.

47. **Holm, S., Maroudas, A., Urban, J. P. G., Selstam, G., and Nachemson, A.,** Nutrition of the intervertebral disc: somite transport and mechanism, *Connect. Tissue Res.,* 8, 107, 1981.

48. **Morgan, J. P.,** Spondylosis deformans in the dog, *Acta Orthop. Scand.,* Suppl. 96, 26, 1967.

49. **Prader, A.,** Die Entwicklung der Zwischenwirbelscheibe beim menschlichen Keimling, *Acta Anat.,* 3, 115, 1947.

50. **Virgin, W. J.,** Anatomical and pathological aspects of the intervertebral disc, *Indian J. Surg.,* 20, 113, 1958.

51. **Maroudas, A. and Stockwell, R. A.,** Factors involved in the nutrition of the human lumbar intervertebral disc; cellularity and diffusion of glucose in vitro, *J. Anat.,* 120, 113, 1975.

52. **Holm, S. and Selstam, G.,** Oxygen tension alterations in the intervertebral disc as a response to changes in arterial blood, *Upsala J. Med. Sci.,* 87, 163, 1982.

53. **Stillwell, D. L.,** The vascular supply of vertebral structures, *Anat. Rec.,* 135, 169, 1959.

54. **Butler, W. F.,** Histological age changes in the ruptured intervertebral disc of the cat, *Res. Vet. Sci.,* 9, 130, 1968.

55. **Butler, W. F.,** unpublished data, 1985.

56. **Charleston, W. A. G.,** Mechanics of the vertebral column of the dog, Ph.D. thesis, University of Bristol, Bristol, England, 1961.

57. **King, A. S. and Smith, R. N.,** Disc protrusion in the cat: ventral protrusions and radial splits, *Res. Vet. Sci.,* 1, 301, 1960.

58. **Smith, R. N.,** Protrusion of the intervertebral disc, *Br. Small Animal Vet. Assoc. Congr. Proc.,* Pergamon Press, Oxford, 1959, 44.

59. **King, A. S. and Smith, R. N.,** Disc protrusions in the cat: distribution of dorsal protrusion along the vertebral column, *Vet. Rec.,* 72, 335, 1960.

60. **Walmsley, R.,** The development and growth of the intervertebral disc, *Edinburgh Med. J.,* 60, 341, 1953.

61. **Scott, N. A., Weiss, J. B. and Bagnall, K. M.**, Quantitative and qualitative observations on changes with age in the outer cellular matrix of the lumbar intervertebral disc of the rabbit, *J. Anat.*, 124, 253, 1977.
62. **Butler, W. F., and Heap, P.**, An ulstrastructural study of glycosaminoglycans associated with collagen and other constituents of the cat annulus fibrosus, *Histochem. J.*, 14, 113, 1982.
63. **Butler, W. F. and Smith, R. N.**, Age changes in the nucleus pulposus of the non-ruptured intervertebral disc of the cat, *Res. Vet. Sci.*, 8, 151, 1967.
64. **Butler, W. F.**, Metachromasia and Alcian Blue staining of the intervertebral disc of the cat, *J. Anat.*, 102, 301, 1986.
65. **Butler, W. F. and Wels, C.**, Glycosaminoglycans of cat intervertebral disc, *Biochem. J.*, 122, 647, 1971.
66. **Hardingham, T. E. and Adams, P.**, A method for the determination of hyaluronate in the presence of other glycosaminoglycans and its application to human intervertebral disc, *Biochem. J.*, 159, 143, 1976.
67. **Ghosh, P., Taylor, T. K. F., Brand, K. G. and Larsen, L. H.**, A comparative chemical and histochemical study of the chondrodystrophoid and non-chondrodystrophoid canine intervertebral disc, *Vet. Pathol.*, 13, 414, 1976.
68. **Adams, P., Eyre, D. R. and Muir, H.**, Biochemical aspects of development and ageing of human lumbar intervertebral discs, *Rheumatol. Rehabil.*, 16, 22, 1977.
69. **Pearce, R. H. and Grimmer, B. J.**, The chemical constitution of the proteoglycans of human intervertebral disc, *Biochem. J.*, 157, 753, 1976.
70. **Adams, P. and Muir, H.**, Qualitative changes with age of proteoglycans in human lumbar discs, *Ann. Rheum. Dis.*, 35, 289, 1976.
71. **Hansen, H. J.**, Comparative views on the pathology of disc degeneration in animals, *Lab. Invest.*, 8, 1242, 1959.
72. **Butler, W. F. and Fujioka, T.**, Fine structure of the annulus fibrosus of the intervertebral disc of the cat, *Anat. Anz.*, 132, 454, 1972.
73. **Pousty, I. and Butler, W. F.**, Staining of glycosaminoglycans of intervertebral disc tissue, *Res. Vet. Sci.*, 25, 182, 1978.
74. **Inoue, H. and Takeda, T.**, Three dimensional observation of the collagen framework of lumbar intervertebral discs, *Acta Orthop. Scand.*, 46, 949, 1975.
75. **Townsend, H. G. G. and Leach, D. H.**, Relationship between intervertebral joint morphology and mobility in the equine thoraco-lumbar spine, *Equine Vet. J.*, 16, 461, 1984.
76. **Watanabe, T.**, The mechanism of transition from notochordal nucleus to fibrocartilaginous nucleus of the disc in young monkey. An electronmicroscope study, *J. Jpn. Orthop. Ass.*, 57, 519, 1983.
77. **Meachim, G. and Cornah, M. S.**, Fine structure of juvenile human nucleus pulposus, *J. Anat.*, 107, 337, 1970.
78. **Meachim, G.**, Meshwork patterns in the ground substance of articular cartilage and nucleus pulposus, *J. Anat.*, 111, 219, 1972.
79. **Trout, J. J., Buckwalter, J. A., Moore, K. C. and Landas, S. K.**, Ultrastructure of the human intervertebral disc: I. Change in notochordal cells with age, *Tissue Cell*, 14, 359, 1982.
80. **Ghosh, P., Taylor, T. K. F., Yarroll, J. M., Braund, K. G. and Larsen, L. H.**, Genetic factors in the maturation of the canine intervertebral disc, *Res. Vet. Sci.*, 19, 304, 1975.
81. **Tondury, G.**, Uber die Diskushernie beim Dackel, *Z. Orthop. Ihre Grenzgeb.*, 83, 184, 1953.
82. **Higachi, M., Kaneda, K. and Abe, K.**, Age-related changes in the nucleus pulposus of intervertebral disc in mice. An electronmicroscope study, *J. Jpn. Orthop. Assoc.*, 56, 321, 1982.
83. **Smith, J. W. and Serafini-Fracassini, A.**, The distribution of the protein-polysaccharide complex in the nucleus pulposus matrix in young rabbits, *J. Cell. Sci.*, 3, 33, 1968.
84. **Butler, W. F. and Fujioka, T.**, Fine structure of the nucleus pulposus of the intervertebral disc of the cat, *Anat. Anz.*, 132, 465, 1972.
85. **Butler, W. F. and Heap, P.**, Correlation between Alcian Blue staining of glycosaminoglycans of cat nucleus pulposus and TEM X-ray probe microanalysis, *Histochem. J.*, 11, 137, 1979.
86. **Cornah, M. S., Meachim, G. and Parry, E. W.**, Banded structures in the matrix of human and rabbit nucleus pulposus, *J. Anat.*, 107, 351, 1970.
87. **King, A. S.**, The anatomy of disc protrusion in the dog, *Vet. Rec.*, 68, 939, 1956.
88. **Hoerlein, B. F.**, Intervertebral disc protrusion in the dog. I. Incidence and pathological lesions, *Am. J. Vet. Res.*, 14, 260, 1953.
89. **Olsson, S. E.**, The dynamic factor in spinal cord compression. A study on dogs with special reference to cervical disc protrusions, *J. Neurosurg.*, 15, 308, 1958.
90. **Wilkinson, G. T.**, *Diseases of the Cat and Their Management*, Wilkinson, G. T., Ed., Blackwell Scientific Publications, Oxford, 1984, 185.
91. **King, A. S., Smith, R. N. and Kon, V. M.**, Protrusions of the intervertebral disc of the cat, *Vet. Rec.*, 70, 1, 1958.

92. **King, A. S. and Smith, R. N.,** Diseases of the intervertebral disc of the cat, *Nature,* 181, 568, 1958.

93. **King, A. S. and Smith, R. N.,** Protrusion of the intervertebral disc in the cat, *Vet. Rec.,* 70, 1, 1958.

94. **King, A. S. and Smith, R. N.,** Disc protrusion in the cat: age incidence of dorsal protrusions, *Vet. Rec.,* 72, 381, 1960.

95. **King, A. S. and Smith, R. N.,** Degeneration of the intervertebral disc in the cat, *Acta Orthop. Scand.,* 34, 139, 1964.

96. **Grabell, I., Hansen, H. J., Olsson, S. E., Orstadius, K. and Thal, E.,** Discospondylitis and arthritis in swine erysipelas, *Acta Vet. Scand.,* 3, 33, 1962.

97. **Key, J. A. and Ford, L. T.,** Experimental intervertebral disc lesions, *J. Bone Jt. Surg.,* 30A, 621, 1948.

98. **Morgan, J. P.,** Spondylosis deformans in the dog, *Acta Orthop. Scand.,* Suppl. 96, 15, 1967.

99. **Beadman, R., Smith, R. N. and King, A. S.,** Vertebral osteophytes in the cat, *Vet. Rec.,* 76, 1005, 1964.

100. **Bane, A. and Hansen, H. J.,** Spinal changes in the bull and their significance in serving inability, *Cornell Vet.,* 52, 362, 1962.

101. **Baker, J. R. and Lyon, D. G.,** A case of intervertebral disc degeneration and prolapse with spondylosis in a sheep, *Vet. Rec.,* 96, 290, 1975.

102. **Kuntze, A.,** Roentgenpathologische Befunde an der Wirbelsaüle von Zootieren, *Monatsh. Veterinäermed.,* 17, 713, 1965.

Chapter 4

VASCULAR ANATOMY RELATED TO THE INTERVERTEBRAL DISC

Henry V. Crock, Miron Goldwasser and Hidezo Yoshizawa

TABLE OF CONTENTS

I. INTRODUCTION

Previous studies on the mechanisms of nutrition of the intervertebral disc and of certain articular cartilages suggest that blood vessels in the adjacent bones are not important in this process[1-3] in the adult.

This inference is based on the interpretation of two sets of experiments:

1.   Biochemical studies on the movement and metabolism of solutes indicated very slow rates of chemical change in the intervertebral disc tissues.
2.   Applied anatomical studies were carried out by McKibbin and Holdsworth[1] based on the injection of dyes into the upper tibial epiphyses of immature and adult rabbits. The experiments were performed after inserting needles into the central area of the epiphyses themselves — individual vessels were not cannulated. The conclusion drawn from these experiments by the authors was that the contribution of subchondral vessels to the nutrition of articular cartilage in adults was negligible.

These conclusions, which have received wide recognition, might reasonably be applied to the interpretation of the relevance of vertebral body circulation to the intervertebral disc nutrition.[4] Both these sets of experiments apparently lead to the same conclusion, namely, that blood vessels in bone have little to do with nutritional mechanisms in the intervertebral disc or articular cartilages.

However, there are a number of observations, the interpretation of which leads to quite different conclusions about the importance of the circulation related to disc metabolism, nutrition, and pathology. For example, the marked diurnal variations in the height of the vertebral column in man are attributed to the movement of fluid into and out of the disc tissues on an hourly basis.

Observations on changes in the appearance of radiopaque substances injected into discs during discography reveal the diffusion of the opaque medium throughout the disc space within minutes and its complete disappearance from the disc within hours. Radiopaque substances may enter the vertebral body veins and fill the internal vertebral venous plexus almost instantaneously during discography.[5] Radio-tracers injected into lumbar discs with chymopapain have been identified within seconds in the pulmonary circulation.[6]

These latter observations cannot be explained on the previously held assumption that the intervertebral disc is relatively inert. Clearly there is a mechanism for the rapid movement of fluids into and out of the intervertebral disc.

The anatomical studies presented in this chapter provide a description of the microcirculation and of its associated complex venous connections which, considered together, provide an understanding of the vascular pathways along which these rapid fluid exchanges can occur. We believe that it is essential for these anatomical findings to be integrated with physiological and biochemical studies, so that a true picture of the mechanisms of nutrition and a clearer picture of the pathological processes of the human intervertebral disc may be developed.

II. DESCRIPTIVE ANATOMY

In the newborn, there is a capillary bed related to the vertebral body in the region of the vertebral end-plate adjacent to the intervertebral disc (Figure 1). This capillary bed is distributed across the cartilage cap of the partly ossified vertebral body. It is made up of vascular terminations in cartilage canals which contain arteriolar vessels and venules (Figure 2). Viewed through the disc surface, these vascular terminations are bulbous and punctate.[7] In the adult, with the final definition of the vertebral end-plate cartilage and the bony sub-

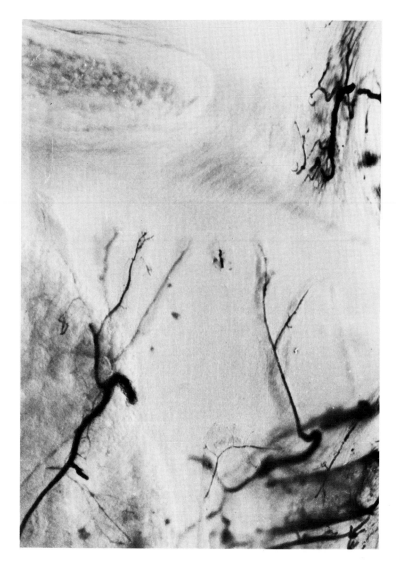

FIGURE 1.   Coronal section in the region of the cartilage cap of the vertebral body in a neonate demonstrating cartilage canals with vascular buds showing the characteristic circulation in developing cartilage.

chondral vertebral end-plate, a clearly defined capillary bed remains within the cartilage end-plate. Changes are then found in the venous drainage of this capillary bed, with the appearance of a horizontal subarticular collecting vein system. Detailed studies of the arterial supply and venous drainage of the human vertebral body have been described by Crock et al.[6] and by Crock and Yoshizawa.[7,8] The descriptions which are now presented are based largely on those earlier works. Added details on vertebral end-plate capillaries have been taken from in vivo injection studies in adult dogs carried out by Crock and Goldwasser.[9]

Taking a typical lumbar vertebra as a model for the description of the arterial supply of the vertebral body, one can build up a picture of the arteries of origin which is both simple and accurate. The pattern of distribution of the major branches of the lumbar arteries to the vertebral bodies is already established at birth and remains unchanged throughout life. However, quite dramatic changes will occur during growth with reference to the vertebral end-plate capillaries and their modes of drainage.

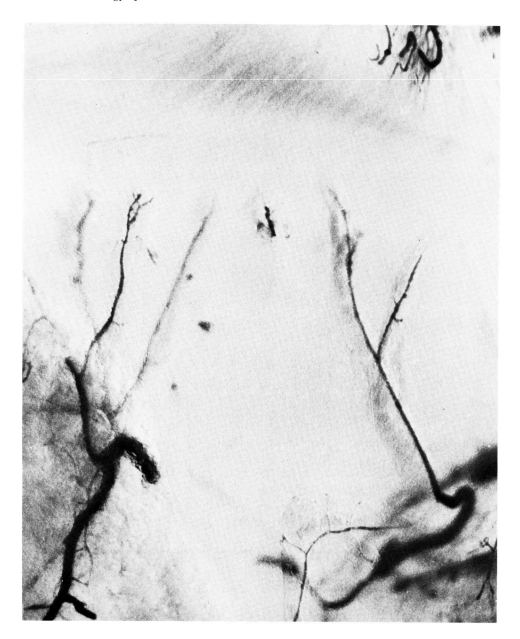

FIGURE 2.   Enlargement of portion of Figure 1, demonstrating that cartilage canals with vascular buds are the characteristic circulation in developing cartilage.

Paired lumbar arteries arise from the posterior wall of the abdominal aorta and each courses around the "waist" or equatorial zone of the vertebral body. These arteries and their multitudinous branches lie "on" and not "in" the periosteum of the vertebra (Figures 3, 4, 5, and 6). Between their origins from the aorta and their point of migration posteriorly away from the vertebral body under the psoas muscles, these arteries give off three sets of branches: (1) the centrum branches (Figures 3 and 4); (2) ascending branches (Figure 7); and (3) descending branches (Figure 7).

Beneath the aorta, and over the anterolateral aspects of the vertebral body, both in children and adults, ascending and descending branches of the lumbar arteries course towards the "metaphyseal" regions of the vertebral body (Figures 5, 6, and 8). Longitudinally oriented

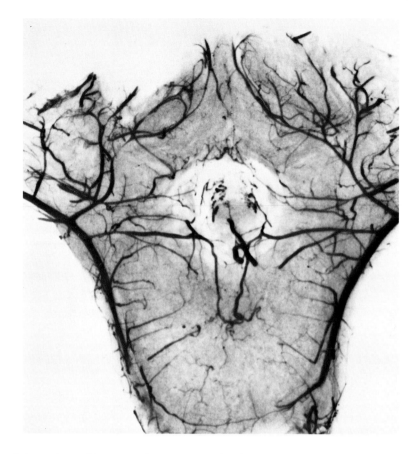

FIGURE 3.   A thin horizontal (transverse) section through the middle of the centrum of an adult human lumbar vertebra showing the arterial supply forming a grid in the centrum of the vertebra.

anastomoses between ascending and descending branches of the lumbar arteries on adjacent vertebrae join in the areolar tissues and on the anterior and posterior surfaces of the anterior longitudinal ligament in front of the intervertebral disc (Figures 5, 6, and 8). We have been unable to identify the intermetaphyseal communicating artery described by Ratcliffe[10] and depicted by him only in diagrams.

As each lumbar artery crosses its related intervertebral foramen, three sets of branches enter the spinal canal. Of these, the anterior spinal canal branches are relevant to the arterial supply of the vertebral body. They form an arcade on the posterior surfaces of the vertebral bodies from which the centrum and metaphyseal branches pass into the vertebral bodies (Figure 9).[7]

Some longitudinal anastomoses also occur between ascending and descending arteries on the posterior surfaces of adjacent vertebral bodies, across the surface of the intervertebral disc. However, these are not as numerous as those on the anterolateral aspects.

The intraosseous distribution of these main branches of the lumbar arteries is as follows: (1) the centrum branches form an arterial grid in the middle of the vertebral body, from which branches pass upwards and downwards to end in arterioles which are oriented vertically at right angles to the middle third of the respective vertebral end-plates (Figures 7 and 10); (2) ascending branches and (3) descending branches penetrate the anterolateral aspects of the vertebral body somewhat obliquely towards its center, dropping vertically oriented arteriolar branches towards their related vertebral end-plates in the outer thirds of the vertebra

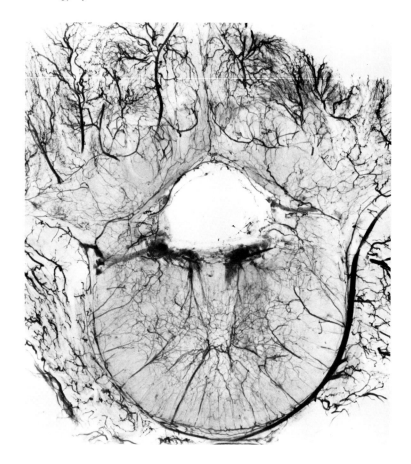

FIGURE 4. A similar transverse section to Figure 3 through an adolescent lumbar vertebra, showing the origins of the arterial supply to the vertebral body and the formation of a grid in the centrum of the vertebra.

(Figures 10 and 11); and (4) the anterior spinal canal branches form an arterial arcade on the posterior surface of the vertebral bodies as described above (Figure 9). From this system, intraosseous branches analogous to those from the centrum and ascending and descending branches of the lumbar arteries on the anterolateral aspects of the vertebral body penetrate the body from behind (Figure 11).

The capillary bed across the area of the vertebral end-plate is fed by arteries based on named branches of the lumbar arteries. Study of specimens of the vertebral body in which the arteries have been incompletely filled suggests that the vertebral end-plate capillary bed may be segmentally supplied by branches from the centrum grid and by metaphyseal branches derived from the ascending and descending branches and from branches of the anterior intraspinal arcade (Figures 7, 8, and 12). While this anatomical account may seem useful in the interpretation of localized destructive lesions in vertebral osteomyelitis,[10] the examination of injections of higher quality suggests that intraosseous anastomoses between small arteries derived from different extraosseous vessels almost certainly exist (Figures 10 and 11).

Conflicting views on this issue highlight a lack of critical analysis of available published information. Resolution of this particular issue is important before the findings of applied anatomical research and physiological and biochemical studies can all be correlated to elucidate the mechanisms of disc nutrition and the deeper understanding of disc pathology.

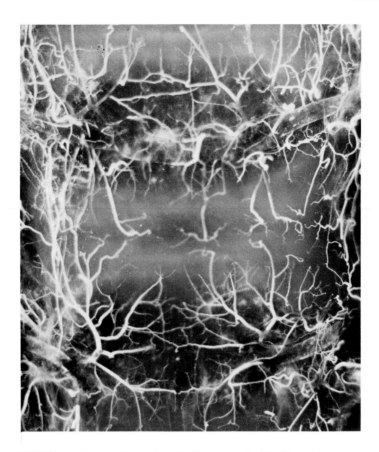

FIGURE 5.   The anterior surface of adjacent vertebral bodies (with the aorta removed) from a neonate showing ascending and descending branches of the lumbar arteries; each of the main stems of four lumbar arteries (two pairs) can be seen on the two adjacent vertebral bodies.

III. DETAILS OF THE VERTEBRAL END-PLATE CAPILLARIES

There is a continuous capillary bed across the bone-disc interface. In the region of the bone-disc interface, over the area of the nucleus pulposus, the capillary terminations are sessile and discoid, like suckers on the tentacles of an octopus (Figure 13). They drain into venules that are at once woven into a plexiform subchondral postcapillary venous network from which drainage into the larger veins of the vertebral body occurs in two ways: (1) some discrete smaller veins enter directly at right angles into the large tributaries of the horizontal subarticular collecting vein system (Figures 13 and 14); and (2) others pass directly into the intricate plexiform veins lining the marrow cavities of the vertebral bodies, from which tributaries emerge to join radicles of the metaphyseal and centrum veins (Figure 15). At the bone-disc interface in the region of the inner annulus, the density of capillaries is lower than in the area related to the nucleus pulposus. The terminations themselves are also smaller. They drain singly or in groups of two or three venules, either into the veins of the marrow spaces or into the subchondral postcapillary network (Figure 16).

Over the area of the bone-disc interface related to the outer annular fibers, the capillary system consists of discrete loop-like terminations. These again drain either directly into the network of veins in subjacent marrow spaces or into the subchondral postcapillary venous network (Figure 17).

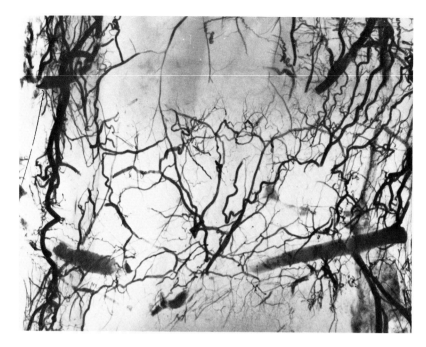

FIGURE 6.   The anterior surface of adjacent vertebral bodies (with the aorta removed) in a young adult showing ascending and descending branches of the lumbar arteries; the main stems of the four lumbar arteries can be seen on two adjacent vertebral bodies.

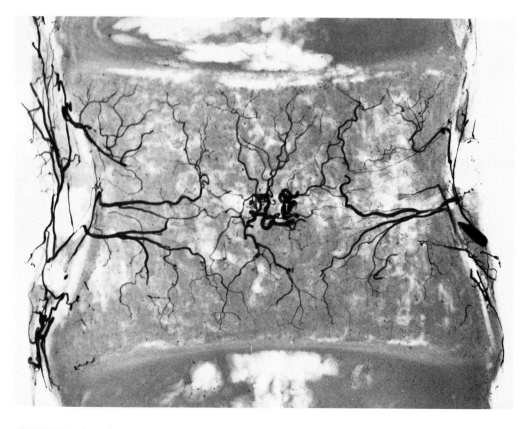

FIGURE 7.   Coronal section of a human lumbar vertebra demonstrating the "incompletely filled" arteries to the metaphyseal region and the centrum of vertebra.

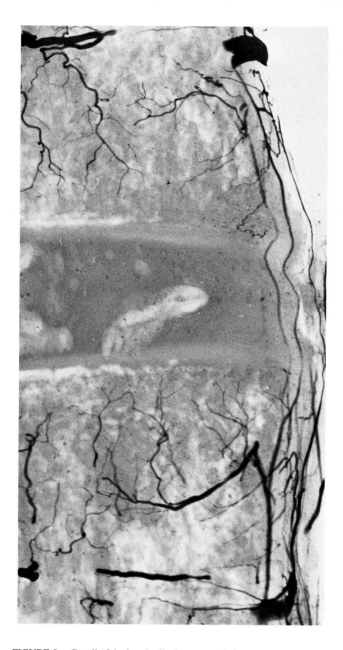

FIGURE 8. Detail of the longitudinal anastamosis between adjacent lumbar arteries shown on coronal section; these vessels pass over the intervertebral disc but do not supply it.

IV. THE VENOUS DRAINAGE OF THE VERTEBRAL END-PLATE

In the newborn, the vertebral end-plate capillaries drain along the cartilage canals (Figure 2). In the adult, a complex postcapillary venous network is established close to the disc-bone interface (Figures 18 A, B, C, D, and 19). This system is described in detail in the legends accompanying Figs. 18 and 19. The postcapillary venous network of the vertebral end-plate drains either directly into the delicate plexiform veins of the marrow spaces of the vertebral body (Figs. 15 and 16), or into a large horizontally oriented subarticular collecting vein system of the vertebral body[6] (Figures 20 and 21).

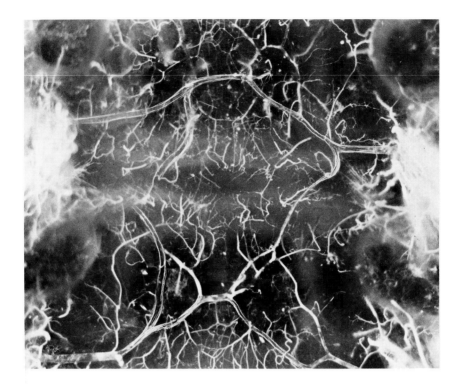

FIGURE 9.   Radiograph of a thin coronal section through two adjacent vertebral bodies in a neonate to show the distribution of anterior spinal branches of the lumbar arteries on the posterior surface of the vertebral bodies. The main intraosseous tributaries from this arcuate system correspond to the ascending and descending branches of the abdominal portion of the lumbar arteries; in the centers of the vertebral bodies, where the right- and left-sided arcades approach each other, centrum branches penetrate the vertebral bodies.

The horizontal subarticular collecting vein system is built up in the central area of the vertebral body by large caliber tributaries of the vertical veins of the centrum. These turn abruptly from their vertical courses to run horizontally, some passing anteriorly, others posteriorly, and still others laterally (Figures 22 and 21). The subarticular collecting vein system can now be recognized in vivo in certain disorders of intervertebral discs by magnetic resonance imaging [5] (Figure 23).

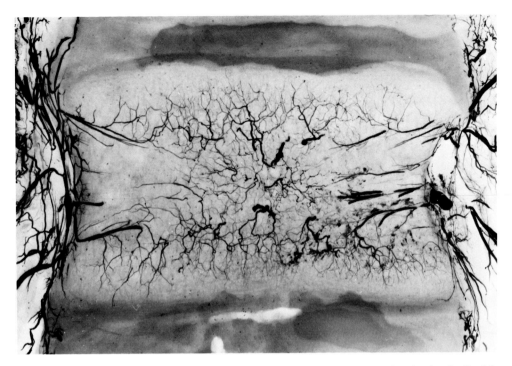

FIGURE 10. Radiograph of a thin coronal section through the center of a lumbar vertebra showing details of the intraosseous distribution of the arteries in the centrum region and, in particular, in the metaphyseal region.

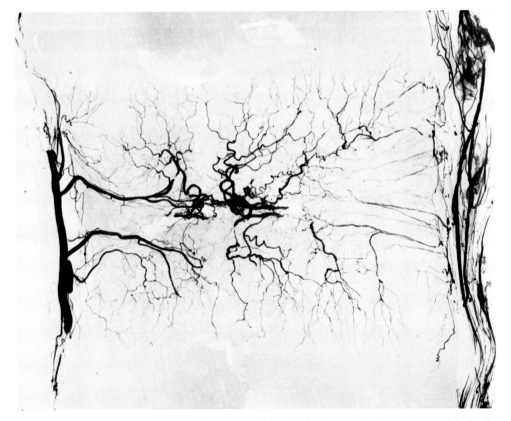

FIGURE 11. Thin sagittal section through the center of the fifth lumbar vertebra from a young adult showing the intraosseous arterial distribution in the region of the vertebral end-plates.

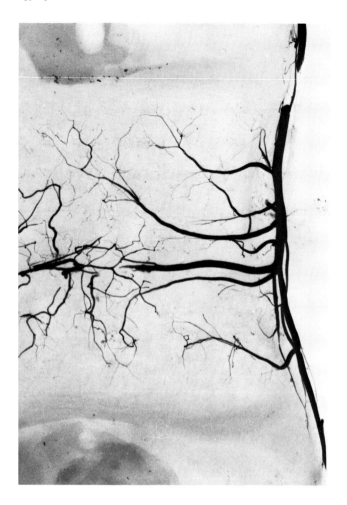

FIGURE 12.   Sagittal section of a lumbar vertebra demonstrating the centrum and metaphyseal arterial branches based on the anterior intraspinal arterial arcade.

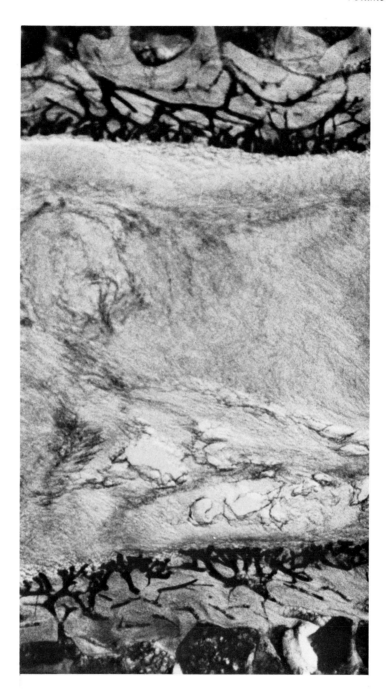

FIGURE 13.   Sagittal section in the region of the nucleus pulposus of a dog lumbar disc showing the capillary circulation with the postcapillary venous network demonstrated on both sides of the disc.

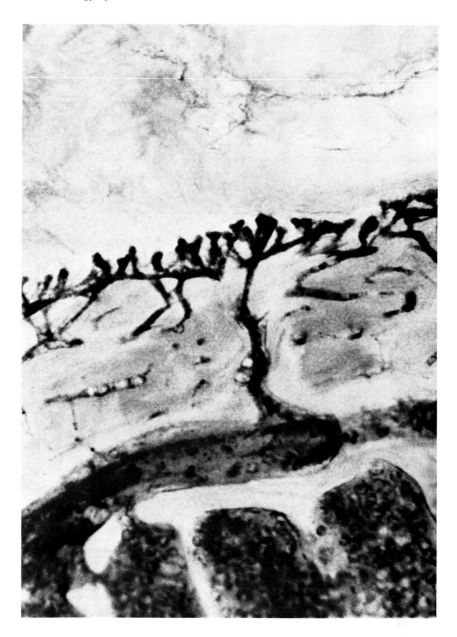

FIGURE 14. Detail of the capillary circulation of the vertebral end-plate cartilage in the region of the nucleus pulposus of a dog lumbar disc; it shows the capillaries draining into the subarticular collecting vein.

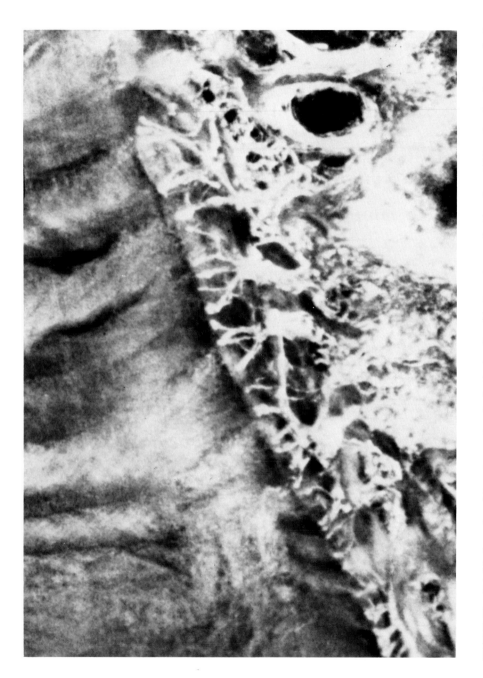

FIGURE 15. Detail in the region of the outer annulus of a dog lumbar disc; this time, photographed in reflected light rather than the transmitted light of the previous figures; it shows the drainage of postcapillary venules directly into the plexiform veins of the marrow spaces.

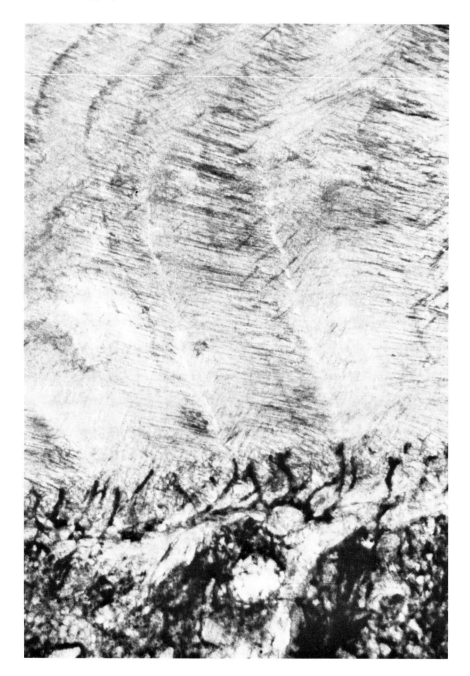

FIGURE 16.   Detail of the capillary circulation of the vertebral end-plate cartilage in the region of the outer annulus of a dog lumbar disc.

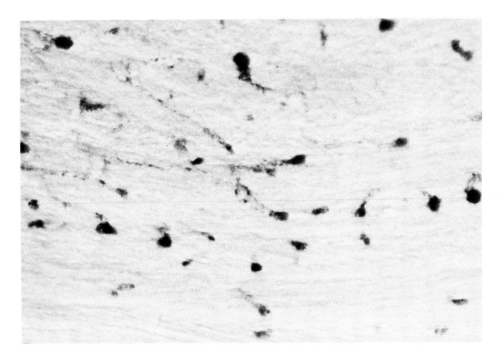

FIGURE 17. Photomicrograph of a transverse section through the vertebral end-plate cartilage showing capillary buds and some radicles of the postcapillary venules; the density of the capillary bed is still high, but the terminations are not quite as bulbous as they are in the capillary bed close to the nucleus pulposus area.

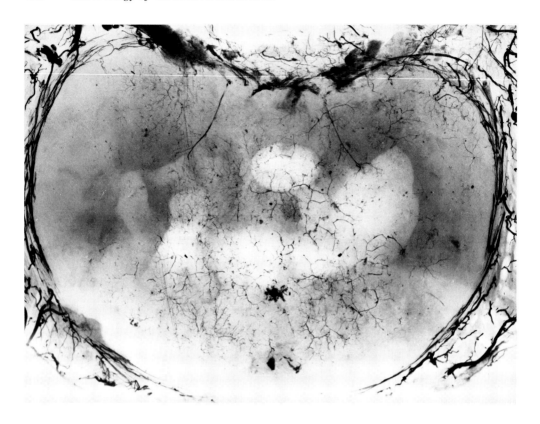

PART I

FIGURE 18.   Part I: A transverse section of a lumbar vertebra from a young adult, cut through the region of the junction of the vertebral end-plate and intervertebral disc. The arteries have been injected with a thin suspension of barium sulfate, which has passed through the capillary bed in the vertebral end-plate partially filling the postcapillary venous network of the vertebral body. The interpretation of the radiographic images in the region of the vertebral end-plate seen in this specimen is facilitated by the accompanying explanatory diagrams A, B, C, and D. Punctate images scattered across the disc surface represent some of the arteriolar and capillary vessels seen end-on in the region of the juntion of the intervertebral disc with the vertebral body. However, images of the postcapillary venous network predominate. These vessels form a spidery network which is oriented horizontally, parallel to the vertebral end-plate. Part II: (A) Drawing of a lumbar vertebral body viewed in a midcoronal section, showing the arterial grid in the centrum from which vertically oriented branches pass through the vertebral end-plate. (B) When a thin section is made in the plane XX of (A) and this section is then viewed from above, the images of the arteriolar and capillary terminations will appear punctate. (C) Drawing of a lumbar vertebral body viewed from a cut in the midsagittal plane viewed from the side. The veins of the vertebral body are represented as a composite with the centrum plexus of Batson in the middle, draining posteriorly into the internal vertebral venous plexus. Vertical veins pass from the region of the vertebral end-plate into Batson's plexus. Oriented parallel to the vertebral end-plate, in close proximity to it, is the horizontal subarticular collecting vein system of the vertebral body.[6] (D) When a thin section YY is made of (C) and viewed from above, the images of the postcapillary venous network will appear as a spidery plexus.

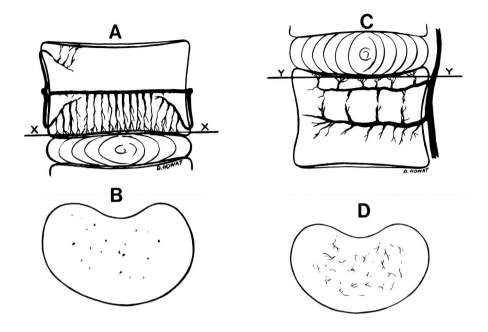

FIGURE 18, Part II

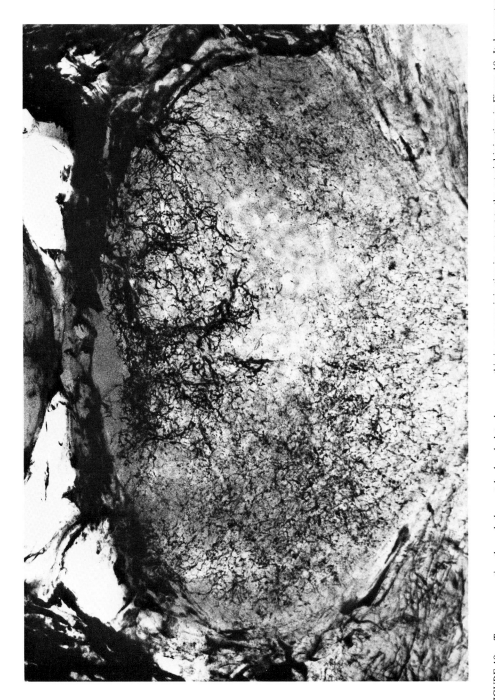

FIGURE 19.   Transverse section through the vertebral end-plate; however, this is a venous injection in contrast to the arterial injection in Figure 18. It demonstrates the postcapillary venous plexus and the subarticular collecting veins draining posteriorly into the internal vertebral venous plexus.

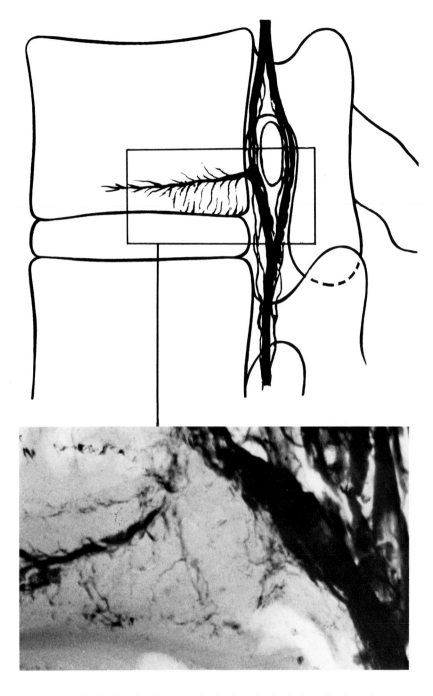

FIGURE 20. Sagittal section demonstrating horizontal subarticular collecting vein system draining into the anterior internal vertebral venous plexus. The postcapillary venules at the vertebral end-plate are shown draining into the horizontal subarticular collecting vein.

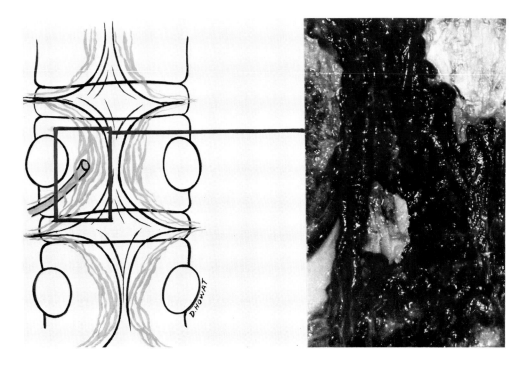

FIGURE 21.   This is a macroscopic figure, a coronal section showing the anterior internal vertebral venous plexus. It demonstrates the relationship of the anterior and posterior venous plexus radicles surrounding an emergent lumbar nerve root. The subarticular collecting venous system drains into these radicles in the region of the vertebral metaphysis. Those vessels behind the nerve root are part of the posterior internal vertebral venous plexus.

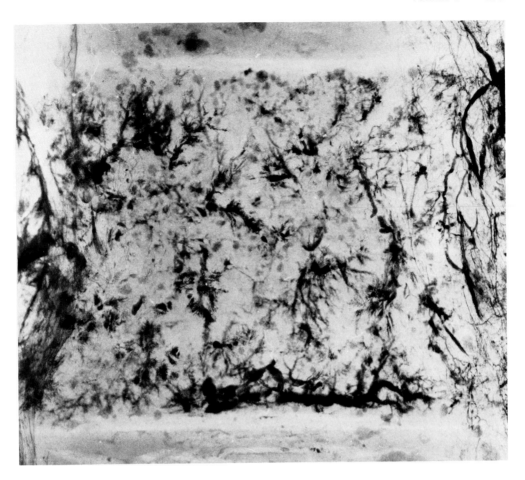

FIGURE 22. Radiograph of a thin coronal section from a thoracic vertebra from a 67-year-old woman; details of the horizontal subarticular collecting vein and its relationship to the intervertebral disc can be seen.

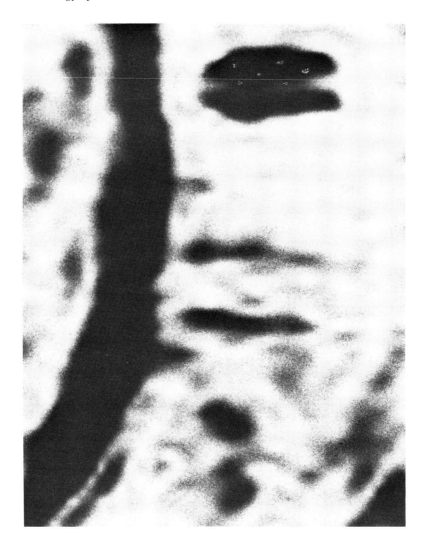

FIGURE 23.   Magnetic resonance imaging (''MRI'') scan showing the appearance of a normal disc (upper) and a disc in a case of traumatic disruption (lower disc), with the reactive circulatory system in the region of the horizontal subarticular veins being demonstrated. (Courtesy P. Schulitz, S. Dohring and J. Assheuer.)

REFERENCES

1. **McKibbin, B. and Holdsworth, F.,** The source of nutrition of articular cartilage, *J. Bone Jt. Surg.,* 50-B, 876, 1968.
2. **Nachenson, A., Lewin, T., Maroudas, A., and Freeman, M. A. R.,** In vitro diffusion of dye through the end-plates and the annulus fibrosus of the human lumbar intervertebral discs, *Acta. Orthop. Scand,* 41, 589, 1970.
3. **Holm, S., Maroudas, A., Urban, J. P. G., Selstram, G., and Nachemson, A.,** Nutrition of the intervertebral disc: solute transport and mechanism, *Connect. Tissue Res.,* 8, 101, 1981.
4. **Freemand, M. A. R.,** Adult Articular Cartilage, Pitman Press, London, 1973.
5. **Schultiz, P., Dohring, S. and Assheuer, J.,** personal communication.
6. **Crock, H. V., Yoshizawa, H., and Kame, S. K.,** Observations on the venous drainage of the human vertebral body, *J. Bone Jt. Surg.,* 55-B, 528, 1973.
7. **Crock, H. V. and Yoshizawa, H.,** The blood supply of the lumbar vertebral column, *Clin. Orthop. Relat. Res.,* 115, 6, 1976.
8. **Crock, H. V. and Yoshizawa, H.,** *The Blood Supply of the Vertebral Column and Spinal Cord in Man,* Springer, New York, 1977.
9. **Crock, H. V. and Goldwasser, M.,** Anatomic studies of the circulation in the region of the intervertebral end-plate in adult greyhound dog, *Spine,* 9, 702, 1984.
10. **Ratcliffe, J. F.,** Anatomic basis for the pathogenesis and radiologic features of vertebral osteomyelitis and its differentiation from childhood discitis. A microangiographic investigation, *Acta Radiol Diag.,* 26, 137, 1985.

Chapter 5

THE INNERVATION OF INTERVERTEBRAL DISCS

Nikolai Bogduk

TABLE OF CONTENTS

I. INTRODUCTION

The question of whether intervertebral discs have a nerve supply has long been a source of controversy and the subject of several investigations and reviews over the last 55 years. The relevance of this question, however, extends beyond simply an issue of anatomy; for while it is has been recognized, since the work of Mixter and Barr,[1] that discs can herniate and cause symptoms by compressing spinal nerve roots, what is less accepted, clinically, is that discs can intrinsically be a source of pain, without herniating. The principal objection to this latter concept is that if discs do not have a nerve supply, then they cannot be a source of pain. It is, therefore, germane to the issue of the etiology of spinal pain to determine whether of not discs are innervated.

Such studies as have been performed have focused principally on the lumbar intervertebral discs; though, recently, data on the cervical discs have become available. The innervation of thoracic discs, in humans, has not been studied, but the data on the lumbar and cervical discs are quite substantial. To appreciate the evolution of this knowledge and the reasons for controversy in this field, it is appropriate to review the literature chronologically. To maintain continuity, the lumbar and cervical discs are considered separately.

II. LUMBAR DISCS

The study of the innervation of the lumbar intervertebral discs has followed two parallel lines of investigation. One has been the search for nerve endings in the discs. The other has been the determination of the source of these endings.

In 1932, Jung and Brunschwig[2] undertook the first search for nerve endings in the lumbar discs. Although they found unmyelinated nerve fibers and nerve endings in both the anterior and posterior longitudinal ligaments, they found neither nerve fibers nor nerve endings within the discs themselves.

In contrast, Tsukada,[3,4] in 1938 and 1939, reported finding both myelinated and unmyelinated nerve fibers in the annulus fibrosus and nerve endings in the notochord and nucleus pulposus. It is noteworthy, however, that of all the studies that have addressed the innervation of the intervertebral discs, those of Tsukada remain the most enigmatic, for no one since has verified the presence of nerve endings in the nucleus pulposus, and, indeed, some authorities[5] have even challenged the accuracy of Tsukada's findings in the annulus fibrosus.

It was in 1940 that Roofe[6] published the first unequivocal evidence of nerve fibers in the annulus fibrosus. He reported "many" unmyelinated fibers in the annulus fibrosus which terminated in "naked nerve endings" and provided photographic evidence of his observations. Although he emphasized that nerve fibers occurred in the annulus fibrosus, Roofe commented that "no nerve tissue was observed within the disc itself." While seemingly contradictory, this was probably meant to imply the absence of nerve fibers in the nucleus pulposus.

Roofe's report[6] was limited to the results of his histological studies, and although suspecting that the nerves he found in the fourth and fifth lumbar discs arose from the third and fourth lumbar spinal nerves, he commented that their origin had still to be determined. However, Spurling and Bradford[7], Spurling and Grantham[8], and later, Bradford and Spurling[9] stipulated that the source of these nerves was the sinuvertebral nerve, which they illustrated as a long descending branch from the L2 spinal nerve (Figure 1A). Roofe was credited with this description,[8] but it was never formally published or endorsed by him.

Lazorthes et al.[10] seized upon this description of the sinuvertebral nerves, for it contradicted those in the classical German[11] and French[12-14] literature. The classical literature maintained that each sinuvertebral nerve arose from two roots: a somatic root from the spinal nerve at each segmental level and an autonomic root from a grey ramus communicans. The nerve

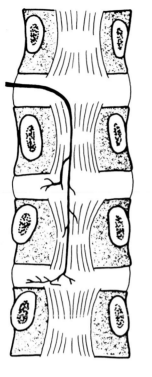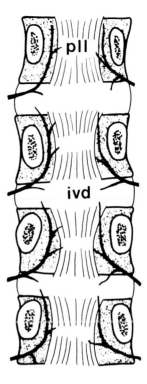

A   B

FIGURE 1.   (A) Erroneous description of the lumbar sinuvertebral nerves as
having a long descending course.[7,8] (B) Actual anatomy of the lumbar sinuvertebral
nerves supplying the intervertebral discs (ivd) at their level of origin and the level
above and the intervening posterior longitudinal ligament (pll).[5,10,34]

so formed passed through the intervertebral foramen to divide into a major ascending branch
and a smaller descending branch, which together supplied the vertebral venous plexuses,
the dura, the vertebral bodies, and the posterior longitudinal ligament. A distribution to
intervertebral discs, however, was never specifically mentioned.

Lazorthes et al.[10] studied 100 nerves in 10 lumbar vertebral columns, and found no
examples of nerves like those described by Spurling and colleagues.[78] Two thirds of the
nerves they dissected were single trunks that ramified at their level of entry and formed an
ascending branch to the level above (Figure 1B). The nerves were distributed to the dura
mater, the posterior longitudinal ligament, the vertebral bodies, and the intervertebral discs
at and above their level of origin. The remaining one third of their specimens were multiple
filaments rather than single nerve trunks, but, nevertheless, with a similar distribution.

Two years later, Herlihy[15] entered the debate on the anatomy of the sinuvertebral nerves,
but without contributing any original work. He simply contrasted the descriptions of Lazorthes et al.[10] with those of Buskirk.[16] Quoting Buskirk, Herlihy claimed that the lumbar
sinuvertebral nerves formed a continuous chain of nerve fibers running longitudinally within
the vertebral canal. This differed from the interrupted, essentially bisegmental distribution
described by Lazorthes et al.[10] Reference to Buskirk's original publication,[16] however, reveals
that what he described was, in fact, the distribution of sympathetic fibers within the vertebral
venous plexus and not the somatic branches of the sinuvertebral nerves. Moreover, his
studies were performed on cats and at thoracic levels. Thus, his data do not constitute a
legitimate challenge to the descriptions of the human lumbar sinuvertebral nerves given by
Lazorthes et al.[10]

Wiberg[17] contributed to this debate in 1949 and illustrated the lumbar sinuvertebral nerves as each ramifying at its level of entry and communicating with the nerves of adjacent levels opposite the middle of the interposed vertebral body, a description similar to that of Lazorthes et al.[10] Wiberg's attempts at histological studies, however, failed to demonstrate any nerve fibers in the annulus fibrosus.

In a paper on the embryology of the vertebral column, published in 1943, Ehrenhaft[18] briefly mentioned the presence of nerve bundles beneath the posterior longitudinal ligament and "within the annulus fibrosus proper". Ikari,[19] on the other hand, in 1954, failed to find any nerve endings in the annulus fibrosus.

In 1956, Stillwell[20] reported an exhaustive study of the innervation of the vertebral column in the monkey, which, while itself not evidence of what occurs in man, nonetheless served to foreshadow what the human anatomy might be. He reported branches from the sinuvertebral nerves to the posterior portions of the annulus fibrosus and branches to the lateral portions from the grey rami communicantes. The anterior longitudinal ligament received branches from the sympathetic trunk and the posterior longitudinal ligament was innervated by the sinuvertebral nerves. Stillwell remarked that the nerves to the annulus fibrosus were confined to the surface of the disc, for he found none within the annulus itself.

In the same year, Pedersen et al.[5] described the lumbar sinuvertebral nerves, in what has become a classical paper in the literature on the lumbar spine. Although apparently unaware of the earlier work of Lazorthes et al.,[10] they confirmed exactly the descriptions of the French investigators (Figure 1B).

At this stage of history, attention briefly changed from the skeletal distribution of the sinuvertebral nerves to their distribution to the dura mater. Bridge[21] described the dural innervation in cats, dogs, and some human specimens, and the study of the dural innervation in humans was later completed by Kimmel[22] and Edgar and Nundy.[23]

The story of the intervertebral discs resumed in 1959 when Malinsky[24] published an exhaustive report on the ontogenetic development of nerve terminations in human lumbar intervertebral discs. He found that the inner part of the annulus fibrosus and the nucleus pulposus were devoid of nerves and nerve endings throughout their whole ontogenetic development. In contrast, he consistently found nerve fibers and nerve endings in the outer zone of the annulus fibrosus and on its surface.

Malinsky's[24] studies demonstrated that, in the prenatal period, nerves are abundant in the annulus fibrosus, where they form simple free endings; and they increase in number in older fetuses. During the postnatal period, various types of nonencapsulated receptors occur, and in adult material five types of nerve terminations can be found: simple and complex free nerve endings; "shrubby" receptors; others that form loops and mesh-like formations; and clusters of parallel free nerve endings. On the surface of the annulus fibrosus, various types of encapsulated and complex unencapsulated receptors occur. They are all relatively simple in structure in neonates, but more elaborate forms occur in older and mature specimens.

Within a given disc, Malinsky[24] reported that receptors are not uniformly distributed. The greatest number of endings occurs in the lateral region of the disc, and nearly all the encapsulated receptors are located in this region. Following postnatal development, there is a relative decrease in the number of receptors in the anterior region, such that in adults, the greatest number of endings occurs in the lateral regions of the disc, a smaller number in the posterior region, and the least number anteriorly.

Having established such a variety of nerve endings, Malinsky[24] speculated as to their function. The free nerve endings associated with blood vessels were ascribed a vasomotor or vasosensory function. Isolated free nerve endings were ascribed a nociceptive function, while the presence of encapsulated receptors implied a proprioceptive function.

Malinsky's[24] contributions were several. Not only did he provide the first definitive evidence of nerve endings deeper than just in the "superficial" layers of the disc, but he also identified a large variety of different types of endings, including complex and encapsulated endings. Moreover, in view of these findings, he was the first to speculate that the innervation of the lumbar discs played more than a nociceptive role. He introduced the concept of an active proprioceptive function for the disc, extending its function beyond its traditional role as a passive hydrodynamic cushion.

While not approaching the detail provided by Malinsky,[24] Hirsch et al.[25] and later Jackson et al.[26] confirmed the presence of free nerve endings in the annulus fibrosus of lumbar intervertebral discs, although they found them only in the most superficial laminae of the annulus. The latter authors also reported finding encapsulated receptors on the ventrolateral surface of the discs in neonates.[26]

In 1976, the first review of the innervation of the lumbar spine was published, based on the data then available. Edgar and Ghadially[27] acknowledged the failure of Jung and Brunschwig,[2] Wiberg,[17] and Ikari[19] to find evidence of nerve fibers in the lumbar intervertebral discs, but they highlighted the detection of nerve fibers in the outer laminae of the annulus fibrosus by Malinsky,[24] Hirsch et al.,[25] and Jackson et al.[26] Their review also encompassed the Japanese literature, including the studies of Tsukada,[3,4] and a lesser known study by Shinohara,[28] who apparently confirmed the presence of nerve fibers in the outer layers of the annulus fibrosus. He also reported that in degenerative discs, nerve fibers could be found accompanying granulation tissue into the deeper layers of the annulus and even into the nucleus pulposus.

Contrasting reviews have been written by Wyke,[29,30] who concluded that nerve terminals in the intervertebral discs "rapidly degenerate and disappear, so that in the mature human spine no nerve endings of any description remain in the nucleus pulposus or annulus fibrosus of the intervertebral discs in any region of the vertebral column." This conclusion was made in spite of the observations of Shinohara,[28] Hirsch et al.,[25] Jackson et al.,[26] and Malinsky.[24] Paradoxically, Malinsky[24] was even cited by Wyke[29,30] to support his negative conclusions.

Apart from misrepresenting the literature, Wyke[29,30] did not consider the possibility that those few studies that failed to demonstrate nerves in the lumbar discs might have been compromised by technical difficulties. Even under the best of conditions, metallic-ion stains for nerves in connective tissue are notoriously capricious. Negative results, therefore, can be false-negative, and as an investigative technique, metallic-ion stains are of value only when positive.

Nevertheless, reviews like those by Wyke[29,30] apparently have not been without influence, for others have stated that the lumbar intervertebral discs lack an innervation.[31,32] However, this conclusion was based more on opinion than on facts, and is unjustified, even given only the literature up until 1976. Fortunately, to dispel such negative conclusions absolutely, additional studies have recently further elaborated the innervation of the lumbar discs.

Prompted by Stillwell's observations in the monkey,[20] Taylor and Twomey[33] and then Bogduk et al.[34] investigated the nerve supply to the human lumbar intervertebral discs. The latter group confirmed that posteriorly, the discs were innervated by the sinuvertebral nerves (Figure 1B) and established that the anterior longitudinal ligament was supplied by recurrent branches of the grey rami communicantes. Their additional revelation was that laterally, the discs were innervated by branches of the grey rami communicantes, and posterolaterally, they receive branches from the grey rami communicantes and direct branches from the ventral rami (Figure 2). The latter finding confirmed the brief report by Taylor and Twomey,[33] and the overall pattern of innervation described by Bogduk et al.[34] is reminiscent of that described by Stillwell[20] in the monkey and has been endorsed by more recent studies.[35]

Although their study was directed principally to determining the sources of innervation of the lumbar discs, Bogduk et al.[34] did report finding nerve fibers within the outer third of the annulus fibrosus, but a contemporary histological study explored this phenomenon in more detail. Yoshizawa et al.[36] studied specimens of intervertebral discs removed at operation

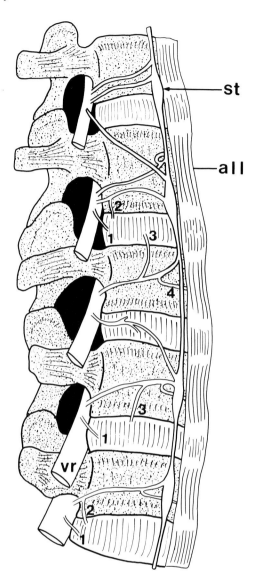

FIGURE 2.   Anterolateral view of the lumbar spine showing
the innervation of the lumbar intervertebral discs; all, anterior
longitudinal ligament; st, sympathetic trunk; vr, ventral ramus;
1, nerve to disc from ventral ramus; 2, nerve to posterolateral
disc from grey ramus communicans; 3, nerve to lateral disc
from grey ramus; and 4, nerve to anterior longitudinal ligament.

for anterior and posterior lumbar interbody fusion and found abundant nerve endings with
various morphologies throughout the outer half of the annulus fibrosus. The varieties of
nerve endings found included free terminals, often ending in club-like or bulbous expansions
or complex sprays, and less commonly, terminal forming convoluted tangles or glomerular
formations that were occasionally demarcated by a "capsule-like" condensation of adjacent
tissue. In contrast to the report of Shinohara,[28] these workers found no evidence of in-growth
of nerve fibers into areas of disc degeneration.

Most recently, Korkala et al.[37] used sophisticated, modern staining techniques to search
for nerves containing substance-P in the lumbar vertebral column. Such nerves were identified

in the longitudinal ligaments, but none were identified in the intervertebral discs. This result, however, does not deny the presence of nerves in the discs. It demonstrates only that either the nerves in the discs do not contain substance-P, or that nerve endings buried deep within the collagenous tissue of the disc are difficult to stain for substance-P.

What is pertinent to the present issue is that coupling the recent studies of Bogduk et al.[34] and Yoshizawa et al.[36] with the earlier literature, there can be no doubt that the outer half of the annulus fibrosus, and thereby the disc, is innervated. Like any ligamentous structure, the lumbar discs receive dissectable nerve branches, and microscopically they are endowed with a variety of nerve endings. The issue is no longer whether the discs are innervated, but rather, what is the function of their nerve supply.

To date, this question has barely been addressed, presumably because of the long-standing and weighty opinion that the disc lacked an innervation. Simply on the basis of morphology, Malinsky[24] postulated a proprioceptive role for the encapsulated receptors on the surface of the disc. Theoretically, this would be a valid, useful role for these receptors, but the only study that has addressed this contention failed to find any evidence in its favor.[38] However, this study was performed on cats which are not suitable models, since they are quadrupedal animals whose vertebral column is not used for weight-bearing. Therefore, it may not be endowed with receptors and reflexes that would be appropriate for an upright vertebral column. In this respect, even monkeys and apes may not be suitable models.

Monkeys are essentially arborial and brachiating, infrequently assuming an upright posture. The lumbar vertebral column of apes differs substantially from that of humans both anatomically and biomechanically.[39] Thus, it may be that further relevant data will only be obtainable from judicious study of humans.

The presumed vasomotor function of nerves to the lumbar discs has not been studied, but there is no doubt about the nociceptive function of other nerve terminals, presumably the isolated free nerve endings. This issue, being the most relevant clinically, however, is readdressed following the description of the cervical intervertebral discs.

III. THE CERVICAL INTERVERTEBRAL DISCS

Compared to the lumbar intervertebral discs, the cervical discs have been less studied. Such descriptions of the innervation of cervical discs as occur in the clinical literature[40,41] have been based on conjecture or extrapolations of data on the lumbar discs. Similarly, statements that deny an innervation of the cervical discs[29,30] are based on extrapolations of incomplete reviews of lumbar data and conspicuously overlook the available literature on the cervical discs.

In 1925 and again in 1927, Hovelacque[12,13] described the cervical sinuvertebral nerves as arising from the so-called vertebral nerve — the sympathetic plexus accompanying the vertebral artery; however, he offered no further description of their distribution within the vertebral canal. Although not describing them in his texts, Hovelacque[12,13] illustrated branches of the vertebral nerve entering the lateral aspects of the cervical discs.

Apart from these two descriptions, however, until recently, there had been no further studies of the cervical sinuvertebral nerves, and indeed, Cloward[41] proclaimed that these nerves were so small as to defy normal anatomical methods.

Again until recently, the only histological study of cervical discs had been an infrequently quoted report by Ferlic[42] who examined human fetal and adult discs obtained at operation. In the fetal material, he found "many nerve fibres...in the anterior and posterior longitudinal ligaments, and in the superficial or most peripheral layers of the annulus fibrosis (sic)."[42] In the adult material he identified nerve fibers in 2 of the 18 sections studied.

Prompted by this limited, though encouraging, literature and by the positive findings of nerves to and within lumbar intervertebral discs, Windsor et al.[43-45] undertook studies of the gross and histological innervation of the cervical discs.

With respect to the cervical sinuvertebral nerves, these investigators established that these nerves at the C3—8 levels resembled those in the lumbar region. (The C1 and C2 sinuvertebral nerves, differed in their anatomy for lack of intervertebral discs at these levels, and their distribution to the atlantoaxial joint complex and the dura mater of the posterior cranial fossa and upper cord has been described elsewhere.[22])

Each of the C3-8 sinuvertebral nerves arises from a somatic and an autonomic root. The somatic root stems from the ventral ramus at each segmental level, while the autonomic roots are derived from the vertebral nerve. At upper cervical levels, the autonomic roots arise from the terminal reaches of the vertebral nerve, while at lower levels they are definitive branches of that sympathetic plexus, which can be traced back, at midcervical levels, to grey rami communicantes from the sympathetic trunk and at lower cervical levels, to branches of the stellate ganglion. The somatic and autonomic roots of each sinuvertebral nerve join medial to the vertebral artery, in the intervertebral foramen.

Once formed, each sinuvertebral nerve runs obliquely upwards and medially through the intervertebral foramen, anterior to the spinal nerve, crossing the back of the intervertebral disc and then the back of the vertebral body above (Figure 3). The principal branch of the nerve then continues rostrally, circumventing the supradjacent pedicle, running parallel to the edge of the posterior longitudinal ligament. This branch finally ramifies in the posterior longitudinal ligament and the peridiscal connective tissue of the segment next above (Figure 3). En route, it furnishes minor branches to the periosteum of the pedicle and vertebral body, the epidural veins, and substantial branches directed dorsally to the dura mater. A major branch consistently arises just above the disc at the level of origin of each sinuvertebral nerve. This passes transversely to end in the posterior longitudinal ligament and supplies small, descending branches to the subadjacent disc (Figure 3).

The C3 sinuvertebral nerve differs somewhat from this typical pattern because of the absence of a disc at the C2 level. As at other levels, this nerve runs obliquely through the intervertebral foramen and forms a transverse branch to the posterior longitudinal ligaments and the intervertebral disc at its level of origin; however, rostrally it continues a prolonged course within the vertebral canal to join the C1 and C2 sinuvertebral nerves to supply the atlantoaxial joints and the craniocervical dura (Figure 3).

In addition to the sinuvertebral nerves, Windsor et al.[43-45] found other branches of the vertebral nerve supplying the cervical discs, in essence confirming the illustrations of Hovelacque.[12,13] These branches include fine filaments running with but distinct from the sinuvertebral nerves, that end in the posterolateral corner of the discs. Other branches include larger definitive nerves passing medially from the vertebral nerve to enter directly the lateral aspect of the adjacent disc (Figure 4).

Because of the intimate relationship between the prevertebral muscles and the front of the cervical discs, Windsor et al.[43-45] included in their study dissections of the prevertebral branches of the cervical ventral rami, which supply the prevertebral muscles, hoping to find branches from them to the discs. This exploration, however, failed to demonstrate any such branches, and the authors concluded that, if they existed, they were too small to be resolved by microdissection.

In their histological studies, Windsor et al.[43-45] were frustrated by technical problems in their attempts to stain nerve fibers in cadaveric discs. However, they did succeed in demonstrating neural tissue in two operative specimens of C5—6 discs. Using a cholinesterase stain, they revealed nerve fibers and nerve endings within the outer third of the annulus fibrosus. The endings included not only free nerve endings but also, what appeared to be, complex unencapsulated endings. The quality of staining achieved, however, precluded any more definitive study or classification of the morphology of these endings.

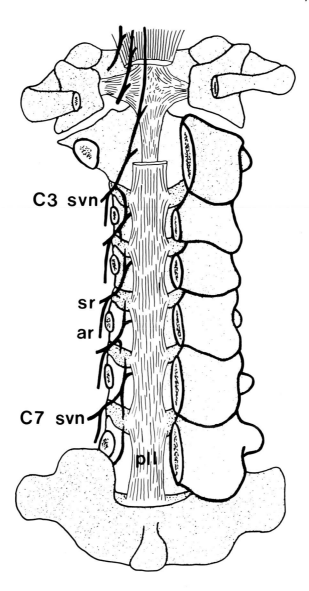

FIGURE 3.   The cervical sinuvertebral nerves in the floor of the
vertebral canal; svn, sinuvertebral nerves; sr, somatic root (from
ventral ramus); ar, autonomic root (from vertebral nerve); pll, posterior longitudinal ligament.

While derived from only a limited number of specimens, these histological observations
were nonetheless clearly positive and corroborated the report of Ferlic.[42] Taken together,
these two studies vindicate the notion that, like the lumbar discs, the cervical discs are
innervated. From the dissection studies of Windsor et al.,[43-45] it would appear that the source
of this innervation is from the cervical sinuvertebral nerves posteriorly and the vertebral
nerve laterally. The existence of any source anteriorly remains conjectural.

One description of cervical sinuvertebral nerves, not based on any formal anatomical
study, maintains that the lower cervical sinuvertebral nerves send long descending branches
to thoracic levels.[46] No such nerves were identified in the studies of Windsor et al.,[43-45] and
it was suggested that this spurious description was based on an extrapolation of the erroneous
description of descending branches of lumbar sinuvertebral nerves made by Spurling and
coauthors,[7-9] which has now been dispelled (see above).

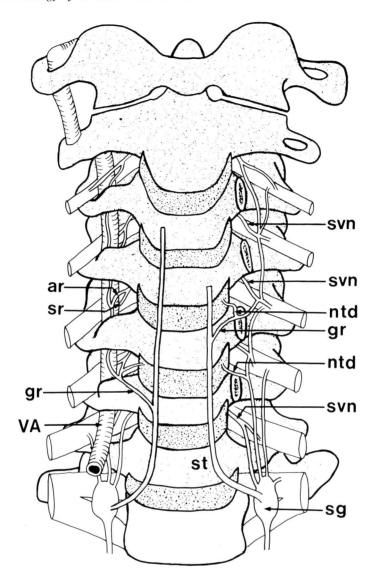

FIGURE 4.   An anterior view of the cervical spine showing the innervation of the
cervical intervertebral discs. The right vertebral artery (VA) is hown *in situ*, accompanied by elements of the vertebral nerve. The autonomic root (ar) of the C5 sinuvertebral nerve is shown arising from the vertebral nerve, while the somatic root (sr)
from the ventral ramus appears from behind the vertebral artery. A grey ramus
communicans (gr) is shown passing into the C5—6 intertransverse space, contributing
to the vertebral nerve, the C6 sinuvertebral nerve, and furnishing a branch to the
C5—6 intervertebral disc. On the left side of the specimen, the anterior roots of the
transverse processes have been resected to reveal the details of the vertebral nerve.
The C4, C5, and C7 sinuvertebral nerves are labeled (svn), as are the nerves to the
C4—5 and C5—6 discs (ntd), arising, respectively, from grey rami (gr) from the
sympathetic trunk (st) and the stellate ganglion (sg).

The fact that the vertebral nerve is predominantly derived from the sympathetic nervous
system[47-52] suggests that the branches from this nerve to the cervical discs would be autonomic
in nature. This may be so, in part, because such vessels as may occur in the discs would
require an efferent innervation, but it is pertinent to note that the vertebral nerve is not
exclusively sympathetic. It has substantial connections with the cervical ventral rami,[52] which

raises the possibility that the vertebral nerve also conveys somatic afferents. Indeed, this has been verified at upper cervical levels, where, in studies of human fetuses, Kimmel[53] traced afferent fibers from the vertebral artery, that ran through the vertebral nerve to the C2 spinal nerve and had cell bodies in the dorsal root ganglion. Thus, it is feasible that a similar phenomenon could occur at lower cervical levels with respect to afferents from the discs using the vertebral nerve to reach the somatic nervous system. Consequently, branches from the vertebral nerve to the cervical discs should not be viewed as exclusively autonomic in nature. Similar arguments have been advanced with respect to the branches to the lumbar discs from grey rami communicantes.[34]

Despite the relative paucity of data on the cervical discs, those studies that have been done are positive, demonstrating that macroscopically and histologically the cervical discs do have an innervation. Thus, the data on cervical discs are in accord with that on the lumbar discs.

IV. DISC PAIN

The presumed vasomotor function and speculative proprioceptive functions of the nerves to the lumbar discs have been discussed above, and one could entertain similar issues with respect to the cervical discs. However, the most pertinent function of the nerves to intervertebral discs, clinically, is their role in nociception. While this function has not been formally studied neurophysiologically in experimental animals, it is evident from clinical practice that discs can be painful, and, therefore, that this pain is mediated by the nerves that innervate the discs.

Clinical studies of lumbar and cervical discography have shown that distention of the annulus fibrosus by intranuclear injections of contrast medium or normal saline provokes pain, and when such injections are made into symptomatic discs, the pain of which a patient complains is reproduced.[54-60] These observations have been invoked as evidence that intervertebral discs can be a primary source of spinal pain, and that because it can occur in the absence of disc herniation, this pain must arise not from nerve root compression, but from the disc itself.

This notion has been challenged on the basis that because the discs lack an innervation, they could not possibly be a source of pain. Given the data covered in this review, however, this challenge cannot be sustained. The intervertebral discs are endowed with the anatomical substrate for nociception, and therefore, must be viewed as potential sources of pain.

Alternative explanations for the pain of discography either have not been offered or have been ambiguous or speculative — like simply "nerve root irritation" or leakage of contrast medium into the vertebral canal. Neither of these alternative mechanisms has been verified; moreover, neither mechanism explains the pain of discography when normal saline is used or when contrast medium is clearly retained wholly within the disc. It is, therefore, an inescapable conclusion that the pain of discography must arise from within the disc and is mediated by the nerves to the disc.

The resolution of the nerve supply to the cervical and lumbar intervertebral discs now permits an elaboration and defense of the rationale of provocation discography, and an explanation of some of its idiosyncrases. As a preface to this end, it should be appreciated that, morphologically and functionally, discs resemble ligaments. Both consist of oriented collagen fibers and both stabilize joints.

In the appendicular skeleton, there is no dispute that straining even a normal ligament to extremes can be painful. Moreover, it is well appreciated that an injured ligament will become painful when subjected to a stress normally tolerated by an uninjured ligament, and this phenomenon is used in various clinical tests to diagnose ligament "strain" clinically. The same principle is applicable to intervertebral discs.

When normal saline or contrast medium is injected into a normal, or an asymptomatic, intervertebral disc, it may or may not be painful. This depends on whether the rise in intranuclear pressure is high enough and whether it is transmitted to the peripheral, innervated portion of the disc at a magnitude sufficient to activate the nerve endings therein.

An injured or diseased disc, on the other hand, is more likely to be painful, or painful at lesser pressures of injection for various possible reasons. First, there may be an injury in the innervated portion of the disc. Under these circumstances stressing the annulus is analogous to stressing an injured ligament in the appendicular skeleton. In some way, presumably because of the presence of latent or subclinical inflammatory responses to injury, the injured site has a lowered threshold for pain when stressed.

Second, the innervated portion of the disc may not be directly involved in a lesion, but other parts of the annulus may be so damaged that the intact portions are required to bear more than their usual share of the normal load on the disc. The otherwise healthy and innervated portions of the disc are, therefore, subjected to greater than normal strains and consequently may become sources of pain. Similar arguments may be raised to account for disc pain in spondylosis, for with degradation of the discs, one or more may be subjected to a greater than normal load and become painful.

Third, if it is accepted that disc degradation, or degeneration, involves an inflammatory-cell-derived proteolytic process within the nucleus, it is conceivable that this process could extend into the annulus. By progressively eroding deeper layers of the annulus, or by extending more rapidly along fissures, this process could eventually reach innervated portions of the annulus. There, the degradation process would provide an abundant supply of enzymes and substances that putatively could excite the nerve endings within the annulus.

Through a combination of any or all of these, albeit theoretical, mechanisms, the production of disc pain can be understood. There is no need to invoke extradiscal explanations for causing the pain when plausible explanations confined to the disc are available, particularly when they are no different from the explanation of pain from ligaments in the appendicular skeleton, about which there is no controversy.

It has been clearly shown that the morphology of discs, as revealed by discography, does not correlate with whether or not they are painful.[61] Rather, the value of discography is the physiological response to the injection: whether or not the injection reproduces the patient's pain. This form of discography has been called provocation discography.[59]

Provocation discography, however, is not without its liabilities, and these, like its rationale, are fundamentally related to the way in which discs are innervated. The rationale of provocation discography is that if a disc is symptomatic, then stressing it should reproduce the patient's pain. However, the primary liability of this rationale stems from how effectively a disc may be stressed by intranuclear injections. If provocation does reproduce the right sort of pain, there is no issue, other than confirming that the patient is not mistaking this pain from the pain of injecting any (normal) disc. This can be done by testing adjacent levels on a single-blind basis and retesting the putatively symptomatic disc.

On the other hand, failure to reproduce pain does not necessarily exclude discs as the source of symptoms, for along the lines outlined above, the test injection may fail to adequately stress an otherwise symptomatic disc. The rise in nuclear pressure may be insufficient to strain the outer laminae of the annulus and therefore fail to activate the nerves to the disc. In this way, provocation discography is liable to false-negative results. However, this does not detract from its value as a diagnostic test when results are clearly positive.

To reinforce their diagnosis, some practitioners add a subsequent injection of local anesthetic — so-called analgesic discography.[62] This test, however, while valuable when positive, is very liable to be falsely negative, and it should be appreciated that the mechanism of analgesic discography differs physically from that of provocation discography.

Provocation discography depends simply on the transmission of induced stress from the nucleus to the innervation portions of the annulus, i.e., the propagation of a force. Analgesic discography, in contrast, depends on the actual material dispersion of local anesthetic from the nucleus to the innervated portions of the annulus. In a disc whose inner annulus is substantially intact, these inner laminae would form a physical barrier to the dispersion of local anesthetic, preventing it from reaching the nerves of the disc, or at least substantially slowing its diffusion. Under such circumstances, the inner annulus might not prevent the transmission of the stress in provocation discography, allowing pain to be provoked, but an injection of local anesthetic might not relieve the pain. Such a paradoxical result should not be viewed as a contradiction, but merely a function of the structure of the disc, the distribution of nerves within it, and the physical differences between inducing a strain and infiltrating a local anesthetic.

On the other hand, advocates of analgesic discography report prompt relief of pain upon injecting local anesthetic, at least in some of their patients. This rapidity cannot be accounted for in terms of rapid diffusion through the dense layers of the inner annulus and implies some difference in anatomy. It is suggested that in such cases, the local anesthetic probably reaches the innervated and symptomatic portions of the annulus along radial fissures or other defects in the inner annulus. Lacking a physical barrier, the anesthetic rapidly disperses to its site of action.

It is acknowledged that these explanations of the idiosyncrasies of provocation and analgesic discography are only theoretical, but they are advanced as logical explanations, based on the known anatomy of discs and their innervation, and are designed to rationalize a field that has so long remained controversial. Fortunately, perhaps with the greater use of computerized axial tomography or axial magnetic resonance imaging during discography, these theories can be evaluated and either vindicated or replaced with clearer explanations of the mechanisms of discogenic pain. However, notwithstanding arguments about the mechanisms and interpretation of discography, the anatomical data are beyond controversy. Regardless of any lingering misconceptions, the evidence clearly demonstrates that the intervertebral discs do have a nerve supply.

REFERENCES

1. **Mixter, W. J. and Barr, J. S.,** Rupture of the intervertebral disc with involvement of the spinal canal, *New Engl. J. Med.,* 211, 210, 1934.
2. **Jung, A. and Brunschwig, A.,** Recherches histologiques des articulations des corps vertebraux, *Presse Med.,* 40, 316, 1932.
3. **Tsukada, K.,** Histologische Studien über die Zwischenwirbelscheibe des Menschen. I. Histologische Befunde des Foetus, *Mitt. Akad. Kioto,* 24, 1057 and 1172, 1938.
4. **Tsukada, K.,** Histologische Studien uber die Zwischenwirbelscheibe des Menschen. II. Altersveranderungen, *Mitt. Akad. Kioto,* 25, 1 and 207, 1939.
5. **Pedersen, H. E., Blunck, C. F. J., and Gardner, E.,** The anatomy of the lumbosacral posterior rami and meningeal branches of spinal nerves (sinu-vertebral nerves), *J. Bone Jt. Surg.,* 38A, 377, 1956.
6. **Roofe, P. G.,** Innervation of annulus fibrosus and posterior longitudinal ligament, *Arch. Neurol. Psychiatry,* 44, 100, 1940.
7. **Spurling, R. G. and Bradford, F. K.,** Neurologic aspects of herniated nucleus pulposus, *JAMA,* 113, 2019, 1939.
8. **Spurling, R. G. and Grantham, E. G.,** Neurologic picture of herniation of the nucleus pulposus in the lower part of the lumbar region, *Arch. Surg.,* 40, 378, 1940.
9. **Bradford, K. and Spurling, R. G.,** *The Intervertebral Disc,* 2nd ed., Charles C Thomas, Springfield, Ill., 1945.
10. **Lazorthes, G., Poulhes, J., and Espagno, J.,** Etude sur les nerfs sinu-vertebraux lombaires. Le nerf de Roofe, existe-t-il?, *C. R. Assoc. Anat.,* 34, 317, 1947.
11. **Luschka, H.,** *Die Nerven des menschlichen Wirbelkanales,* Laupp, Tubingen, The Netherlands, 1850.

12. **Hovelacque, A.,** Le nerf sinuvertebral, *Ann. Anat. Pathol. Anat. Norm., Med.-Chir.,* 2, 435, 1925.

13. **Hovelacque, A.,** *Anatomie des Nerfs Craniens et Rachidiens et du Systeme Grande Sympathique,* Doin, Paris, 1927.

14. **Soulie, A.,** Nerfs rachidiens, in *Traite d'Anatomie Humaine,* Vol. 3, 2nd ed., Poirier, P. and Charpy, A., Eds., Masson, Paris, 1905.

15. **Herlihy, W. F.,** The sinu-vertebral nerve, *N. Z. Med. J.,* 48, 214, 1949.

16. **Buskirk, C.,** Nerves in the vertebral canal, *Arch. Surg.,* 43, 427, 1941.

17. **Wiberg, G.,** Back pain in relation to the nerve supply of intervertebral discs, *Acta Orthop. Scand.,* 19, 211, 1949.

18. **Ehrenhaft, J. L.,** Development of the vertebral column as related to certain congenital and pathological changes, *Surg. Gynecol. Obstet.,* 76, 282, 1943.

19. **Ikari, C.,** A study on the mechanism of low back pain. The neurohistological examination of the disease, *J. Bone Jt. Surg.,* 36A, 195, 1954.

20. **Stillwell, D. L.,** The nerve supply of the vertebral column and its associated structures in the monkey, *Anat. Rec.,* 125, 139, 1956.

21. **Bridge, C. J.,** Innervation of spinal meninges and epidural structures, *Anat. Rec.,* 133, 553, 1959.

22. **Kimmel, D. L.,** Innervation of spinal dura mater and dura mater of the posterior cranial fossa, *Neurology,* 10, 800, 1961.

23. **Edgar, M. A. and Nundy, S.,** Innervation of the spinal dura mater, *J. Neurol. Neurosurg. Psychiatry,* 29, 530, 1966.

24. **Malinsky, J.,** The ontogenetic development of nerve terminations in the intervertebral discs of man, *Acta Anat.,* 38, 96, 1959.

25. **Hirsch, C., Ingelmark, B. E., and Miller, M.,** The anatomical basis for low back pain, *Acta Orthop. Scand.,* 33, 1, 1963.

26. **Jackson, H. C., Winkelmann, R. K., and Bickel, W. M.,** Nerve endings in the human lumbar spinal column and related structures, *J. Bone Jt. Surg.,* 48A, 1272, 1966.

27. **Edgar, M. A. and Ghadially, J. A.,** Innervation of the lumbar spine, *Clin. Orthop.,* 115, 35, 1976.

28. **Shinohara, H.,** A study on lumbar disc lesions, *J. Jpn. Orthop. Assoc.,* 44, 553, 1970.

29. **Wyke, B.,** Neurological aspects of low back pain, in *The Lumbar Spine and Back Pain,* Jayson, M. I. V., Ed., Grune & Stratton, New York, 1976, 189.

30. **Wyke, B.,** The neurology of low back pain, in *The Lumbar Spine and Back Pain,* 2nd ed., Jayson, M. I. V., Ed., Pitman, Tunbridge Wells, England, 1980, chap. 11.

31. **Lamb, D. W.,** The neurology of spinal pain, *Phys. Ther.,* 59, 971, 1979.

32. **Anderson, J.,** Pathogenesis of back pain, in *Low Back Pain,* Vol. 2, Grahame, R. and Anderson, J. A. D., Eds., Eden Press, Westmount, Quebec, 1980, chap. 4.

33. **Taylor, J. R. and Twomey, L. T.,** Innervation of lumbar intervertebral discs, *Med. J. Aust.,* 2, 701, 1979.

34. **Bogduk, N., Tynan, W., and Wilson, A. S.,** The nerve supply to the human lumbar intervertebral discs, *J. Anat.,* 132, 39, 1981.

35. **Paris, S. V.,** Anatomy as related to function and pain, *Orthop. Clin. N. Am.,* 14, 475, 1983.

36. **Yoshizawa, H., O'Brien, J. P., Thomas-Smith, W., and Trumper, M.,** The neuropathology of intervertebral discs removed for low-back pain, *J. Pathol.,* 132, 95, 1980.

37. **Korkala, O., Gronblad, M., Liesi, P., and Karaharju, E.,** Immunohistochemical demonstration of nociceptors in the ligamentous structures of the lumbar spine, *Spine,* 10, 156, 1985.

38. **Kumar, S. and Davis, P. R.,** Lumbar vertebral innervation and intra-abdominal pressure, *J. Anat.,* 114, 47, 1973.

39. **Farfan, H. F.,** The biomechanical advantage of lordosis and hip extension for uopright activity. Man as compared with other anthropoids, *Spine,* 3, 336, 1978.

40. **Cloward, R. B.,** Cervical diskography. A contribution to the aetiology and mechanism of neck, shoulder and arm pain, *Ann. Surg.,* 130, 1052, 1959.

41. **Cloward, R. B.,** The clinical significance of the sinu-vertebral nerve of the cervical spine in relation to the cervical disk syndrome, *J. Neurol. Neurosurg. Psychiatry,* 23, 321, 1960.

42. **Ferlic, D. C.,** The nerve supply of the cervical intervertebral discs in man, *Bull. Johns Hopkins Hosp.,* 113, 347, 1963.

43. **Windsor, M., Inglis, A., and Bogduk, N.,** The innervation of the cervical intervertebral discs, in Proceedings of the Anatomical Society of Australia and New Zealand, *J. Anat.,* 142, 218, 1985.

44. **Bogduk, N., Windsor, M., and Inglis, A.,** The innervation of the human cervical intervertebral discs, presented at the XIIth Int. Anat. Congr., London, August 17 to 22, 1985.

45. **Bogduk, N., Windsor, M., and Inglis, A.,** The innervation of the cervical intervertebral discs, *Spine,* in press.

46. **Wyke, B.,** The neurological basis of thoracic spinal pain, *Rheumatol. Phys. Med.,* 10, 356, 1970.

47. **Guerrier, Y.,** Les nerfs vertebraux, *Acta Anat.,* 8, 62, 1949.
48. **Laux, G. and Guerrier, Y.,** Innervation de l'artere vertebral, *Ann. Anat. Pathol. Anat. Norm. Med-Chir.,* 16, 897, 1939.
49. **Laux, G. and Guerrier, Y.,** Innervation de l'artere vertebrale, *C. R. Assoc. Anat.,* 298, 1947.
50. **Lazorthes, G. and Cassan, J.,** Essai de schematisation des ganglions etoile et intermediare, *C. R. Assoc. Anat.,* 193, 1939.
51. **Monteiro, H. and Rodrigues, A.,** Sur les variations du nerf vertebral, *C. R. Assoc. Anat.,* 406, 1931.
52. **Bogduk, N., Lambert, G. A., and Duckworth, J. W.,** The anatomy and physiology of the vertebral nerve in relation to migraine, *Cephalalgia,* 1, 11, 1981.
53. **Kimmel, D. L.,** The cervical sympathetic rami and the vertebral nerve plexus in the human foetus, *J. Comp. Neurol.,* 112, 141, 1959.
54. **Hirsch, C.,** An attempt to diagnose the level of a disc lesion clinically by disc puncture, *Acta Orthop. Scand.,* 18, 132, 1949.
55. **Lindblom, K.,** Technique and results in myelography and disc puncture, *Acta Radiol.,* 34, 321, 1950.
56. **Collis, J. S. and Gardner, W. J.,** Lumbar discography — an analysis of 1,000 cases, *J. Neurosurg.,* 19, 452, 1962.
57. **Wiley, J. J., MacNab, I., and Wortzman, G.,** Lumbar discography and its clinical applications, *Can. J. Surg.,* 11, 280, 1968.
58. **Simmons, E. H. and Segil, C. M.,** An evaluation of discography in the localisation of symptomatic levels in discogenic disease of the spine, *Clin. Orthop.,* 108, 57, 1975.
59. **Park, W.,** The place of radiology in the investigation of low back pain, *Clin. Rheumatic Dis.,* 6, 93, 1980.
60. **Kikuchi, S., MacNab, I., and Moreau, P.,** Localisation of the level of symptomatic cervical disc degeneration, *J. Bone Jt. Surg.,* 63B, 272, 1981.
61. **Holt, E. P.,** The fallacy of cervical discography, *JAMA,* 188, 799, 1964.
62. **Roth, D. A.,** Cervical analgesic discography. A new test for the definitive diagnosis of the painful-disk syndrome, *JAMA,* 235, 1713, 1976.

Chapter 6

PROTEOGLYCANS OF THE INTERVERTEBRAL DISC

Cahir A. McDevitt

TABLE OF CONTENTS

I. INTRODUCTION

Proteoglycans and collagens constitute the two major classes of macromolecules in the nucleus pulposus, annulus fibrosus, and hyaline lamina (end-plate) of the intervertebral disc (See earlier reviews in References 1 through 8). The proteoglycans play a critical role in the load-carriage function of the disc. They are mainly responsible for the high water content of the gel-like nucleus[9] and changes in their quantity or quality, such as occurs in acquired disc generation[10,11] or induced chemonucleolysis,[12,13] will compromise the shock absorption function of the tissue.

The intervertebral disc is a particularly attractive structure for investigations of the structure/function relationships of proteoglycans in developmental, aging, and pathological processes. The nucleus pulposus has a low concentration of cells,[14] probably the lowest of any connective tissue, yet the morphological integrity of the tissue is maintained up to about the end of the 3rd decade in life.[15] It would appear, therefore, that the cell-matrix communication mechanisms for maintenance and repair of the extracellular matrix are particularly effective in the nucleus pulposus. The proteoglycan gel of the nucleus must play a key role in these communication mechanisms. The nucleus pulposus also represents an interesting structure for investigations of extracellular processing of proteoglycans: unusual in-vivo degradation products survive in the disc in a manner quite different from those in articular cartilage (discussed in this chapter). The topographical complexity of the disc, with varying radial distributions in the proportions of types I and II collagen (see Chapter 7) and in the quantities and quality of proteoglycan, poses important questions with respect to the relationship between the molecular anatomy and biomechanical properties of the disc.

The developmental changes that the disc undergoes in early childhood, the most dramatic of any connective tissue, involve the replacement of notochordal cells with chondrocyte-like cells.[2] The genetic and biochemical events regulating that process have yet to be established, despite interesting preliminary biochemical studies. Finally, and perhaps most challenging of all, the molecular changes in proteoglycans in the programmed senescence of the disc and in pathological processes in aging, such as disc degeneration, have yet to be elucidated.

Research in proteoglycans has developed in the last 5 years to an extent that the structural/ functional relationship of these intriguing molecules are now being actively explored in intracellular organelles[16] and cell surfaces[17] of various cells, as well as tissues as diverse as muscle, bone, nerve, and ligaments.[18] The proteoglycans of hyaline cartilage have, perhaps, received more attention than those of any other tissue and, as they bear some structural homologies with those of the disc, they serve as a useful prototype for the latter. In this chapter the properties of hyaline cartilage proteoglycans will be summarized: the proteoglycans of the disc will then be discussed in detail.

II. PROTEOGLYCANS: DEFINITION, CLASSIFICATION, AND NOMENCLATURE

Proteoglycans are now considered a subclass of glycoconjugate. A glycoconjugate is a peptide/protein (glycoprotein) or lipid (glycolipid) to which carbohydrate is covalently attached. The proteoglycans are therefore a subclass of glycoprotein distinguished by the presence of one or more glycosaminoglycan chains (see below). Glycoproteins were formerly classified by the nature of the carbohydrate-amino acid linkage they contained. This classification is now considered overly simplistic, as any one glycoprotein may contain several types of carbohydrate linkage. Indeed, three major types of glycoprotein linkages are found in cartilage proteoglycans.

The major types of linkages found in mammalian glycoproteins are:

Table 1
COMPOSITION OF PREDOMINANT DISACCHARIDE
IN EACH GLYCOSAMINOGLYCAN FAMILY

Modern name	Amino sugar	Uronic acid	Sulfate
Hyaluronate	Glucosamine	Glucuronic acid	
Chondroitin 4-sulfate	Galactosamine	Glucuronic acid	O-sulfate
Chondroitin 6-sulfate	Galactosamine	Glucuronic acid	O-sulfate
Dermatan sulfate	Galactosamine	Iduronic acid	O-sulfate
		Glucuronic acid	
Keratan sulfate	Glucosamine	(Galactose)	O-sulfate
Heparan sulfate	Glucosamine	Iduronic acid	N-sulfate
		Glucuronic acid	O-sulfate
Heparin	Glucosamine	Iduronic acid	N-sulfate
		Glucuronic acid	O-sulfate

1. Asn-GlcNAc (*N*-acetylgluctosamylasparagine): this link (referred to as an N-link as it involves the amide nitrogen of asparagine) is most commonly found in globular glycoproteins, including the hyaluronate binding site of cartilage proteoglycans. Oligosaccharides bearing this linkage usually have the same starting sugar sequence (Asn-GlcNAc-GlcNAc-Man), with subsequent branching into "antennae" after the first mannose. The first oligosaccharide sugar sequence is attached via a dolichol lipid intermediate in its biosynthesis, a process that is inhibited by the drug tunicamycin.[19]
2. Ser (Thr)-GalNAc (*N*-acetylgalactosamylserine): this type of link "(O-link)" is characteristic of mucins secreted by epithelial cells. It is also found in globular glycoproteins such as thyroglobin and on the protein core of cartilage proteoglycans in the attachment of keratan sulfate and O-linked oligosaccharides.
3. Ser(Thr)-Xyl-Gal-Gal (xylosylserine): this is the linkage that attaches and chondroitin sulfates to their core proteins.
4. Hyl-Gal and Hyl-Gal-Glc (galactosylhydroxylysine): this appears to be restricted to the triple helical domains of collagens.

A. Definition

Proteoglycans are now defined as a protein or peptide (the "core protein") to which one or more glycosaminoglycan chains are covalently attached. Note that this definition includes not only the proteoglycans with many glycosaminoglycan chains that, as a consequence, have a high buoyant density, but also those with one or few chains that would band in the low density portions of a density gradient.

Glycosaminoglycans are heteropolysaccharides composed of repeating disaccharide groups in which an N-acetylated hexosamine is linked by a glycosidic bond to a nitrogen-free monosaccharide, usually a uronic acid. The hexosamine bears a sulfate group, the sole exception to this rule being hyaluronate, where the *N*-acetylglucosamine does not have an acidic group. The distinctive feature of glycosaminoglycan chains, therefore, is their high fixed charged density, with each disaccharide usually bearing a sulfate and a carboxyl group.

The glycosaminoglycans may be classified by composition into subfamilies (Table 1): hyaluronate; chondroitin 4- and 6- sulfate; dermatan sulfate; keratan sulfate, heparin, and heparan sulfate. The chondroitin sulfates, keratan sulfate, and hyaluronate are the major glycosaminoglycans of the intervertebral disc.

The term proteoglycan replaces the former terms of mucoprotein, mucopolysaccharide, mucopolysaccharide-protein complex, and protein polysaccharide. Kennedy[20] has reviewed the historical development of the nomenclature for glycosaminoglycans and proteoglycans and has discussed the rationale for the modern terminology. Comprehensive reviews on the distribution of glycosaminoglycans in different species[22] as well as their interactions with other molecules[22,23] have been published.

B. Classification

1. General

Proteoglycans from different tissues and cells show enormous diversity with respect to size and composition.[21] The large amount of carbohydrate in most types of proteoglycans has frustrated attempts to sequence their core proteins by classical Edman procedures, although the progressive integration of cDNA technology into proteoglycan structural studies should fill this void in the foreseeable future. The absence of such sequence data means that the assignment of proteoglycans to gene families is not yet feasible. Nevertheless, a classification is possible based on the known properties of the molecules and their location in tissues or cells.

Hassell et al. have proposed the following classification[18] (their review and that of Poole[21] should be referred to for detailed discussions):

1. Major proteoglycans in cartilage (i.e., those aggregable with hyaluronate).
2. Small proteoglycans in collagenous connective tissues (bone, skin, cornea, etc.)
3. Cell surface proteoglycans
4. Basement membrane proteoglycans
5. Intracellular vesicle proteoglycans
6. Type IX collagens

2. Classification of Proteoglycans of Hyaline and Fibrous Cartilage and the Intervertebral Disc

There is now sufficient information on the proteoglycans of cartilage and the intervertebral disc to permit a preliminary subclassification.

1. **Large proteoglycans that aggregate with hyaluronate** — These proteoglycans are most abundant in young hyaline cartilage (such as bovine nasal septum)[18,24-27] and the immature intervertebral disc.[28] The distinctive properties of these proteoglycans are their high buoyant density, large hydrodynamic size (Kdaltons on Sepharose® 2B is about 0.2; length is about 350 nm), their high content of chondroitin sulfate, and their capacity to aggregate specifically with hyaluronate (HA) via a disulfide-stabilized globular protein portion of the core protein. The core protein of bovine nasal septum proteoglycans bears about 100 chondroitin sulfate chains, each with an average molecular weight of about 20,000, and 30 to 60 keratan chains, each with molecular weight of 4000 to 8000.[26] Proteoglycans can attach themselves along chains of hyaluronate by means of a noncovalent interaction between the hyaluronate-binding site and a small portion of the HA chain[25,29] to form proteoglycan aggregates (Figure 1).[25-27] The capacity to aggregate proteoglycans is a specific property of hyaluronate, as other polyelectrolytes such as chondroitin sulfate, dextran sulfate, DNA, sodium alginate or desulfated chondroitin sulfate are ineffective.[29,30] Fragments containing the HA-binding site have been isolated from mild proteinase digests of the aggregated proteoglycans and have a molecular weight of about 65,000.[31] Rotary shadowing suggests the presence of another globular domain between the binding site and the glycosaminoglycan attachment region of the molecule.[32] The average molecular weight of the composite proteoglycan molecule in nasal cartilage is about 2.5×10^6.[33,34] The structurally distinct domains of the proteoglycan molecule are discussed later.

    The proteoglycan binding sites are protected from enzymatic attack and the aggre-

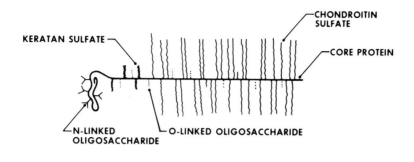

A

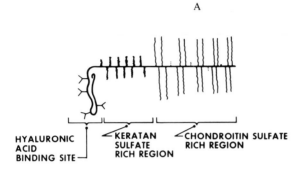

B

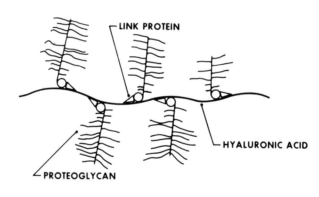

C

FIGURE 1. Models of structures for proteoglycans and proteoglycan aggregate. (A) Proteoglycan molecule of fetal or young hyaline cartilage. (B) Proteoglycan molecule of hyaline cartilage of skeletally mature tissues. This molecule is smaller than that in A and has a dintinctive keratan sulfate-rich region. (C) Proteoglycan aggregate. Individual proteoglycans associative nonconvalently with chains of hyaluronate acid through their hyaluronate acid binding sites (here depicted as a circle). The link proteins (triangles) stabilize the interaction.

gates stabilized by link proteins (mol wt: 41 to 45 Kdaltons) that bind to both the binding site and the hyaluronate chains.[35,36,37,38,39]

A more thorough description of the critical experiments in the development of the current model of the proteoglycan aggregate may be found in the reviews of Hascall,[26] Hascall and Heingard,[27] Muir,[40] and Muir and Hardingham.[25]

2. **Moderate size and small proteoglycans that aggregate with hyaluronate** — These proteoglycans predominate in older articular[41,42,43,44] and meniscal[45,46] cartilage. They are different from Group 1 in having a smaller hydrodynamic size, an enriched keratan-

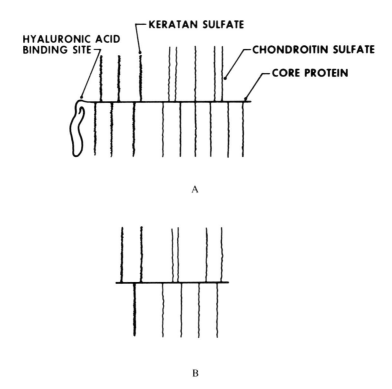

FIGURE 2.   Models for structures of aggregable (A) and nonaggregable (B) proteoglycans of the mature nucleus pulposus.

sulfate content and a smaller chondroitin sulfate-rich region.[41,45,47] It should be emphasized that these proteoglycans may be proteolytically derived from the larger molecules. Alternatively, they may represent a distinct subclass of proteoglycan with a unique protein core.

3.   **Large and moderately sized proteoglycans that do not aggregate with hyaluronate (Figure 2)** — These molecules are present in cartilage to a small extent[49] and are the major proteoglycans in the mature nucleus pulposus (discussed later).

4.   **Small proteoglycans that do not aggregate with hyaluronate** — These proteoglycans are a minor species in young hyaline cartilage. They may be subclassified into the chondroitin sulfate[48] and dermatan sulfate[50] proteoglycans, respectively.

5.   **Type IX collagen** — The identification of at least one glycosaminoglycan chain in Type IX collagen allows this interesting molecule to be defined as a proteoglycan. It constitutes a minor proportion of the total collagen in hyaline cartilage[51] and the intervertebral disc (see chapter 7).

C. Structural Domains of Cartilage Proteoglycans

The large proteoglycans of young hyaline cartilage (Group 1) are composed of structurally distinct domains: (1) the hyaluronate binding site that is predominantly protein in composition but bears significant amounts of N-linked nonsulfated oligosaccharides;[52] (2) the keratan sulfate-rich region of the protein core which contains about 60% of the keratan sulfate of the nasal septum proteoglycan but only 10% of the chondroitin sulfate;[53] (3) the chondroitin sulfate-rich region that contains about 90% of the chondroitin sulfate chains and about 20% of the keratan sulfate (Figure 1).[53] The relative locations of the core protein of the keratan sulfate and chondroitin sulfate-rich regions were determined by degradative experiments of bovine nasal and tracheal cartilage proteoglycans.[53] Monomeric proteoglycans were digested with chondroitinase (which removes all but short stubs of the chondroitin sulfate chains) followed by trypsin and chymotrypsin (that digest the binding site and the core protein of the chondroitin sulfate-rich region) and the digestion products chromatographed on a Sepharose® CL-6B column. A fraction composed mainly of protein and keratan sulfate separated from another fraction composed mainly of protein and chondroitin sulfate degradation products.[53] This experiment demonstrated that the chondroitin sulfate and keratan sulfate of proteoglycans were each concentrated on different regions of the protein core. Hydroxylamine digestion of proteoglycan aggregates liberated a large peptide enriched in chondroitin sulfate from a protein and a keratan sulfate-enriched fragment attached to hyaluronate. The large keratan sulfate complex eluted in the void volume of a Sepharose® 2B column, while the chondroitin sulfate-enriched region was retarded on the column. The keratan sulfate-enriched region was isolated from the large complex after the chondroitinase-trypsin-chymotrypsin procedure described above. Thus, the hydroxylamine cleaved the protein core, possibly at an asparagine-glycine bond,[54] between the keratan sulfate- and chondroitin sulfate-rich regions. The experiment demonstrated that the keratan sulfate-enriched region was located next to the hyaluronate-binding site.[53]

The chondroitin sulfate chains are grouped in clusters along the chondroitin sulfate-enriched region of the proteoglycan.[55,56] Separation and characterization of proteolytic digests of nasal septum of tracheal cartilage proteoglycans demonstrated that 100 chondroitin sulfate chains in the molecule are grouped in about 25 clusters, containing 1 to 8 chains per cluster.[56,57] O-Linked, nonsulfated oligosaccharides are located on the glycosaminoglycan attachment region of the molecule.[58]

It should be emphasized that the domain structure outlined above is purely a hypothetical model. More recent work suggests that a second globular domain exists between the binding site and the keratan sulfate-rich region,[32] and a third globular domain may reside at the distal end of the chondroitin sulfate-rich region, at least in unprocessed molecules.[130]

D. Nomenclature for Identification of Isolated Proteoglycans (A1, D1, and A1-D1 Fractions)

Heinegard[59] introduced a nomenclature based exclusively on operational conditions that has been widely used to identify proteoglycan fractions isolated by density gradient procedures. The term A1 (A for associative; 1 for the first, most dense fraction) is used to identify the most dense fraction of a density gradient generated in an associative solvent such as 0.5 M guanidinium chloride. Fractions of progressively lower density in the gradient are referred to as A2, A3, etc., depending on the number of fractions cut. The bottom fraction of a density gradient generated under dissociative conditions (e.g., in 4 M guanidinium chloride) is referred to as the D1 fraction. If a two-step gradient procedure is used, employing first associative with subsequent dissociative centrifugation of the A1 fraction, the most dense fraction of the dissociative gradient is identified as A1-D1.

E. Electron Microscopy

Rosenberg and colleagues[60] imaginatively applied the Kleinschmidt technique of coating polyanions with cytochrome c for visualization of proteoglycans in monomolecular layers. Cytochrome c binds to all glycosaminoglycans.[61] The technique enables evaluation of individual proteoglycan molecules and proteoglycan aggregates. Cartilage proteoglycans are visualized in this technique as bottle-brush structures,[60,62] while in the aggregate, the proteoglycans project laterally at fairly regular intervals from both sides of an "elongated filamentous structure," the dimensions of which are consistent with it being hyaluronate.[62]

This technique, therefore, permits statistical distributions to be determined on the length of the monomeric proteoglycans, the length of the hyaluronate, and the density of distribution of proteoglycans in the individual aggregates. Large proteoglycans have a length of 100 to

400 nm by this technique, with mean values of 249 nm[63] and 343 nm[64] recorded in separate studies. The large, high density proteoglycans that have about 100 chondroitin sulfate chains display about 25 side extensions about 11 nm apart and 45 nm in length[65] in the electron microscope. Each extension, therefore, apparently represents 4 chondroitin sulfate chains condensed together, perhaps in the clusters that can be isolated from trypsin digests of the molecule.[56]

Marked polydispersity is evident in the length of the hyaluronate chains in cartilage proteoglycan aggregates[62] with mean lengths of 1037 nm[63] and 1998 nm[64] for chains in aggregates reconstituted from bovine nasal septum.

F. Heterogeneity

Proteoglycans are normally too large to penetrate conventional polyacrylamide gels. They will, however, penetrate gels composed of a low percentage of acrylamide and agarose, the function of the agarose in the composite gel being mechanical support.[66] Chondroitin sulfate or other glycosaminoglycan chains that show marked polydispersity in size by gel chromatography migrate in these gels as relatively sharp bands.[66] Articular cartilage proteoglycans showed an even more surprising result when similarly analyzed and migrated as two relatively sharp bands that were clearly distinguishable in densitometric scans.[66] This unanticipated finding has been reproduced in many laboratories with cartilage proteoglycans derived from a wide variety of anatomical sites and species.[67-72]

The mobilities of proteoglycans on polyacrylamide-agarose gels is a function of charge, size, and possibly some interaction with the gel matrix.[66] The proteoglycans therefore contain a structural difference to which the gel electrophoretic system is sensitive. It is notable that no other separation system is known that can similarly resolve proteoglycans.

Heinegard et al.[72] employed rate-zonal centrifugation to separate two bovine nasal septum cartilage proteoglycan populations to electrophoretic homogeneity. The larger proteoglycan (weight average M_R: 3.5 × 10^6) had a slower electrophoretic mobility and apparently lacked a well-defined keratan sulfate-rich region, but had a chondroitin sulfate-rich region. This proteoglycan appeared similar to that found in immature cartilage or in osteoarthritic cartilage[47] of mature tissues. The smaller proteoglycan isolated by Heinegard et al.[72] (weight average M_R: 1.3 × 10^6) had both keratan sulfate and chondroitin sulfate-rich regions and was of faster mobility than the larger species. The two proteoglycans were labeled with radioactive iodine, digested with trypsin, and the resulting populations of peptide were mapped by thin-layer chromatography.[72] Most peptides were common to both proteoglycans, but a few were unique to one population, suggesting that the two molecules contained small regions that were not identical and large regions that were identical. Sequencing studies should resolve the issue as to whether the populations are products of different genes.

The structural models for the proteoglycan molecule depicted in Figure 1 are clearly simplistic as models for all the aggregating proteoglycans in cartilage, particularly tissue of skeletally mature animals. The structurally different proteoglycan molecules may arise from the biosynthesis of core proteins that differ in specific subregions in their respective amino acid sequences. Alternatively, identical core proteins may undergo different posttranslational glycosylation. Catabolic events in the extracellular matrix may also be responsible, solely or in part, for the different proteoglycan subpopulations. The phenomenon of heterogeneity in proteoglycans is discussed again later in relation to the intervertebral disc.

III. PROTEOGLYCANS OF THE INTERVERTEBRAL DISC

A. The Glycosaminoglycans of Disc: Identity and Distribution

Histology of cat,[73,74] dog, horse, ox, sheep, and pig[75,76] intervertebral disc revealed an abundant sulfated glycosaminoglycan in the extracellular matrix of the nucleus pulposus, with a tendency towards heavier staining in the center of the tissue. The staining in the annulus fibrosus was most intense between the collagenous lamellae, except near the nucleus pulposus where the lamellae themselves also stained.[74] More specific staining procedures with human discs suggested that chondroitin sulfate, keratan sulfate, and hyaluronate[77,78] were the major glycosaminoglycans.

Beard et al.[79] employed polyclonal antibodies against pig proteoglycan and Types I and II collagen to localize these molecules in young and mature porcine discs. Proteoglycans and Type I collagen were located in different regions of the annulus fibrosus, in agreement with the histology described above.

Biochemical analyses of separated glycosaminoglycan fractions established that chondroitin sulfate, keratan sulfate, and hyaluronate were present in old human discs.[80] As anticipated, the water content of the disc correlates well with the glycosaminoglycan content being highest in the center of the nucleus pulposus.

B. Glycosaminoglycans of Disc Proteoglycans

Early work on disc proteoglycans established that they were composed of the glycosaminoglycan chains chondroitin sulfate and keratan sulfate.[82-86] Different fractions of isolated proteoglycans invariably contained both chondroitin sulfate and keratan sulfate, suggesting the both glycosaminoglycans were probably attached to the same protein core.[83-86]

The classical experiments of Sajdera and Hascall[87] introduced a new technology for extraction and isolation of proteoglycans. The discovery of reversible aggregation,[26] the role of hyaluronate[29,30] and the hyaluronate-binding site[25,26] in that phenomenon, and the application of Sepharose® 2B chromatography to separate nonaggregated and aggregated proteoglycans[29] provided a technology for investigations of a specific, functional property of proteoglycans. These important technological developments were subsequently applied to disc proteoglycans.

Despite the homology in structure that they apparently share, hyaline cartilage and disc proteoglycans are different in two notable respects: the proportion of proteoglycan aggregates in both tissues and the size and quantity of their respective keratan sulfate chains.

C. Aggregation of Disc Proteoglycans with Hyaluronate

The proportion of proteoglycans that can be isolated as aggregates from hyaline cartilage is usually about 85%.[26] This proportion is lower in aged human articular cartilage,[43] due apparently to the presence of increased quantities of free hyaluronate binding sites that compete for the hyaluronate chains.[88] The composite proteoglycans of aged cartilage appear to have functional binding sites, suggesting that any cleaved glycosaminoglycan-rich regions are rapidly removed from the extracellular matrix.[44] The proportion of the total proteoglycans isolated as aggregates from mature human discs[89,90] was, in striking contrast, only about 30 to 40%, despite the presence of adequate quantities of hyaluronate in the tissue.[91,92] These proteoglycans do not have functional binding sites as the addition of exogenous hyaluronate did not increase the proportion of aggregated molecules.[96]

Canine and human[89,96,97] annulus fibrosus proteoglycans contained a higher proportion of aggregable proteoglycans than that of nucleus pulposus. The center of the nucleus pulposus contains the higher proportion of nonaggregable proteoglycans.[121] This low proportion of nucleus aggregates is not an artifactual degradative phenomenon, because labeled cartilage proteoglycans do not lose their capacity to aggregate when introduced into the extraction milieu.[92] Moreover, the lower proportion of aggregates is demonstrable by different techniques, such as gel chromatography,[90] analytical ultracentrifugation,[90] and electron microscopy.[28] Biosynthetic studies (see below) confirm that the genesis of nonaggregable proteoglycans is an event that occurs in vivo.

D. Metabolism

The cells of all three tissues in the intervertebral disc actively incorporate radioactive sulfate into extracellular proteoglycans.[93-95] Young mice (30-day-old) synthesize a large aggregable chondroitin sulfate-containing proteoglycan that apparently lacks keratan sulfate, and smaller quantities of a small, nonaggregable proteoglycan.[95] The large proteoglycan still retained its capacity to aggregate with hyaluronate 6 weeks after synthesis. These molecules appeared to be similar to those isolated by Buckwalter et al. from new-born human discs.[28] In-vivo[96,97] and in-vitro[98] studies of canine and human nucleus pulposus, respectively, however, reveal a strikingly different fate for the proteoglycans in the extracellular matrix of the mature disc. Both the canine and human nuclei synthesize a large aggregable proteoglycan.[96-98] With time, in the extracellular matrix, these proteoglycans become progressively smaller in hydrodynamic size, with a loss of their aggregating ability.[97] Structural studies suggest that the nonaggregable proteoglycans lack a hyaluronate binding site,[99-101] presumably because of enzymatic scission of the core-protein. The change in the manner in which extracellular proteoglycans are processed appears to occur in the 1st year of human life: large aggregable proteoglycans that persist extracellularly in the new-born are apparently processed to a nonaggregable species by 6 to 8 months of life.[28]

The mechanisms responsible for the extracellular processing of mature nucleus proteoglycans are unknown. Turnover in young mice[95] and guinea pigs[102] is quite rapid, in contrast to the mature disc.[104] However, young and old articular cartilage proteoglycans also have markedly different half lives,[103] without the generation of significant quantities of nonaggregable molecules in the older tissues.[98] The link proteins in the disc do not apparently protect aggregates from dissociation by hyaluronate oligosaccharides, and the aggregate may be less stable than that of hyaline cartilage.[105] The binding site may be more vulnerable to enzymatic attack as a consequence.

E. Keratan Sulfate of Disc Proteoglycans

The mature nucleus pulposus has the highest concentration of keratan sulfate of any connective tissue.[106-108] There is extensive documentation in the literature that the keratan sulfate chains of the nucleus pulposus are longer than those of articular cartilage or cornea (e.g., see references in References 109 and 110). The difference is striking when tissues are matched for species and age. The keratan sulfate of bovine nasal septum cartilage had a number average molecular weight of 4100, while those from bovine nucleus pulposus in the same study had number average molecular weights of 12,900 to 14,000.[110,111]

A keratan sulfate-rich region has been isolated from porcine,[111] human,[101] and bovine[110] nucleus proteoglycans by the chondroitinase-trypsin-chymotrypsin proceudre of Heinegard and Axelsson.[53] Stevens et al.[111] estimated that the keratan sulfate-rich region thus isolated from pig nucleus proteoglycans contained 60% of the total glucosamine and 40% of the total galactose of the starting preparation. The fragment contained minimal amounts of xylose, confirming that it bore few chondritin sulfate chains. A noteworthy feature of the keratan sulfate peptides isolated from bovine nucleus pulposus was its biomodal separation on Sepharose® Cl-6B.[110] The larger fragment bore longer keratan sulfate chains (mol wt$_n$: 14,100) than those of the smaller one (mol wt$_n$: 12,900). The two fragments may be derived from structurally distinct proteoglycan molecules. Alternatively, each disc proteoglycan may have more than one keratan sulfate-rich region.

Both aggregable and nonaggregable proteoglycans of bovine[110] and human[101] nucleus proteoglycans contain a keratan sulfate-rich region, although the fragment has a larger hydrodynamic size in the aggregable molecules.[100]

F. Electron Microscopy

The cytochrome c spreading technique has been applied by Buckwalter and colleagues[28] to disc proteoglycans in an elegant study, examples of which are shown in Figures 3 and

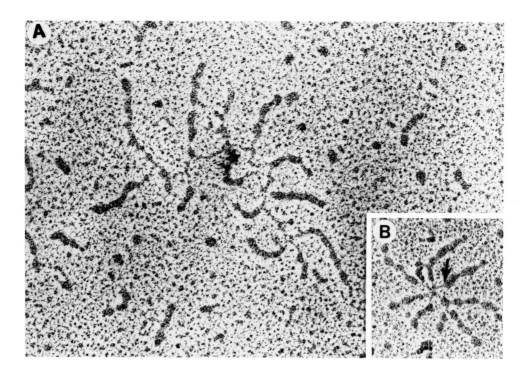

FIGURE 3. Electron micrograph of proteoglycan aggregates extracted from human infant nucleus pulposus under associative conditions and purified as A1 fractions by associative density gradient centrifugation. (A) Long proteoglycan aggregate with large distances between attached proteoglycans; (B) short proteoglycan with closely spaced proteoglycans. (From Buckwalter, J. A., Pedrini-Mille, A., Pedrini, V., and Tudisco, C., *J. Bone Jt. Surg.*, 67, 284, 1985. With permission.)

4. They isolated proteoglycans from newborn, 6-month and 8-month human discs. Proteoglycans were extracted from the nucleus pulposus under associative conditions and would therefore be attached to hyaluronate chains in proteoglycan aggregates as they were in the tissue. Two populations of aggregates were evident in the nucleus samples. The newborn specimens had a greater proportion of aggregates with long hyaluronate chains (mean length, 1096 nm) with widely spaced proteoglycans attached (Figure 3A). The older infant discs had a higher proportion of aggregates with shorter chains along which the proteoglycans were more closely spaced (Figure 3B).

Aggregates contained from 8 to 18 proteoglycans, irrespective of their size. Individual proteoglycans were revealed as thick projections, each of which was attached to the hyaluronate by a thin filament. The thin filaments presumably represent, in part, the hyaluronate binding site and, perhaps, all or some of the keratan sulfate-rich region. These thin sections observed with human disc proteoglycans were shorter (mean length, 25 nm) than those in proteoglycans derived from skeletally mature (mean length, 36 nm) or immature (mean length, 69 nm) bovine nasal cartilage.[28]

Annulus fibrosus proteoglycans and proteoglycan aggregates of infant human discs (Figure 4A and B) were similar to those of the nucleus,[28] but tended to have longer hyaluronate chains.

G. Heterogeneity

Early pioneering work by Pedrini[112] established that human disc proteoglycans could be separated by cellulose acetate electrophoresis. Subsequent studies employed the sensitive extraction and isolation techniques, introduced by Sajdera and Hascall,[87] that minimized

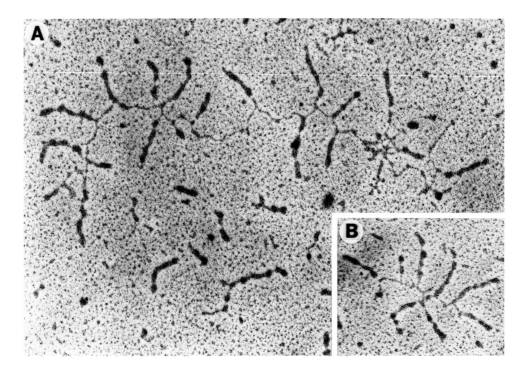

FIGURE 4.   Electron micrographs from human infant annulus fibrosus. These proteoglycans were extracted under dissociative conditions, reaggregated under associative conditions, and then purified as A1. (A) Large proteoglycan aggregates (as in 3A). (B) Small aggregate with broadly spaced proteoglycans.

artifactual degradation of the molecules. The large-pore agarose-acrylamide electrophoresis of McDevitt and Muir,[66] successful as it was in resolving the total extractable population of cartilage proteoglycans into two or more relatively sharp bands, did not produce the same quality of separated bands with unfractionated disc proteoglycans. Gel electrophoresis of unfractionated or partially fractionated baboon,[68] canine,[97] and human[101] nucleus pulposus proteoglycans produce fairly diffuse bands. Whether the two bands represent the aggregable and nonaggregable proteoglycans, respectively, is unclear. Annulus fibrosus proteoglycans, in contrast, migrate as two relatively sharp bands.[68]

Are the proteoglycans that have functional hyaluronate binding sites in the disc electrophoretically heterogeneous as they are in cartilage? Jahnke and McDevitt[100,101] first separated the aggregable from the nonaggregable population of radiologically normal human nuclei pulposi. The electrophoretic separation of the total aggregable population of nucleus proteoglycans thus prepared was of poor quality. Further separation of the aggregable proteoglycans into fractions of varying hydrodynamic size by dissociative chromatography yielded two sharp electrophoretic bands (*F* and *S*) for each fraction analyzed.[100,101] Not only did this experiment confirm that the aggregable proteoglycans of the nucleus were heterogeneous, it also demonstrated that each electrophoretically distinct population was polydisperse in hydrodynamic size, a property that obscured electrophoretic separation of unfractionated material. Removal of the hyaluronate binding site with hydroxylamine demonstrated that the structural feature responsible for the electrophoretic heterogeneity was in the main glycosaminoglycan attachment region of the molecule. Further isolation of the proteoglycans by dissociative density grandient centrifugation indicated the presence of three electrophoretically distinct populations in the human nucleus pulposus: (1) a large proteoglycan, uronate-rich and of high buoyant density Band F-1; (2) a smaller proteoglycan of lower buoyant density, greater protein content and slower mobility than the first (Band S); and (3) a very small proteoglycan of low buoyant density and slightly faster in electrophoretic mobility than the Band F-1 proteoglycans (Band F-2).[101]

The two smaller proteoglycans may, of course, represent in-vivo degradation products of the larger species. Alternatively, their respective protein cores could also represent products of different genes. Only amino acid sequencing studies can unequivocably resolve that issue.

The nonaggregable proteoglycans of normal 20-year-old nuclei pulposi, in contrast to the aggregable molecules, showed only one electrophoretic band throughout the entire hydrodynamic size spectrum of the molecules.[101] When similar nonaggregable proteoglycans were isolated from donors age 64, 67, and 72 years, however, the population migrated electrophoretically as three distinct subpopulations.[113] It is of interest that the distinct nonaggregable bands observed by DiFabio et al.[113] were only evident after fractionation by gel chromatography, as were the gel electrophoretic subpopulations of aggregable proteoglycans identified by Jahnke and McDevitt.[101]

Thus, each subpopulation of the nonaggregable proteoglycans of the aged disc was apparently itself polydisperse in size. Aging and, perhaps, subtle pathological changes in the nucleus appear to be associated with the generation of three nonaggregable proteoglycan subpopulations, while only one is detectable in the normal young adult disc.

H. Proteoglycans in Development and Aging of the Disc

The cells of the human nucleus pulposus are notochordal at birth and are gradually replaced by chondrocyte-like cells in childhood.[2,114] The microanatomical changes of the disc during early development, skeletal maturation, and subsequent middle and old age have been extensively reviewed.[114-116] It should, however, be noted that genetic factors critically influence the rate of this developmental process in certain subsets of a particular species. The chondrodystrophoid breeds of dogs,[117] to which the beagle has been assigned,[118] demonstrate a chondroid metamorphosis in the nucleus pulposus that occurs much more rapidly than in the nonchondrodystrophoid breeds and is completed by the 1st year of life.

The dramatic and continuing changes in the human disc throughout life prompt two notes of caution in interpreting the literature on ''aging'' of disc proteoglycans. First, the prevalence of notochordal cells in animal discs suggests that direct extrapolation of data on the structure and metabolism of animal disc proteoglycans to those of mature human tissue may not always be valid. Second, as anatomical pathological changes are very frequent in the human disc in and after the 4th decade of life, the distinction between changes due to programmed senescence and those due to an underlying pathology may be difficult to discern. Recent studies on human disc proteoglycans[100,101,119] have addressed this issue by morphologically grading the spines prior to study of their disc proteoglycans.

The human nucleus pulposus, a highly hydrated tissue at birth with water accounting for 88% of its dry weight, progressively loses water during development and aging. Water accounts for about 80% and 65% of its dry weight at 18 and 77 years, respectively.[120] The annulus fibrosus is about 78% water at birth, declining to 70% water at 38 years of age. This loss of water is consistent with the progressive decrease in the glycosaminoglycan content of the human[89] and canine[122] nucleus and annulus. Proteins that bind to glycosaminoglycan chains in the disc could also influence the water content of the tissue. Lysozyme is a constituent of the normal nucleus pulposus,[123] and as it binds to chondroitin sulfate chains, any accummulation of the protein with age could diminish the water-binding capacity of the proteoglycans. During maturation and aging, the change in composition in the nucleus pulposus is far more pronounced than that of the annulus fibrosus.[89] Galactosamine and glucosamine comprise 9.2% and 3.5%, respectively, of the dry weight of the $4^1/_2$-year nucleus pulposus; by 76 years of age these values drop to 1.7% (galactosamine) and 2.6% (glucosamine).[86] Assuming that the nonsulfated oligosaccharides contribute minimally to the overall hexosamine content of proteoglycans, the available evidence suggests that the proteoglycans of neonatal and postneonatal nuclei and annuli are predominantly chondroitin sulfate proteoglycans, and development and aging is associated with the progressive acquisition of molecules that contain both chondroitin and keratan sulfate.[89,122,124] In this respect, development and aging of disc tissues is similar to that of articular cartilage.[3]

Most of the proteoglycans of the nuclei pulposi of human and mouse neonates and early-post neonates, as noted earlier, exist as aggregates with hyaluronic acid in the tissue.[28,95] Buckwalter and colleagues demonstrated that the predominance of nonaggregating proteoglycans in the nucleus, a characteristic feature of adult disc, becomes evident by 6 months of age.[28] While 52% of the proteoglycans of neonate nuclei were isolated as aggregates, this proportion dramatically dropped to 28% in the 6-month old tissue.[28] These changes in the neonates are accompanied by a sharp decrease in the length of the hyaluronate chain in aggregates from a length at birth of 1096 nm to 274 nm at 6 months of age.[28] A further slight decrease in the proportion of aggregates of the human nucleus is evident from 8 to 44 years of age.[89,90] Moreover, maturation and aging is associated with an increase in the relative proportion of small nonaggregated proteoglycans at the expense of large nonaggregated molecules.[89] It should be stressed that these changes are found in discs with no detectable pathology and should be considered a feature of the normal programmed senescence of the tissue.[101] The changes in development and aging in the annulus fibrosus are similar, but far less marked, than those of the nucleus pulposus.

IV. PROTEOGLYCANS IN DISC DEGENERATION

Although studies of the quantity of proteoglycan of the degenerated disc suggest that the pathological process resembles that of a marked acceleration of aging, it probably should be viewed as a pathological process distinct from that of programmed senescence. The most consistent change observed in degeneration is a loss of proteoglycan in both nucleus pulposus[99,125] and annulus fibrosus.[125] This loss is usually accompanied by a loss of water.[124,125]

Studies with a rabbit model, in which degeneration was induced by surgical ventral herniation,[126,127] demonstrated that the disc cells respond to depletion of their extracellular matrix by initiating a repair mechanism. The repair potential of the nucleus pulposus was dramatically illustrated in a chemonucleolysis experiment in dogs by Bradford[128] and colleagues. In vivo injection of chymopapain into dog discs produced a loss of proteoglycans and disc narrowing.[128] By 3 months after injection, however, nuclear material and disc height had been regained somewhat, and by 6 months, the proteoglycans of the injected discs were identical to those of normal tissues. The human disc also seems capable of responding to degeneration by an active synthesis of proteoglycans. The proteoglycans of the degenerate human disc had a larger size and a larger proportion had more functional hyaluronate binding sites than those of normal tissue.[99] These proteoglycans presumably represent proteoglycans synthesized as part of a repair process, analogous to the proteoglycans with larger chondroitin sulfate-rich regions found in osteoarthritic articular cartilage.[47] The proteoglycans of degenerate nuclei have higher keratan sulfate to chondroitin sulfate ratios than those of normal tissue.[99,129] This again is consistent with an active repair process, as aggregable disc proteoglycans are enriched in keratan sulfate and nonaggregable proteoglycans are rich in chondroitin sulfate. It should be emphasized that the experiments of Lyons et al.[99] and Lipson and Muir[126,127] employed modern sensitive procedures for the isolation of proteoglycans, in contrast to earlier work where marked degradation of proteoglycans in degeneration was implied.[124]

Pearce at al.[119] attempted to correlate the proteoglycan changes in the disc with degenerative changes by assigning grades to the disc that were based on their morphological appearance, including degenerate and nondegenerate ones within the same spine. Their findings suggest that morphologically recognizable degeneration occurs only if a low proteoglycan concentration is present throughout the lumbar spine. They proposed the hypothesis that low proteoglycan concentrations in all the discs of a spine precede degeneration. It would be interesting to test this hypothesis in animal models of degeneration that permitted systematic studies of the molecular events in the pathologic process.

In summary, the early stages of disc degeneration appear to involve excessive degradation of proteoglycans with an accompanying response on the part of the cells to repair their matrix. The later stages of degeneration involve further loss of proteoglycans, although some ineffective repair process may still be operative. The interesting hypothesis of Pearce et al.[119] suggests that the degenerative process is not confined to the degenerate discs, but is widespread, although at different stages of the pathological process, throughout the lumbar spine.

V. CONCLUSION

It is evident from this chapter that the recent remarkable advances in our knowledge of disc proteoglycans in normal and pathological discs have initiated the beginning of what should be a productive era in disc proteoglycan research. Indeed, as noted in the introduction to this chapter, the study of the proteoglycans of the disc should provide insights into other areas of connective tissue biology.

ACKNOWLEDGMENTS

I wish to thank Dr. Joseph A. Buckwalter for providing the electron micrographs in Figures 3 and 4, Laurie Micco for help in preparing the bibliography, and Drs. Richard Pearce and Peter Ghosh for providing manuscripts prior to publication. Drs. Richard Pearce, Peter Roughley, and Victor Stanescu kindly proofread the manuscript and their advice and suggestions are acknowledged. The limitations of this chapter are exclusively the responsibility of the author.

REFERENCES

1. **Rosenberg, L., Haberman, E. T., Pal, S., Tang, L. H., and Choi, H. U.**, Structure of intervertebral disc proteoglycans, in *The American Academy of Orthopaedic Surgeons: Symp. Idiopathic Low Back Pain,* White, A. A. and Gordon, S. L., Eds., C. V. Mosby, St. Louis, 1982, chap. 17.
2. **Buckwalter, J. A.**, The fine structure of human intervertebral disc, in *The American Academy of Orthopaedic Surgeons: Symp. Idiopathic Low Back Pain,* White, A. A. and Gordon, S. L., Eds., C. V. Mosby, St. Louis, 1982, 108.
3. **McDevitt, C. A.**, The proteoglycans of cartilage and the intervertebral disc in aging and osteoarthritis, in *Handbook of Inflammation,* Vol. 3, Glynn, L. E., Ed., Elsevier-North Holland, New York, 1981, 111.
4. **Urban, J. and Maroudas, A.**, The chemistry of the intervertebral disc in relation to its physiological function, *Clin. Rheum. Dis.,* 6, 51, 1980.
5. **Eyre, D.**, Biochemistry of the interbertebral disc, *Int. Rev. Connect. Tissue Res.,* 8, 227, 1979.
6. **Bushell, G. R., Ghosh, P., Taylor, T. F. K., and Akeson, W. H.**, Proteoglycan chemistry of the intervertebral disc, *Clin. Orthop. Relat. Res.,* 129, 115, 1977.
7. **Ghosh, P., Bushell, G. R., Taylor, T. F. K., and Akeson, W. H.**, Collagens, elastin and non-collagenous protein of the intervertebral disk, *Clin. Orthop. Relat. Res.,* 129, 124, 1977.
8. **Eyring, E. J.**, The biochemistry and physiology of the intervertebral disk, *Clin. Orthop. Rel. Res.,* 67, 16, 1969.
9. **Urban, J., and Maroudas, A.**, Swelling of the intervertebral disc in vitro, *Connect. Tissue Res.,* 9, 1, 1981.
10. **Taylor, T. K. and Akeson, W. H.**, Intervertebral disc prolapse: a review of morphologic and biochemical knowledge concerning the nature of prolapse, *Clin. Orthop. Relat. Res.,* 76, 54, 1971.

11. **Naylor, A.,** Intervertebral disc prolapse and degeneration. The biochemical and biophysical approach, *Spine,* 1, 108, 1976.

12. **Nordby, E. J. and Brown, M. D.,** Present status of chymopapain and chemonucleolysis, *Clin. Orthop. Relat. Res.,* 129, 79, 1977.

13. **Bradford, D. S., Cooper, K. M., and Oegema, T. R. Jr.,** Chymopapain, chemonucleolysis, and nucleus pulposus regeneration, *J. Bone Jt. Surg.,* 65, 1220, 1983.

14. **Maroudas, A., Stockwell, R. A., Nachemson, A., and Urban, J.,** Factors involved in the nutrition of the human lumbar intervertebral disc: cellularity and diffusion of glucose in vitro, *J. Anat.,* 120, 113, 1975.

15. **Bywaters, E.,** The pathology of the spine, in *The Joints and Synovial Fluid,* Vol. 2, Sokoloff, L., Ed., Academic Press, New York, 1980, chap. 9.

16. **Stevens, R. L. and Austen, K. F.,** Proteoglycans of the mast cell, in *Biochemistry of the Acute Allergic Reactions,* Alan R. Liss, New York, 1981, 69.

17. **Hook, M., Kjellen, L., and Johansson, S.,** *Annu. Rev. Biochem.,* 53, 847, 1984.

18. **Hassell, J. R., Kimura, J. H., and Hascall, V. C.,** Proteoglycan core proteins, *Annu. Rev. Biochem.,* 55, 539, 1986.

19. **Montreuil, J.,** Primary structure of glycoprotein glycans: basis for the molecular biology of glycoproteins, *Advances in Carbohydrate Chemistry and Biochemistry,* Vol. 37, Academic Press, New York, 1980, 157.

20. **Kennedy, J. F.,** Chemical and biochemical aspects of the glycosaminoglycans in health and disease, *Adv. Clin. Chem.,* 18, 5, 1976.

21. **Poole, A. R.,** Proteoglycans in health and disease: structures and functions, *Biochem. J.,* 236, 1, 1986.

22. **Mathews, M. B.,** *Connective Tissue: Macromolecular Evolution and Function,* Springer-Verlag, Heidelberg, 1975.

23. **Lindahl, V. and Hook, M.,** Glucosaminoglycans and their binding to biological macromolecules, *Annu. Rev. Biochem.,* 47, 385, 1978.

24. **Kuettner, K. E. and Kimura, J. H.,** Proteoglycans: an overview, *J. Cell. Biochem.,* 27, 327, 1985.

25. **Muir, H. and Hardingham, T. E.,** The role of hyaluronic acid in proteoglycan aggregation, in *Glycoconjugate Research,* Vol. 1, Gregory, J. D. and Jeanloz, R. W., Eds., Academic Press, New York, 1979, 375.

26. **Hascall, V. C.,** Interaction of cartilage proteoglycans with hyaluronic acid, *J. Supramol. Struct.,* 7, 101, 1977.

27. **Hascall, V. and Heinegard, D.,** Structure of cartilage proteoglycans, in *Glycoconjugate Research,* Vol. 1, Gregory, J. and Jeanloz, R., Eds., Academic Press, New York, 1979, 341.

28. **Buckwalter, J. A., Pedrini-Mille, A., Pedrini, V., and Tudisco, C.,** Proteoglycans of human infant intervertebral disc, *J. Bone Jt. Surg.,* 67, 284, 1985.

29. **Hardingham, T. E. and Muir, H.,** The specific interactions of hyaluronic acid with cartilage proteoglycans, *Biochim. Biophys. Acta,* 279, 401, 1972.

30. **Hascall, V. C. and Heinegrad, D.,** Aggregation of cartilage proteoglycans. II. Oligosaccharide competitors of the proteoglycan-hyaluronic acid interaction, *J. Biol. Chem.,* 249, 4242, 1974.

31. **Hascall, V. C. and Heinegard, D.,** Aggregation of cartilage proteoglycans. I. The role of hyaluronic acid, *J. Biol. Chem.,* 249, 4232, 1974.

32. **Wiedman, H., Paulsson, M., Timpl, R., Engel, J., and Heinegard, D.,** Domain structure of cartilage proteoglycans revealed by rotary shadowing of intact and fragmented particles, *Biochem. J.,* 223, 587, 1984.

33. **Hascall, V. and Sajdera, S.,** Physical properties and polydispersity of proteoglycans from bovine nasal cartilage, *J. Biol. Chem.,* 245, 4920, 1970.

34. **Pasternack, S. V., Veis, A., and Breen, M.,** Solvent-dependent changes in proteoglycan sub-unit conformation in aqueous guanidine hydrochloride solutions, *J. Biol. Chem.,* 249, 2206, 1974.

35. **Heinegard, D. and Hascall, V. C.,** Aggregation of cartilage proteoglycans. III. Characteristics of the proteins isolated from trypsin digests of aggregates, *J. Biol. Chem.,* 249, 4250, 1974.

36. **Caterson, B. and Baker, J.,** The interaction of link proteins with proteoglycan monomers in the absence of hyaluronic acid, *Biochem. Biophys. Res. Commun.,* 80, 496, 1978.

37. **Baker, J. and Caterson, B.,** The isolation and characterization of the link proteins from proteoglycan aggregates of bovine nasal cartilage, *J. Biol. Chem.,* 254, 2387, 1979.

38. **Hardingham, T. E.,** The role of link-protein in the structure of cartilage proteoglycan aggregates, *Biochem. J.,* 177, 237, 1979.

39. **Roughley, P. J., Poole, A. R., and Mort, J. S.,** The heterogeneity of link proteins isolated from human articular cartilage proteoglycan aggregates, *J. Biol. Chem.,* 257, 11, 908, 914, 1982.

40. **Muir, H.,** Proteoglycans: state of the art, *Semin. Arthritis Rheum.,* 9, 7, 1981.

41. **Thonar, E. J. and Sweet, M. B. E.,** Maturation-related changes in proteoglycans of fetal articular cartilage, *Arch. Biochem. Biophys.,* 208, 535, 1981.

42. **Bayliss, M. T. and Ali, S. Y.,** Age related changes in the composition and structure of human articular cartilage proteoglycans, *Biochem. J.,* 176, 683, 1978.

43. **Roughley, P. J. and White, R. J.,** Age-related changes in the structure of the proteoglycan subunits from human articular cartilage, *J. Biol. Chem.,* 255, 217, 1980.
44. **Inerot, S. and Heinegard, D.,** Bovine tracheal cartilage proteoglycans. Variations in structure and composition with age, *Collagen Relat. Res.,* 3, 245, 1983.
45. **Roughley, P. J., McNicol, D., Santer, V., and Buckwalter, J.,** The presence of a cartilage-like proteoglycan in the adult human meniscus, *Biochem. J.,* 197, 77, 1981.
46. **Adams, M. E., McDevitt, C. A., Ho, A., and Muir, H.,** Isolation and characterization of high-buoyant density proteoglycans from semi-lunar menisci, *J. Bone Jt. Surg.,* 68, 55, 1986.
47. **Cox, J. M., McDevitt, C. A., Arnoczky, S. P., and Warren, R. F.,** Changes in the chondroitin sulfate-rich region of proteoglycans in experimental osteoarthritis, *Biochim. Biophys. Acta,* 850, 228, 1985.
48. **Heinegard, D., Paulsson, M., Inerot, S., and Carlstrom, C.,** A novel low-molecular-weight chondroitin sulfate proteoglycan isolated from cartilage, *Biochem. J.,* 197, 355, 1981.
49. **Heinegard, D. K. and Hascall, V. C.,** Characteristics of the nonaggregating proteoglycans isolated from bovine nasal cartilage, *J. Biol. Chem.,* 254, 927, 1979.
50. **Rosenberg, L. C., Choi, H. U., Tang, L. H., Johnson, T. L., Pal, S., Webber, C., Reiner, A., and Poole, A. R.,** Isolation of dermatan sulfate proteoglycans from mature-bovine articular cartilages, *J. Biol. Chem.,* 260, 6304, 1985.
51. **Noro, A., Kimata, K., Oike, Y., Shinomura, T., Maeda, N., Yano, S., Takahashi, N., and Suzuki, S.,** Isolation and characterization of a third proteoglycan (PG-LT) from chick embryo cartilage which contains disulfide-bonded collagenous polypeptide, *J. Biol. Chem.,* 258, 9323, 1983.
52. **De Luca, S., Lohmander, S., Nilsson, B., Hascall, V. C., and Caplan, A. I.,** Proteoglycans from chick limb bud chondrocyte cultures: keratan sulfate and oligosaccharides which contain mannose and sialic acid, *J. Biol. Chem.,* 255, 6077, 1980.
53. **Heinegard, D. and Axelsson, I.,** Distribution of keratan sulfate in cartilage proteoglycans, *J. Biol. Chem.,* 252, 1971, 1977.
54. **Bornstein, P. and Balian, G.,** Cleavage at Asn-Gly bonds with hydroxylamine, in Methods in Enzymology, Vol. 47, Hirs, C. H. W. and Timasheff, S. N., Eds., Academic Press, New York, 1977, 132.
55. **Mathews, M. B.,** Comparative biochemistry of chondroitin sulphate-proteins of cartilage and notochord, *Biochem. J.,* 125, 37, 1971.
56. **Heinegard, D. and Hascall, V. C.,** Characterization of chondroitin sulfate isolated from trypsin-chymotrypsin digests of cartilage proteoglycans, *Arch. Biochem. Biophys.,* 185, 427, 1974.
57. **Roughley, P. J. and Barrett, A. J.,** The degradation of cartilage proteoglycans by tissue proteinases. Proteoglycans structure and it susceptibility to proteolysis, *Biochem. J.,* 167, 629, 1977.
58. **Lohmander, L. S., De Luca, S., Nilsson, B., Hascall, B. C., Caputo, C. C., Kimura, J. H., and Heinegard, D.,** Oligosaccharides on proteoglycans from the swarm rat chondrosarcoma, *J. Biol. Chem.,* 225, 6084, 1980.
59. **Heinegard, D.,** Extraction, fractionation and characterization of proteoglycans from bovine tracheal cartilage, *Biochim. Biophys. Acta,* 285, 181, 1972.
60. **Rosenberg, L., Hellman, W., and Kleinschmidt, A. K.,** Macromolecular models of protein-polysaccharide from bovine nasal cartilage based on electron microscopic studies, *J. Biol. Chem.,* 245, 4123, 1970.
61. **Sampson, P. M., Heimer, R., and Fishman, A. P.,** Detection of glycosaminoglycans at the one-nanogram level by I — cytochrome C, *Anal. Biochem.,* 151, 304, 1985.
62. **Rosenberg, L., Hellman, W., and Kleinschmidt, A. K.,** Electron microscopic studies of proteoglycan aggregates from bovine articular cartilage, *J. Biol. Chem.,* 250, 1877, 1975.
63. **Heinegard, D., Lohmander, S., and Thyberg, J.,** Cartilage proteoglycan aggregates. Electron-microscopic studies of native and fragmented molecules, *Biochem. J.,* 175, 913, 1978.
64. **Kimura, J. H., Osbody, P., Caplan, A. I., and Hascall, V. C.,** Electron microscopic and biochemical studies of proteoglycan polydispersity in chick limb bud chondrocyte cultures, *J. Biol. Chem.,* 253, 4721, 1978.
65. **Thyberg, J., Lohmander, S., and Heinegard, D.,** Electron-microscopic studies on isolated molecules, *Biochem. J.,* 151, 157, 1975.
66. **McDevitt, C. A. and Muir, H.,** Gel electrophoresis of proteoglycans and glycosaminoglycans on large-pore composite polyacrylamide-agarose gels, *Anal. Biochem.,* 44, 612, 1971.
67. **Stanescu, V., Maroteaux, P., and Sobczak, E.,** Gel electrophoresis of the proteoglycans of the growth and of articular cartilage from various species, *Biomedicine,* 19, 460, 1973.
68. **Stanescu. B., Maroteaux, P., and Sobczak, E.,** Proteoglycan populations of baboon (Papio papio) cartilages from different anatomical sites. Gel electrophoretic analysis of dissociated proteoglycans and of fractions obtained by density gradient centrifugation, *Biochim. Biophys. Acta,* 629, 371, 1980.
69. **Roughley, P. J. and Mason, R. M.,** The electrophoretic heterogeneity of bovine nasal cartilage proteoglycans, *Biochem. J.,* 157, 357, 1976.

70. **Roughley, P. J. and White, R. J.,** Age-related changes in the structure of the proteoglycan subunits from human articular cartilage, *J. Biol. Chem.,* 255, 217, 1980.

71. **Schwartz, E. R., Leveille, C. R., Stevens, J. W., and Oh, W. H.,** Proteoglycan structure and metabolism in normal and osteoarthritic cartilage of guinea pigs, *Arthritis Rheum.,* 24, 1528, 1981.

72. **Heinegard, D., Wieslander, J., Sheehan, J., Paulsson, M., and Sommarin, Y.,** Separation and characterization of two populations of aggregating proteoglycans from cartilage, *Biochem. J.,* 225, 95, 1985.

73. **Butler, W. F.,** Metachromasia and alcian blue staining of the intervertebral disc of the cat, *J. Anat.,* 102, 301, 1968.

74. **Butler, W. F. and Heap, P. F.,** Correlation between Alcian Blue staining of glycosaminoglycans of cat nucleus pulposus and TEM x-ray probe microanalysis, *Histochem. J.,* 11, 137, 1979.

75. **Pousty, I. and Butler, W. F.,** Staining of glycosaminoglycans of intervertebral disc tissue, *Res. Vet. Sci.,* 25, 182, 1978.

76. **Braund, K., Ghosh, P., Taylor, T., and Larsen, L.,** The qualitative assessment of glycosaminoglycans in the canine intervertebral disc using a critical electrolyte concentration staining technique, *Res. Vet. Sci.,* 21, 314, 1976.

77. **Kitahara, H.,** Histochemical study of the human intervertebral disc, *J. Jpn. Orthop. Assoc.,* 53, 77, 1979.

78. **Ghosh, P., Bushell, G. R., Taylor, R. K. F., Pearce, R. H., and Grimmer, B. J.,** Distribution of glycosaminoglycan across the normal and the scoliotic disc, *Spine,* 5, 99, 1977.

79. **Beard, H., Ryvar, R., Brown, R., and Muir, H.,** Immunochemical localization of collagen types and proteoglycan in pig intervertebral disc, *Immunology,* 41, 491, 1980.

80. **Antonopoulos, C., Fransson, L., Heinegrad, D., and Gardell, S.,** Chromatography of glycosaminoglycans on ECTEOLA-cellulose columns, *Biochim. Biophys. Acta,* 148, 158, 1967.

81. **Urban, J. and Maroudas, A.,** The measurement of fixed charge density in the intervertebral disc, *Biochim. Biophys. Acta,* 586, 166, 1979.

82. **Davidson, A. and Woodhall, B.,** Biochemical alterations in herniated intervertebral discs, *J. Biol. Chem.,* 234, 2951, 1959.

83. **Lowther, D. A. and Baxter, E.,** Isolation of a chondroitin sulphate protein complex from bovine intervertebral disks, *Nature (London),* 211, 585, 1966.

84. **Heinegard, D. and Gardell, S.,** Studies on proteinpolysaccharide complex from human nucleus pulposus. I. Isolation and preliminary characterization, *Biochim. Biophys. Acta,* 148, 164, 1967.

85. **Rosenberg, L. and Schubert, M.,** The protein polysaccharides of bovine nucleus pulposus, *J. Biol. Chem.,* 242, 4691, 1967.

86. **Gower, W. E. and Pedrini, V.,** Age-related variations in protein-polysaccharides from human nucleus pulposus, annulus fibrosus and costal cartilage, *J. Bone Jt. Surg.,* 51, 1154, 1969.

87. **Sajdera, S. W. and Hascall, V. C.,** Proteinpolysaccharide complex from bovine nasal cartilage. A comparison of low and high shear extraction procedures, *J. Biol. Chem.,* 255, 77, 1969.

88. **Roughley, P. J., White, A. R., and Poole, A. R.,** Identification of a hyaluronic acid-binding protein that interferes with the preparation of high-buoyant-density proteoglycan aggregates from adult human articular cartilage, *Biochem. J.,* 231, 129, 1985.

89. **Adams, P. and Muir, H.,** Qualitative changes with age of human lumbar discs, *Ann. Rheum. Dis.,* 35, 289, 1976.

90. **Emes, J. and Pearce, R. H.,** The proteoglycans of the human intervertebral disc, *Biochem. J.,* 145, 549, 1975.

91. **Hardingham, T. E. and Adams, P.,** A method for the determination of hyaluronate in the presence of other glycosaminoglycans and its application to human intervertebral disc, *Biochem. J.,* 159, 143, 1976.

92. **Stevens, R. L., Dondi, P. G., and Muir, H.,** Proteoglycans of the intervertebral disc. Absence of degradation during the isolation of proteoglycans from the intervertebral disc, *Biochem. J.,* 179, 573, 1979.

93. **Souter, W. and Taylor, T.,** Acid mucopolysaccharide metabolism in the rabbit intervertebral disc, *J. Bone Jt. Surg.,* 51, 385, 1969.

94. **Souter, W.,** Sulphated acid mucopolysaccharide metabolism in the rabbit intervertebral disc, and autoradiographic study, *Ann. Rheum. Dis.,* 30, 202, 1971.

95. **Venn, G. and Mason, R. M.,** Biosynthesis and metabolism in vivo of intervertebral-disc proteoglycans in the mouse, *Biochem. J.,* 215, 217, 1983.

96. **McDevitt, C. A., Billingham, M., and Muir, H.,** In-vivo metabolism of proteoglycans in experimental osteoarthritic and normal canine articular cartilage and the intervertebral disc, *Semin. Arthritis Rheum.,* 11, 17, 1981.

97. **Cole, T., Burkhardt, D., Frost, L., and Ghosh, P.,** The proteoglycans of the canine intervertebral disc, *Biochim. Biophys. Acta,* 832, 127, 1985.

98. **Oegema, T. Jr., Bradford, D., and Cooper, K.,** Aggregated proteoglycan synthesis in organ cultures of human nucleus pulposus, *J. Biol. Chem.,* 245, 10579, 1979.

99. **Lyons, G., Eisenstein, S., and Sweet, M.,** Biochemical changes in intervertebral disc degeneration, *Biochim. Biophys. Acta,* 673, 443, 1981.

100. **Jahnke, M.,** Heterogeneity of human intervertebral disc proteoglycans, University Microfilms International, Ann Arbor, 1983.
101. **Jahnke, M. and McDevitt, C.,** Proteoglycans of the intervertebral disc: electrophoretic heterogenity of the aggregating proteoglycans of the nucleus pulposus, *Biochem. J.,* in press, 1988.
102. **Lohmander, S., Antonopoulos, C. A., and Friberg, U.,** Chemical and metabolic heterogeneity of chondroitin sulfate and keratan sulfate in guinea pig cartilage and nucleus pulposus, *Biochim. Biophys. Acta,* 304, 430, 1973.
103. **Maroudas, A.,** Nutrition and metabolism of the intervertebral disc, in *The American Academy of Orthopaedic Surgeons: Symp. Idiopathic Low Back Pain,* White, A. A. and Gordon, S. L., Eds., C. V. Mosby Co., St. Louis, 1982, 370.
104. **Maroudas, A.,** Glycosaminoglycan turn-over in articular cartilage, *Philos. Trans. R. Soc. London Ser. B,* 271, 293, 1975.
105. **Tengblad, A., Pearce, R., and Grimmer, B.,** Demonstration of link protein in proteoglycan aggregates from human intervertebral disc, *Biochem. J.,* 222, 85, 1984.
106. **Antonopoulous C., Fransson, L., Gardell, S., and Heinegard, D.,** Fractionation of keratan sulfate from human nucleus pulposus, *Acta Chem. Scand.,* 1, 23, 1969.
107. **Axelsson, L.,** Keratan sulfate proteoglycans, Ph.D. thesis, University of Lund, Lund, 1977.
108. **Pearce, R. H. and Grimmer, B. J.,** The chemical constitution of the proteoglycan of human intervertebral disc., *Biochem. J.,* 157, 753, 1973.
109. **Choi, H. and Meyer, K.,** The structure of keratan sulphates from various sources, *Biochem. J.,* 151, 543, 1975.
110. **Heinegard, D., Axelsson, I., and Inerot, S.,** Skeletal keratan sulfate peptides from different tissues. Characterization and alkaline degradation, *Biochim. Biophys. Acta,* 581, 122, 1979.
111. **Stevens, R. L., Ewins, R. J. F., Revell, P. A., and Muir, H.,** Proteoglycans of the intervertebral disc. Homology of structure with laryngeal proteoglycans, *Biochem. J.,* 179, 561, 1979.
112. **Pedrini, V.,** Electrophoretic heterogeneity of proteinpolysaccharides, *J. Biol. Chem.,* 244, 1540, 1969.
113. **DiFabio, J., Pearce, R., Caterson, B., and Hughes, H.,** The heterogeneity of the non-aggregation proteoglycans of the human intervertebral disc, *Biochem. J.,* 244, 27, 1986.
114. **Buckwalter, J. A.,** The fine structure of human intervertebral disc, in *The American Academy of Orthopaedic Surgeons: Symp. Idiopathic Low Back Pain,* White, A. A. and Gordon, S. L., Eds., C. V. Mosby, St. Louis, 1982, 108.
115. **Peacocks, A.,** Observations on the postnatal structure of the intervetebral disc in man, *J. Anat.,* 86, 162, 1952.
116. **Pritzker, K.,** Ageing and degeneration in the lumbar intervertebral disc, *Orthop. Clin. N. Am.,* 8, 65, 1977.
117. **Hansen, H.,** Comparative views on the pathology of disk degeneration in animals, *Lab. Invest.,* 8, 1242, 1959.
118. **Braund, K., Ghosh, P., Taylor, T., and Larsen, L.,** Morphological studies on the canine intervertebral disc. the assignment of the beagle to the achondroplastic classification, *Res. Vet. Sci.,* 19, 167, 1975.
119. **Pearce, R., Grimmer, B., and Adams, M.,** Degeneration of the chemical composition of the human intervertebral disc, *J. Orthop. Res.,* 5, 198, 1987.
120. **Naylor, A.,** The biochemical changes in the human intervertebral disc in degeneration and nuclear prolapse, *Orthop. Clin. N. Am.,* 2, 343, 1971.
121. **Chiang, Y.,** A study on topographical change of proteoglycans in human lumbar discs, *J. Jpn. Orthop. Ass.,* 57, 539, 1983.
122. **Ghosh, P., Taylor, T., and Braund, K.,** Variation of the intervertebral disc with aging. II. Non-chondrodystrophoid breed, *Gerontology.,* 23, 99, 1977.
123. **Sorce, D., McDevitt, C., Greenwals, R., and Moak, S.,** Protein and lysozyme content of adult human nucleus pulposus, *Experientia,* 42, 1157, 1986.
124. **Lyons, H., Jones, E., Quinn, F., and Sprunt, D.,** Changes in the protein-polysaccharide fraction of nucleus pulposus from human intervertebral disc with age and disc herniation, *J. Lab. Clin. Med.,* 68, 930, 1966.
125. **Stevens, R., Ryvar, R., Robertson, W., O'Brien, J., and Beard, H.,** Biological changes in the anulus fibrosus in patients with low-back pain, *Spine,* 7, 223, 1982.
126. **Lipson, S. and Muir, H.,** Experimental intervertebral disc degeneration: morphologic and proteoglycan changes over time, *Arthritis Rheum.,* 24, 12, 1981.
127. **Lipson, S. and Muir, H.,** 1980, Volvo award in basic science. Proteoglycans in experimental intervertebral disc degeneration, *Spine,* 6, 194, 1981.
128. **Bradford, Oegema, T. Jr., Cooper, K., Wakano, K., and Chao, E.,** Chymopapain, chemonucleolysis, and nucleus pulposus regeneration. A biochemical and biomechanical study, *Spine,* 9, 135, 1984.

129. **Lehtonen, A., Viljanto, J., and Karkkainen, J.,** The mucopolysaccharides of herniated human intervertebral discs and semilunar cartilages, *Acta Chir. Scand.,* 133, 303, 1967.
130. **Oldberg, A., Antonsson, P., and Heinegard, D.,** The partial amino acid sequence of bovine cartilage proteoglycan, deduced from a cDNA clone, contains numerous Ser-Gly sequences arranged in homologous repeats, *Biochem. J.,* 243, 255, 1987.

Chapter 7

COLLAGENS OF THE DISC

David R. Eyre

TABLE OF CONTENTS

This chapter summarizes current knowledge of the genetically distinct types of collagen and reviews what is understood about collagen biochemistry in the tissues of the intervertebral disc.

The unique fibrous organization of the disc has clearly evolved to meet unusual mechanical demands.[1] As more is learned about the molecular heterogeneity within this collagen architecture, the more the notion is reinforced that the disc is best considered as a unique connective tissue, certainly a very specialized form of cartilage.

After it was learned that the fibrous framework of the intervertebral disc embodied two principal types of collagen, types I and II,[2] several new, genetically distinct collagens were discovered, and the list of known collagen types in the disc has increased. Seven molecular species of collagen, types I, II, III, V, VI, IX, and XI, are now known to be present in the disc, of which types I and II account for about 80% by weight.

I. OVERVIEW OF COLLAGEN TYPES

Eleven genetically distinct types of collagen have been assigned type numbers (Table 1). All fit the definition of a collagen in being structural components of the extracellular matrix and having (a) collagen triple-helical domain(s) for a significant portion of their native molecular conformation.[3] They represent the products of 18 or more genes. These individual types of collagen molecule have been segregated into three groups or classes.[4] Class 1 collagens include all the 67-nm-banded fibril-forming molecules. These collagens share a very similar molecular conformation, consisting of a single, 300-nm long uninterrupted triple-helix. Short telopeptide sequences at both ends, on each of the three α-chains, provide the lysine and hydroxylysine side-chains that are the substrates for lysyl oxidase in forming the aldehydes that initiate intermolecular covalent cross-linking.[5] Class 2 collagen molecules are at least as long as class 1 molecules, but they have nontriple-helical domains interrupting the triple-helix, and in the case of type IV collagen, globular extension sequences.[6] Class 3 molecules, or the short-chain collagens, have a much shorter helical domain than class 1 molecules, globular extensions at one or both ends, and the helix may be interrupted along its length. The relative sizes and conformations of molecules in these various collagen classes are illustrated in Figure 1.

Although class 1 molecules can be classified in this scheme confidently, those in classes 2 and 3 may interchange or become members of new classes as more knowledge of their molecular topology, properties, and functions emerges. Indeed, the distribution of collagen types in Table 1 differs from that of Miller,[4] because recent work suggests that type VIII collagen is a short-helix molecule.[7] Clearly this classification, though useful, is somewhat arbitrary at present. It can be refined as the evolutionary and functional relationships of the various molecular types are established.

A. Types I, II, and III

These molecules form the bulk collagen fibrils of the body. They share very similar molecular dimensions and conformations. Only the telopeptide sequences of about 10 to 15 amino acid residues lack a triple-helical conformation at both ends of the three α-chains, each of which is about 1020 amino acids long.

B. Types V and XI

These collagens appear to be a subclass of the fibril-forming class 1 collagens.[4] Type V collagen[8] is codistributed everywhere that type I collagen appears at about 3% of the concentration of type I. Similarly, type XI (1α2α3α) collagen,[9] a close relative of type V, is codistributed with type II collagen at about 3% of the amount of type II.[10] Both type V and

Table 1
A SUMMARY OF CLASSES AND TYPES OF COLLAGEN MOLECULE

Collagen Classes

Class 1: The molecules are 290 nm of uninterrupted triple helix; all types can form 67-nm-banded fibrils: types I, II, III, V, and XI

Class 2: The molecules are at least 300 nm of interrupted helical domains; nonfibrillar: types IV and VII

Class 3: The molecules are much shorter than 300 nm; polymeric structures vary: types VI, VIII, IX, and X

Individual Types

Type	Synonyms	Molecular formula	Polymeric form	Tissue distribution
I	—	$[\alpha 1(I)]_2 \alpha 2(I)$	67-nm-banded fibril	Abundant and widespread
II	Cartilage collagen	$[\alpha 1(II)]_3$	67-nm-banded fibril	Hyaline cartilage, intervertebral disc, vitreous humor, notochordal sheath
III	Reticulin collagen	$[\alpha 1(III)]_3$	67-nm-banded fibril	Widespread; conc in vascular tissue
IV	Basement membrane collagen	$[\alpha 1(IV)]_2 \alpha 2(IV)$	"Chicken-wire" lattice	Basal laminae
V	AB collagen	Principal form: $[\alpha 1(V)]_2 \alpha 2(V)$	67-nm-banded fibril	Widespread in low conc with type I
VI	Intima collagen, GP 140	$[\alpha 1(IV)\alpha 2(VI)\alpha 3(VI)]$?	110-nm-banded microfibril	Widespread in small amounts; interfibrillar location
VII	Anchoring fibril protein	$[\alpha 1(XI)]_3$	800-nm long centrosymmetric fibril	Anchors ectodermal basement membranes
VIII	Endothelial cell collagen		Hexagonal lattice?	Descemet's membrane; other endothelial basement membranes
IX	M collagen, PG-Lt	$\alpha 1(IX)\alpha 2(IX)\alpha 3(IX)$	Unknown	Hyaline cartilage, intervertebral disc, vitreous humor
X	G or short-chain collagen	$[\alpha 1(X)]_3$	Unknown	Hypertrophic zone of ossifying cartilage; codistributed in low conc with type II
XI	$1\alpha 2\alpha 3\alpha$ collagen	$[1\alpha 2\alpha 3\alpha]$ or $\alpha 1(XI)\alpha 2(XI)\alpha 3(XI)$	67-nm-banded fibril	

CLASS 1 —Fibril forming

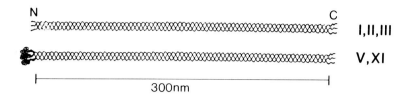

CLASS 2—Interrupted helix

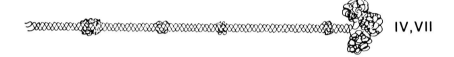

CLASS 3 —Short helix

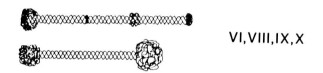

FIGURE 1.   A comparison of the basic molecular forms of the three different classes of collagens.

XI collagens apparently function in the extracellular matrix with their N-propeptides retained.[11,12]

C. Type IV

This collagen forms the scaffold of basement membranes. The molecules polymerize and become chemically cross-linked by their ends to form a 3-dimensional open network that resembles a chicken-wire in its structure.[6]

D. Type VI

Type VI collagen was called GP-140, intima collagen, or short-chain collagen in some of the earlier studies of the protein.[13-18] The molecule consists of a short triple-helical domain with large globular extensions at both ends.[19] It is widely distributed, usually in relatively small amounts, has been detected in most connective tissues, and is particularly abundant in large vessels, kidney, skin, liver, and muscle.[20] Ultrastructurally, type VI collagen seems to form an array of beaded filaments distributed between the banded collagen fibrils.[20,21] It also seems to be a component of distinctive fibrillar structures having a repeating period of about 110 nm formed by lateral clustering of the beaded filaments, that have been noted for many years by electron microscopists in various connective tissues and tumor matrices.[21,22]

E. Type VII

Type VII collagen is quantitatively a very minor ingredient of tissues that contain basement membranes of ectodermal origin.[23,24] Type VII is believed to be the protein component of structures known from electron microscopy as anchoring fibrils, which underly certain kinds of basal laminae, apparently linking them to their matrix substratum.

Table 2
CHROMOSOMAL LOCATION OF HUMAN
COLLAGEN GENES

Procollagen Chain	Chromosome	Region	Ref.
α1(I)	17	q21—q22	42
α2(I)	7	q21—q22	43, 44
α1(II)	12	q131—q132	44, 45, 46
α1(III)	2	q31—q323	46, 47
α1(IV)	13	q34	46, 48
α2(V)	2	q24-q31	47

F. Type VIII

This protein, originally identified as a product of bovine aortic endothelial cells[25] and rabbit corneal endothelial cells[26] in culture, is a structural component of Descemet's membrane[27] and perhaps of other endothelial basal laminae. Recent data point to a molecule consisting of a triple-helix that is about half the length of that in types I, II, and III collagens.[7]

G. Type IX

This collagen was originally called type M collagen after its discovery in pepsin digests of hyaline cartilage.[28] Independent work that set out to screen a cDNA library constructed from chondrocyte mRNA for collagenous gene products discovered two genes that coded for previously unknown collagenous polypeptides.[29] They turned out to encode the α1(IX) and α2(IX) chains of type IX collagen, and virtually the complete amino acid sequences coded by these genes have been determined.[29,30] Protein sequence data confirmed their identities as type IX collagen genes.[31] One of the type IX chains (α2(IX)) was shown to contain a covalently attached glycosaminoglycan chain.[32] The protein seems to be identical to a quantitatively minor form of proteoglycan (PG-Lt) that had been isolated earlier from chick cartilage and shown to have a collagenous composition.[33] The function of type IX collagen in cartilage matrix is unknown, though a linking function between collagen fibrils and proteoglycans is an attractive hypothesis, if only by virtue of the dual status of the molecule as a collagen and a proteoglycan.

H. Type X

The single triple-helical domain of the type X collagen molecule is half the length of that of type I collagen, with a globular domain at one end and short nontriple-helical sequences at the other end.[34-41] The protein is highly restricted in its tissue distribution, being found only in the hypertrophic zone of the epiphyseal plate of growing animals. Chondrocytes switch their phenotype in this region from making type II to type X collagen. The function of type X in the tissue is unknown, but speculations include roles in matrix calcification, vascular invasion, and matrix destruction.

I. Collagen Genes

Table 2 summarizes current knowledge of the distribution of collagen genes among human chromosomes.[42-48] The most striking feature of the structure of genes encoding the class 1 collagen chains is the highly interrupted nature of the coding domains, which for the proα2(I) chain, for example, are divided by introns into 52 exons or coding sequences. The commonest exon size is 54 bases coding for 18 amino acids, believed to be a carry-over by multiple duplications of an ancestral collagen gene to form the fibrillar collagen genes, which are now highly conserved in length and exon structure.[49] The genes for collagen chains in class

Table 3
COLLAGEN TYPES IN THE INTERVERTEBRAL DISC

	Molecular formula	Tissue distribution	% of total collagen
Class 1: Fibril forming			
Type I	$[\alpha 1(I)]_2\alpha 2(I)$	Annulus fibrosus	Radial increase of <0-80% from transition zone to outer rim
Type II	$[\alpha 1(II)]_3$	Annulus fibrosus and nucleus pulposus	Radial increase of 0-80% from outer rim to transition zone
Type III	$[\alpha 1(III)]_3$	Possible traces in the nucleus and annulus	—
Type V	$[\alpha 1(V)]_2\alpha 2(V)$	Annulus fibrosus	~3%
Type XI	$1\alpha 2\alpha 3\alpha$ or $[\alpha 1(XI)\alpha 2(XI)\alpha 3(XI)]$	Nucleus pulposus	~3%
Class 3: Short helix collagens			
Type VI		Annulus fibrosus	~10%
		Nucleus pulposus	15—20%
Type IX		Annulus fibrosus	1—2%
		Nucleus pulposus	1—2%

2 and 3 molecules, however, tend to have fewer, larger exons, or coding sequences, and so do not fit this highly interrupted structure of the class 1 collagen genes.[41]

II. DISC COLLAGEN TYPES

The collagen content of the disc steadily increases from the center of the nucleus pulposus to the outer annulus.[1] In some adult human discs, collagen can represent as little as 6 to 8% of the dry weight of the very central region of the nucleus, with a range of 6 to 25% of the dry weight.[50] The content seems to vary between individuals and between discs, with no obvious correlation with degree of degeneration. In the outer annulus, collagen reaches 70% or more of the dry weight. These values are all based on hydroxyproline weights converted to collagen by a factor of 7.5.

All seven molecular types of collagen that in aggregate occur in hyaline cartilage and a fibrous tissue such as skin or tendon can be found in the annulus and nucleus of the intervertebral disc (Table 3). The nucleus pulposus contains types II, VI, IX, and XI and the annulus, types I, II, III, V, VI, IX, and XI.

A. Fibrillar Collagens
1. Types I and II
The fibrous framework of the intervertebral disc is built from types I and II collagen fibrils. These two collagen types are distributed radially in opposing concentration gradients, with type II exclusively in the nucleus pulposus and type I most concentrated in the exterior of the annulus fibrosus, where it provides the tough lamellar sheets that are anchored into the bone of the vertebral bodies above and below. This distribution was demonstrated originally by SDS-polyacrylamide gel electrophoresis of CNBr-digests of serial tissue samples taken radially across anterior segments of pig[51] and human[52] lumbar intervertebral discs. Using polyclonal antibodies specific for types I and II collagens, the same opposing radial concentration gradients were evident by fluorescence immunohistochemistry.[53] This latter study also revealed local patterns of heterogeneity, with type II collagen appearing to be concentrated in more homogeneous and proteoglycan-rich pockets between the coarse, striated fiber bundles of type I collagen. Small amounts of type III collagen were similarly detected by immunohistochemistry and located pericellularly in the nucleus and inner annulus fibrosus.[54]

Presumably, types I and II collagen molecules are each restricted to their own homopolymeric fibrils. However, this has not been confirmed, for example, using type-specific antibodies and immunogold labeling under the electron microscope. Biochemical analyses designed to test for possible molecular intermingling, by seeking intertype cross-linked collagen peptides in protease digests of bovine annulus fibrosus, have so far failed to turn up any type I-type II hybrids.[55] Nevertheless, it remains possible that hybrid fibrils, which are copolymers of types I and II collagen molecules, are present in the annulus fibrosus.

In degree of posttranslational modifications, disc type I collagen contains more hydroxylysine and hydroxylysine glycosides than type I collagen in other tissues including skin, tendon, and bone.[1,52,56] It resembles type I collagen of meniscus fibrocartilage in this respect. Similarly, type II collagen of adult human nucleus pulposus was richer in hydroxylysine and hydroxylysine glycoside residues than type II collagen of adult human articular cartilage.[1,52,56] The significance of these chemical differences is unknown.

2. Types V and XI

Ayad et al.[57-59] have isolated and fractionated the pool of minor collagens from bovine intervertebral disc tissues. Type XI collagen ($1\alpha2\alpha3\alpha$) was a major component of this fraction.[57] In individual analyses of annulus fibrosus and nucleus pulposus, type XI collagen was found predominantly in the 1.2 M NaCl fraction from the nucleus, but type V collagen was predominant in that fraction from the annulus.[59,60] The distributions of types V and XI collagens thus seem to follow those of types I and II collagens, respectively.

The polymeric form and ultrastructural distribution of types V and XI collagens are unclear. In cornea, using very well-characterized monoclonal antibodies to type V collagen, types I and V collagens were shown to be intimately associated. The results suggested that these two collagen types may be copolymerized within the same fibril network.[61] This may be how type V collagen, and by implication its close relative type XI collagen, are laid down in all tissues. Thus, in the disc, type V collagen may be copolymerized with type I collagen and type XI with type II collagen.

In understanding the function of these minor collagens, the finding may also be relevant that type XI collagen binds firmly to various sulfated polysaccharides, including chondroitin sulfate-proteoglycans, under conditions when type II collagen shows no binding.[62]

B. Type VI Collagen

Several studies have noted unusual banded structures that have about a 110-nm periodicity on electron microscopy of nucleus pulposus.[22,63,64] The incidence of similar structures in other tissues has been reviewed.[21,22] They were suspected to be a form of collagen, though having a different organization to the usual 64- to 67-nm banded fibrils formed by types I, II, and III collagens. The 110-nm banded structures appeared to be lateral aggregates formed from fine microfibrils that had electron-dense nodes at regular intervals providing the periodicity and the sites of interaction. Variations on these structures in various fields of matrix in human nucleus pulposus are shown in Figure 2. Recent electron microscopic work now strongly indicates that such structures in cell cultures, tumors, tendons, and other tissues are aggregated forms of type VI collagen.[17,19-21]

Electrophoresis after disulfide-cleavage of extracts of bovine nucleus pulposus or annulus fibrosus in 4 M guanidine HCl shows an abundant protein band at 140 kdaltons with three or four associated bands at about 25 kdaltons (Figure 3A). This pattern is characteristic of type VI collagen. Pepsin digests of disc tissue also yield prominent type VI fragments in the 1.8 M NaCl precipitate at acid pH (Figure 3B).[65] The recoveries show that type VI collagen is remarkably abundant in disc tissue. Estimates from fraction weights and gel electrophoresis yields indicate that in calf nucleus pulposus, the type VI content is about 20% of the type II collagen content by weight or 5% or more of the tissue dry weight. In

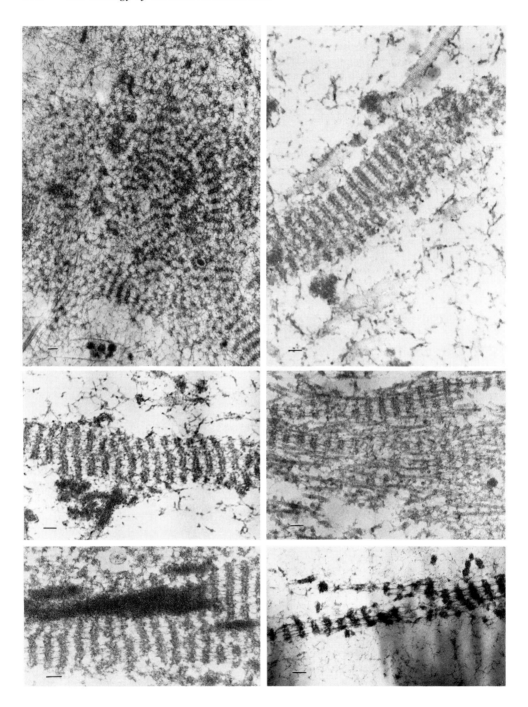

FIGURE 2.   Electron microscopic appearance of novel-banded structures in the human nucleus pulposus, which are believed to be due to a polymeric form of type VI collagen. Several different fields are shown; some include typical 67-nm-banded type I or II fibrils intermingled with the 110-nm-banded type VI structures. The bar in the lower left of each figure is 100 nm. Individual electronmicrographs were generously supplied by Dr. Joseph A. Buckwalter.

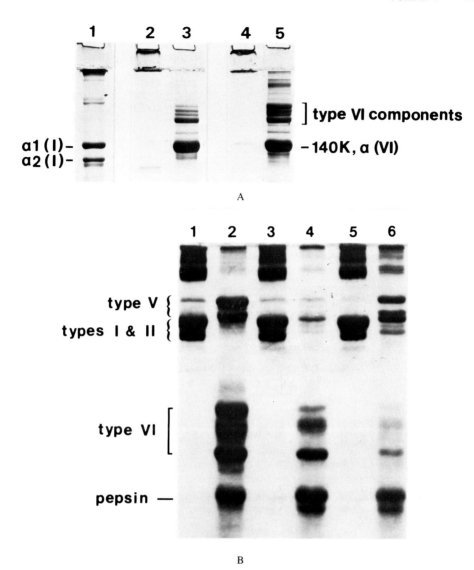

FIGURE 3.   Electrophoresis in SDS 8%-polyacrylamide of type VI collagen chains from bovine interv-ertebral disc. (A) Native-sized molecules extracted without protease treatment. Lane 1, type I collagen standard (4 *M* guanidine HCl extract); lanes 2 and 3, type VI collagen extracted from nucleus pulposus; lanes 4 and 5, type VI collagen extracted from annulus fibrosus. Lanes 2 and 4 were run without and lanes 3 and 5 with disulfide reduction. (B) Pepsin-solubilized collagens. Lane 1, 0.9 *M* NaCl (pH3) precipitate from a digest of bovine annulus fibrosus that contains mainly types I and II collagen chains; lane 2, 2.0 *M* NaCl (pH 3) precipitate from a pepsin digest of bovine annulus fibrosus that contains mainly types V and VI collagens. Lanes 3,4 and 5,6 contain similar pairs of 0.9 *M* and 2.0 *M* NaCl fractions, respectively, from bovine meniscus fibrocartilage and Achilles tendon for comparison. All lanes were run with dithioth-reitol to reduce disulfides. The positions of the three main α(VI) pepsin-derived chains are indicated, and also the pepsin remaining in the sample.[115]

the annulus, where fibrillar collagens account for more of the dry weight (40 to 60%), type VI also accounts for 5% of the tissue dry weight. Cornea is another tissue that appears to be unusually rich in type VI collagen, where it is estimated to make up a quarter of the tissue's dry weight, the other collagens being types I and V.[66] Type VI, therefore, appears not to be distributed among tissues with restriction to any particular phenotype of fibrillar collagens.

The function of type VI collagen is unknown. It is unlikely that it performs an equivalent tensile-strengthening job to that of types I and II collagens. No aldehyde-mediated cross-links have been found in type VI collagen, and most if not all of the protein is quantitatively extracted from disc tissue by the protein denaturant, 4 *M* guanidine HCl.[60,65] A matrix-organizing function between or on the surface of the common types of collagen fibril is one possibility. Type VI collagen is a constituent of most connective tissues, including skin, tendon, aorta, and cartilage and is synthesized by fibroblasts in culture.[19-21,67] The unusual abundance of type VI collagen throughout the intervertebral disc implies a function that is particularly important to the material or biological properties of its tissues.

C. Type IX Collagen

In nucleus pulposus, the concentration of type IX collagen relative to type II collagen (1 to 2% by weight) is similar to that in hyaline cartilages.[60] In the annulus fibrosus, the concentration of type IX appears to be lower than in the nucleus and consistent with it being present roughly in proportion to type II collagen.[60] In hyaline cartilages, type IX collagen seems to be more abundant during development than in the adult tissue,[28] and this may also be true in the nucleus pulposus.

The first immunohistochemical work on locating type IX in hyaline cartilage, using polyclonal antibodies, showed an enrichment pericellularly in the lacunar rim of the chondrocytes.[68,69] More recently, well characterized monoclonal antibodies have shown that type IX collagen is spread throughout the extracellular matrix in close association with type II collagen.[70] Immunogold localization under the electronmicroscope showed an apparent concentration of type IX molecules at intersections between type II fibrils.[71] It was concluded that type IX might function in some way as a fibril adhesion protein. Cross-linking analyses had also raised this concept: it was observed with articular cartilage that the same kind of hydroxypyridinium residues that cross-link type II collagen molecules were even more abundant in pepsin-solubilized type IX collagen.[72] Since no polymeric structure has yet been ascribed to type IX collagen, it is not known whether these aldehyde-mediated cross-links are used solely for selfpolymerization or perhaps for linking type IX molecules to the surface of type II fibrils or to other matrix macromolecules.

Type IX collagen resembles types I, II, V, and XI collagens in the disc in apparently being totally inextractable in 4 *M* guanidine HCl, in contrast to type VI collagen, which appears to be largely extracted by this solvent.

D. Species Variations

Human annulus fibrosus is richer in type II collagen than bovine or porcine annulus fibrosus. The ratio of type II to type I collagens in whole annulus segments dissected from human lumbar discs is about 1.5 compared with 0.25 in similar segments from the quadruped discs.[2,52] This higher proportion of type II in man is presumably related to the altered anatomy and greater thickness of human discs, which in turn are an adaptation to accommodate the mechanical loads imposed by an upright, bipedal posture.

III. CROSS-LINKING

Two main pathways of aldehyde-mediated cross-linking operate in the common collagens of vertebrates, one based on lysine aldehydes, which in skin and cornea is the dominant pathway, and the other on hydroxylysine aldehydes.[5,73] The fibrous collagens of annulus and nucleus are cross-linked largely by the hydroxylysine aldehyde route, in keeping with the collagens of most skeletal connective tissues.[56]

The earliest studies were on the borohydride-reducible intermediate cross-links of the disc.[75,76] As fibrils mature, these cross-links rapidly disappear and are replaced by mature, nonreducible cross-links, which on the hydroxylysine aldehyde pathway are hydroxypyridinium residues.[5,56,73] The concentrations of these cross-links in human disc collagens, however, are the highest observed of any vertebrate connective tissue.[5,56,73,77] This is most evident in the nucleus pulposus, where the density of hydroxypyridinium (HP) cross-linking residues can reach 3 mol/mol of collagen in the young mature tissue.[78] Mature bovine articular cartilage in comparison contains a maximum of 2 mol of HP residue per mole of collagen.[72,73,77] It may seem puzzling that a tissue which in the young is a gel with no intrinsic tensile strength should need such highly cross-linked collagen. One explanation may be that the relatively sparsely distributed type II fibrils in the proteoglycan-rich watery gel of the nucleus individually need to be highly cross-linked to withstand the frictional forces they must take in providing fiber reinforcement to the gel. The degree of cross-linking of the fibrous component of a fiber-reinforced gel is related to the material properties of the composite.[79] In this context, potential functions of type VI and type IX collagens in mediating interactions between the surface of type II fibrils and the interfibrillar proteoglycan domain of the nucleus pulposus will be important to evaluate.

No differences in basic mechanism of cross-linking between types I and II collagens of annulus fibrosus have been noted.[80] However, the degree of cross-linking of type I collagen may be less than that of type II collagen, though hydroxypyridinium residues are the major form of cross-link in both.[78] In general, tissues based on type I collagen that employ the hydroxylysinealdehyde route attain a maximum of about 1 mol/mol of collagen of hydroxypyridinium residues, about half that of type II collagen.[5,73] This may be related to the presence in the molecule of the $\alpha 2(I)$ chain, which lacks a lysine at the aldehyde site in its carboxytelopeptide and may impose other restrictions on the cross-linking of the type I molecule.[35]

There is growing attention on the effects of nonenzymic glycosylation on connective tissues.[81] With increasing age, long-lived proteins such as collagen accumulate covalently-bound glucose residues on their amine side-chains (lysine and hydroxylysine).[82,83] This chemical addition by the carbonyl group of the glucose, followed by an Amadori or ketoamine rearrangement, is significantly enhanced in diabetic patients[84] and is the start of the series of still poorly defined spontaneous reactions known as ''browning'' or Maillard reactions that occur in protein hydrolysates, aging foods, and animal tissues.[85] Recent work in vitro indicates that these glycation reactions lead to covalent links between polypeptide chains.[86] One compound has been identified which is fluorescent and has the structure, 2-(2-furoyl)-4(5)-(2-furanyl)-imidazole (FFI), the condensation product of 2 glucose molecules and two lysine side-chains.[86] It is notable that human intervertebral discs and other connective tissues, such as articular cartilage, develop a pronounced yellow to markedly brown color in elderly individuals. This pigmentation used to be described by pathologists as aging pigment or lipofuscin, thought to be derived from the oxidation products of lipids.[88] However, it now seems likely that much of this coloration may be due to the ensuing products of nonenzymic glycosylation reactions in collagen and in other long-lived protein components of the disc. The significance of such progressive cross-linking, by what appears to be a physiologically artifactual process, in terms of increased brittleness of collagen fibrils and perhaps deteriorating mechanical properties of intervertebral discs, deserves attention.

IV. SUPRAMOLECULAR ORGANIZATION

A. X-ray and Neutron Diffraction

X-ray diffraction has given useful insights on the packing of fibrillar collagen in the disc at two levels of organization: (1) the packing of molecules within fibrils and (2) the arrangement of fibrils in adjacent annular lamellae.

Preliminary results of an X-ray and neutron diffraction study of bovine intervertebral disc observed a unique meridional pattern of intensities from the collagen fibrils compared with those of tendon.[89] Further work on the relative intensities of the meridional diffraction lines at low angle suggested an intimate and orderly association of another molecule aligned along the collagen fibrils at the axial level of the gap region in the nucleus pulposus.[90] Trypsin digestion altered these relative intensities, presumably by removing the superimposed molecules. The predicted size from the diffraction data of the associated molecule of 16 kdaltons suggested it might be a chondroitin or keratan sulfate chain. Another study on human nucleus pulposus showed a lower angle for the main equatorial reflection from type II collagen, compared with type I collagen in specimens of outer annulus, indicating that the average lateral spacing between collagen molecules packed in type II fibrils was greater than that in type I collagen fibrils.[91] The difference was 16 to 17Å vs. 14Å. The findings implied that type II collagen fibrils are more hydrated than type I collagen fibrils, perhaps because they contain more covalently bound sugar residues. This may be important in understanding basic differences in the function of the two collagen types.

X-ray diffraction has also proved useful for determining the collective mean-tilt angle of collagen fibers in alternate lamellae of the annulus fibrosus.[92-96] This was done for discs that were unloaded or while deformed in compression, bending, or torsion (see Chapter 1 for details). In the relaxed disc the mean angle of collagen fibers to the spinal axis was found to be 60 to 65°C, with no change going from fetus to adult.[92] Thus, the angular inclination to the spinal axis of collagen fibers in the annular lamellae, which alternates from side to side from one lamella to the next, is laid down in the fetus as it will appear in the adult. Also, small changes in the angle of this fiber tilt were detected when bending,[93] torsional,[93] or compressive[94,95] strains were applied to the disc.

B. Electron Microscopy

Electron microscopy of specimens of human annulus showed a continuous increase with increasing age in the mean diameter of the collagen fibrils and an increasing proportion of larger fibrils.[97,98] In another ultrastructural study, a peculiar sheathing of fibrils by electron-dense cylinders of material was consistently noted around a small proportion of the collagen fibrils seen in electron micrographs of both the annulus and nucleus of human discs.[99] The chemical nature of this material, for example, whether it represented aggregates of proteoglycans or of protein, was unknown. However, the consistency of the observations and a related report[100] suggests it was a normal feature, perhaps peculiar to the disc.

The three-dimensional organization of collagen in the disc has also been studied thoroughly by scanning electronmicroscopy.[101,102]

V. METABOLISM AND TURNOVER

All the evidence would suggest that collagen fibers in the disc are very long lived. No specific measurements of their turnover rates in the disc have been published. However, Maroudas[103] extrapolated from studies on articular cartilage and unpublished preliminary results on intervertebral disc tissue, using hydroxyproline incorporation rates from radio-labeled proline given systemically to adult dogs. The results indicated mean turnover times for the collagen of over 100 years. This means that most of the collagen fibers laid down during development and growth remain in the tissue throughout life. However, since there are at least seven molecular types of collagen in the disc, all contributing to the hydroxyproline pool, the relative turnover rate of each type needs to be evaluated to appreciate fully the meaning of gross turnover rates of radiolabeled hydroxyproline. For instance, if a quantitatively minor collagen, such as type VI, is turned over more rapidly than are other collagen types, then the actual half-life of the fibrous collagens may be even longer than the overall mean for hydroxyproline would suggest.

It seems likely that different cell types are responsible for synthesizing different subsets of the seven known molecular types of collagen in the disc. Thus, cells of fibroblastic, chondrocytic, and notochordal appearance are all reported to be in the disc.[1,104] Furthermore, the known collagen phenotype expressed by hyaline chondrocytes, i.e., types II, IX, and XI collagens, together with that expressed by fibroblasts, i.e., types I, III, V, and VI collagens, add up to the overall profile of collagen types seen in the disc.

The percentage of necrotic cells in the human nucleus pulposus has been reported to increase with age from 2% or less in fetal specimens, to over 50% in adults.[105] This electron microscopic study also noted a buildup with increasing age in the abundance of distinctive pericellular nests made up of collagen fibrils, filaments, dense particles, and the 110-nm-banded structures, surrounding both viable and necrotic cells. Their occurrence may be related to the abundance in the nucleus pulposus of type VI collagen, which is the protein component of the 110-nm-banded structures.

Neutral proteases have been extracted from human intervertebral disc tissue that could degrade collagen, gelatin, and elastin[106] (see also Chapter 8). Both latent and active collagenase activities were demonstrated. That the collagenolytic activity could degrade native collagen molecules into three fourths and one fourth fragments, the hallmark of an animal collagenase, was however, not established.

VI. DEVELOPMENT, AGING, AND DISEASE

No dramatic changes were noted in the relative amounts of types I and II collagens in human lumbar discs from individuals aged 5, 16, 59, and 66 years.[1,52] The results of this limited study, however, suggested a possible increase in the proportion of type II collagen in the anterior annulus fibrosus between 5 and 16 years. Subsequently, very detailed measurements were reported of the collagen contents, type I/type II collagen ratios. and relative amounts of borohydride-reducible cross-links in individual lamellae dissected from the four separate quadrants of human discs.[107] Twenty-seven discs from six patients aged 13 to 78 years were dissected in this way and each piece was analyzed. The results showed that the proportion of type I collagen relative to type II collagen increased in the outer lamellar region of the posterior quadrant of the annulus fibrosus between adolescence and mature adulthood. Conversely, type II collagen increased relative to type I collagen in the outer lamellae of the anterior quadrants.

A smaller number of similar analyses were made on the collagen type distribution in discs removed from patients with idopathic scoliosis.[108] In individual discs from the apex of the scoliotic curve, the ratio of type I to type II collagens in the annulus fibrosus was different on the convex side compared with the concave side. Type I collagen was enriched in the compressed, concave side of the annulus. An altered distribution in the overall quantity of collagen in scoliotic discs had previously been noted.[108] The results on normal and scoliotic discs were taken as evidence that disc tissue can respond metabolically to changing mechanical forces and so alter the local composition of the extracellular matrix to better suit the new loading patterns. Thus, the increased type I collagen content of the posterior wall of the annulus fibrosus during skeletal growth and maturation and the increased type I collagen content in the compressed lateral half of a scoliotic disc were presumably the effects of metabolic responses of the tissue to altered mechanical forces. Such remodeling of a soft connective tissue in response to altered mechanical loading was likened to an expression of Wolff's Law, originally formulated for the remodeling ability of bone.[107] Potential variations in disc composition due to loading history during growth and adolescence may, therefore, be a factor in determining which discs and individuals are predisposed to disc degeneration in adult life.

In a related observation, possible changes were noted in the collagen content of human discs removed by anterior excision to correct spondylolisthesis.[109] Less type I and III collagen seemed to be present in the outer annulus layers as observed by immunofluorescence, perhaps resulting from biochemical changes caused by the mechanical trauma.

Chemonucleolysis, in which chymopapain is injected into herniated human discs to cure the symptoms of nerve root compression, has become an accepted alternative to surgery for many orthopedic surgeons and was approved for use by the Food and Drug Administration in the U.S. in 1982 (see Chapter 12). Some enthusiasts have injected bacterial collagenase, presumably on the premise that this enzyme may be a more potent and effective treatment with fewer side effects. In one study in Germany, 11 patients with low-back and sciatic pain were so treated.[110,111] Eight of the eleven needed open surgery to correct the failed chemonucleolysis, and the tissues removed were examined histologically. Two patients showed severe disabling vertebral bone necrosis. In four, the dorsal intervertebral ligament was destroyed, and in all, the cartilaginous end-plates were said to be destroyed to varying degrees. It was concluded that the enzyme had caused the extensive tissue damage to the surrounding structures of the disc, including end-plates, ligaments, bone, and epidural fat, as well as to the annulus fibrosus and nucleus pulposus. This interpretation has been questioned based on the surgical findings in 82 of 412 patients previously given intradiscal collagenase,[112] but the observations nevertheless are consistent with the potent ability of collagenase to destroy collagen in all its forms, which in itself is a reason for caution (see Chapter 12 for further discussion on this point).

VII. FUTURE DIRECTIONS

To understand the unique material properties[113,114] and functioning of the disc, more basic knowledge is needed at the molecular level about how collagen fibrils interact with each other and with the proteoglycan molecules that keep the collagen network inflated. In the annulus, particularly towards its outer edge, the coarse fiber bundles in adjacent lamellae that are anchored into vertebral bone may need to be ''lubricated'' or linked elastically so that they can slide relative to each other. In the nucleus pulposus and the annulus fibrosus, the type II fibrils may be coated with specific molecules to provide adhesion rather than lubrication. More work is needed on the minor types of collagen in the disc as potential mediators of interactions between collagen fibrils and between collagen fibrils and the proteoglycan domain. Such questions of supramolecular assembly and bonding are keys to understanding how the distinctive material properties of all connective tissues are regulated at the molecular level. The intervertebral disc presents for study an unusually complex yet organized range of textures and molecular mix of ingredients in its collagenous framework.

ACKNOWLEDGMENTS

Work described in the author's laboratory was supported in part by U.S. Public Health Service grants AM36794 and AM37245. Dr. Joseph Buckwalter generously supplied original electronmicrographs of fibrillar structures in human nucleus pulposus.

REFERENCES

1. **Eyre, D. R.,** Biochemistry of the intervertebral disc, *Int. Rev. Connect. Tissue Res.,* 8, 227, 1979.
2. **Eyre, D. R. and Muir, H.,** Collagen polymorphism: two molecular species in pig intervertebral disc, *FEBS Lett.,* 42, 192, 1974.
3. **Piez, K. A.,** Molecular and aggregate structures of the collagens, *Extracellular Matrix Biochemistry,* Piez, K. A. and Reddi, A. H., Eds., Elsevier, New York, 1984, chap. 1.

4. **Miller, E. J.,** The structure of fibril-forming collagens, *Ann. N.Y. Acad. Sci.,* 460, 1, 1985.
5. **Eyre, D. R.,** Collagen cross-linking amino acids, *Methods Enzymol.,* in press, 1986.
6. **Kuhn, K., Glanville, R. W., Babel, W., Qian, R., Dieringer, H., Voss, T., Siebold, B., Oberbaumer, I., Schwarz, U., and Yamada, Y.,** The structure of type IV collagen, *Ann. N.Y. Acad. Sci.,* 460, 14, 1985.
7. **Benya, P. D. and Padilla, S. R.,** Isolation and characterization of type VIII collagen synthesized by cultured rabbit corneal endothelial cells, *J. Biol. Chem.,* 261, 4160, 1986.
8. **Burgeson, R. E., El Adli, F. A., Kaitila, I. I., and Hollister, D. W.,** Fetal membrane collagens: identification of two new collagen alpha chains, *Proc. Natl. Acad. Sci. U.S.A.,* 73, 2579, 1976.
9. **Burgeson, R. E. and Hollister, D. W.,** Collagen heterogeneity in human cartilages: identification of several new collagen chains, *Biochem. Biophys. Res. Commun.,* 87, 1124, 1979.
10. **Eyre, D. R. and Wu, J. J.,** Type XI collagen ($1\alpha 2\alpha 3\alpha$), in *Structure and Function of Collagen Types,* Mayne, R., and Burgeson, R. E., Eds., *Biology of Extracellular Matrix,* Vol. I, Mecham, R. P., Ed., Academic Press, New York, 1987, 261.
11. **Broek, D. L., Madri, J., Eikenberry, E. F., and Brodsky, B.,** Characterization of the tissue form of type V collagen from chick bone, *J. Biol. Chem.,* 260, 555, 1985.
12. **Broek, D. L.,** Isolation and characterization of the intact forms of type V and 1α 2α 3α collagen, Ph.D. dissertation, Rutgers University, The State University of New Jersey, and the University of Medicine and Dentistry of New Jersey, Piscataway, 1984.
13. **Furoto, D. K. and Miller, E. J.,** Isolation of a unique collagenous fraction from limited pepsin digests of human placental tissue, *J. Biol. Chem.,* 255, 290, 1980.
14. **Gibson, M. A. and Cleary, E. G.,** A collagen-like glycoprotein from elastin-rich tissue, *Biochem. Biophys. Res. Commun.,* 105, 1288, 1982.
15. **Heller-Harrison, R. A. and Carter, W. G.,** Pepsin-generated type VI collagen is a degradation product of GP-140, *J. Biol. Chem.,* 259, 6858, 1984.
16. **Jander, R., Troyer, D., and Rauterberg, J.,** A collagen-like glycoprotein of the extracellular matrix is the undegraded form of type VI collagen, *Biochemistry,* 23, 3675, 1984.
17. **Furthmayr, H., Wiedemann, H., Timpl, R., Odermatt, E., and Engel, J.,** Electron-microscopical approach to a structural model of intima collagen, *Biochem. J.,* 211, 303, 1983.
18. **Trueb, B. and Bornstein, P.,** Characterization of the precursor form of type VI collagen, *J. Biol. Chem.,* 259, 8597, 1984.
19. **Engel, J., Furthmayr, H., Odermatt, E., von der Mark, H., Aumailley, M., Fleischmajer, R., and Timpl, R.,** Structure and macromolecular organization of type VI collagen, *Ann. N.Y. Acad. Sci.,* 460, 25, 1985.
20. **von der Mark, H., Aumailley, M., Wick, G., Fleischmajer, R., and Timpl, R.,** Immunochemistry, genuine size and tissue localization of collagen VI, *Eur. J. Biochem.,* 142, 493, 1984.
21. **Bruns, R. R.,** Beaded filaments and long-spacing fibrils: relation to type VI collagen, *J. Ultrastruct. Res.,* 89, 136, 1984.
22. **Buckwalter, J. A., Maynard, J. A., and Cooper, R. R.,** Banded structures in human nucleus pulposus, *Clin. Orthop.,* 139, 259, 1979.
23. **Bentz, H., Morris, N. P., Murray, L. W., Sakai, L. Y., Hollister, D. W., and Burgeson, R. W.,** Isolation and partial characterization of a new human collagen with an extended triple-helical structural domain, *Proc. Natl. Acad. Sci. U.S.A.,* 80, 3168, 1983.
24. **Burgeson, R. E., Morris, N. P., Murray, L. W., Duncan, K. G., Keene, D. R., and Sakai, L. Y.,** The structure of type VII collagen, *Ann. N.Y. Acad. Sci.,* 460, 47, 1985.
25. **Sage, H., Pritzl, P., and Bornstein, P.,** A unique, pepsin-sensitive collagen synthesized by aortic endothelial cells in culture, *Biochemistry,* 19, 5747, 1980.
26. **Benya, P. D.,** EC collagen: biosynthesis by corneal endothelial cells and separation from type IV without pepsin treatment or denaturation, *Renal Physiol.,* 3, 30, 1980.
27. **Labermeier, U. and Kenney, M. C.,** The presence of EC collagen and type IV collagen in bovine Descemet's membrane, *Biochem. Biophys. Res. Commun.,* 116, 619, 1983.
28. **Shimokomaki, M., Duance, V. C., and Bailey, A. J.,** Identification of a new disulphide bonded collagen from cartilage, *FEBS Lett.,* 121, 51, 1980.
29. **Ninomiya, Y. and Olsen, B. R.,** Synthesis and characterization of cDNA encoding a cartilage-specific short collagen, *Proc. Natl. Acad. Sci. U.S.A.,* 81, 3014, 1984.
30. **Ninomiya, Y., van der Rest, M., Mayne, R., Lozano, G., and Olsen, B. R.,** Construction and characterization of cDNA encoding the $\alpha 2$ chain of chicken type IX collagen, *Biochemistry,* 24, 4223, 1985.
31. **van der Rest, M., Mayne, R., Ninomiya, Y., Seidah, N. G., Chretien, M., and Olsen, B. R.,** The structure of type IX collagen, *J. Biol. Chem.,* 260, 220, 1985.
32. **Bruckner, P., Vaughan, L., and Winterhalter, K. H.,** Type IX collagen from sternal cartilage of chicken embryo contains covalently bound glycosaminoglycans, *Proc. Natl. Acad. Sci. U.S.A.,* 82, 2608, 1985.

33. **Noro, A., Kimata, K., Oike, Y., Shinomura, T., Maeda, N., Yano, S., Takahashi, N., and Suzuki, S.,** Isolation and characterization of third proteoglycan (PG-Lt) from chick embryo cartilage which contains disulfide-bonded collagenous polypeptide, *J. Biol. Chem.,* 258, 9323, 1983.

34. **Schmid, T. M. and Conrad, H. E.,** A unique low molecular weight collagen secreted by cultured chick embryo chondrocytes, *J. Biol. Chem.,* 257, 12444, 1982.

35. **Gibson, G. J., Schor, S. L., and Grant, M. E.,** Effects of matrix macromolecules on chondrocyte gene expression: synthesis of a low molecular weight collagen species by cells cultured within collagen gels, *J. Cell Biol.,* 93, 767, 1982.

36. **Schmid, T. M. and Linsenmayer, T. F.,** Developmental acquisition of type X collagen in embryonic chick tibiotarsus, *Develop. Biol.,* 107, 373, 1985.

37. **Grant, W. T., Sussman, M. D., and Balian, G.,** A disulfide-bonded short chain collagen synthesized by degenerative and calcifying zones of bovine growth plate cartilage, *J. Biol. Chem.,* 260, 3798, 1985.

38. **Remington, M. C., Bashey, R. I., Brighton, C. T., and Jimenez, S. A.,** Biosynthesis of a disulphide-bonded short chain collagen by calf growth-plate cartilage, *Biochem. J.,* 224, 227, 1984.

39. **Schmid, T. M., Mayne, R., Bruns, R. R., and Linsenmayer, T. F.,** Molecular structure of short-chain (SC) cartilage collagen by electron microscopy, *J. Ultrastruct. Res.,* 86, 186, 1984.

40. **Schmid, T. M., Mayne, R., Jaffrey, J. J., and Linsenmayer, T. F.,** Type X collagen contains two cleavage sites for a vertebrate collagenase, *J. Biol. Chem.,* 261, 4184, 1986.

41. **Ninomiya, Y., Gordon, M., van der Rest, M., Schmid, T., Linsenmayer, T., and Olsen, B. R.,** The developmentally regulated type X collagen gene contains a long open reading frame without introns, *J. Biol. Chem.,* 261, 5041, 1986.

42. **Church, R. C., Sundar Raj, C. V., and McDougall, J. K.,** Regional chromosomal mapping of the human skin type I procollagen gene using adenovirus 12-fragmentation of human/mouse somatic cell hybrids, *Cytogenet. Cell Genet.,* 27, 24, 1980.

43. **Solomon, E., Hiorns, L., Dalgleish, R., Tolstoshev, P., Crystal, R., and Sykes, B.,** Regional localization of the human α2(I) collagen gene on chromosome 7 by molecular hybridization, *Cytogenet. Cell Genet.,* 35, 64, 1983.

44. **Huerre-Jeanpierre, C., Mattel, M., Weil, D., Grzeschik, K. H., Chu, M., Sangiorgi, F. O., Sobel, M. E., Ramirez, F., and Junien, C.,** Further evidence for the dispersion of the human fibrillar collagen genes, *Am. J. Hum. Genet.,* 38, 26, 1986.

45. **Strom, C. M., Eddy, R. L., and Shows, T. B.,** Localization of human type II procollagen gene (COL2A1) to chromosome 12, *Somat. Cell. Mol. Genet.,* 10, 651, 1984.

46. **Solomon, E., Hiorns, L. R., Spurr, N., Kurkinen, M., Barlow, D., Hogan, B. L. M., and Dalgleish, R.,** Chromosomal assignments of the genes coding for human types II, III and IV collagen: a dispersed gene family, *Proc. Natl. Acad. Sci., U.S.A.,* 82, 330, 1985.

47. **Emanuel, B. S., Cannizzano, L. A., Seyer, J. M., and Myers, J. C.,** Human α1(III) and α2(V) procollagen genes are located on the long arm of chromosome 2, *Proc. Natl. Acad. Sci. U.S.A.,* 82, 3385, 1985.

48. **Emanuel, B. S., Sellinger, B. T., Gudas, L. J., and Myers, J. C.,** Localization of the human procollagen α1(IV) gene to chromosome 13q34 by in situ hybridization, *Am. J. Hum. Genet.,* 38, 38, 1986.

49. **de Crombrugghe, B., Liau, G., Setoyama, C., Schmidt, A., McKeon, C., and Mudryj, M.,** Structural and functional studies on the interstitial collagen genes, in *Fibrosis,* Ciba Foundation Symposium 114, Pitman, London, 1985, 20.

50. **Eyre, D. R.,** unpublished results,

51. **Eyre, D. R. and Muir, H.,** Types I and II collagens in intervertebral disc: interchanging radial distributions in annulus fibrosus, *Biochem. J.,* 157, 267, 1976.

52. **Eyre, D. R. and Muir, H.,** Quantitative analysis of types I and II collagens in human intervertebral discs at various ages, *Biochim. Biophys. Acta,* 492, 29, 1977.

53. **Beard, K. H., Ryvar, R., Brown, R., and Muir, H.,** Immunochemical localization of collagen types and proteoglycan in pig intervertebral discs, *Immunology,* 41, 491, 1980.

54. **Beard, H. K., Roberts, S., and O'Brien, J. P.,** Immunofluorescent staining for collagen and proteoglycan in normal and scoliotic intervertebral discs, *J. Bone Jt. Surg.,* 63B, 529, 1981.

55. **Eyre, D. R., Wu, J. J., and Apone, S.,** unpublished results.

56. **Eyre, D. R.,** Collagen structure and function: its relevance to spinal disease, in *Symp. Idiopathic Low Back Pain,* White, A. A. and Gordon, S. L., Eds., C. V. Mosby, St. Louis, 1982, 357.

57. **Ayad, S., Abedin, M. Z., Grundy, S. M., and Weiss, J. B.,** Isolation and characterisation of an unusual collagen from hyaline cartilage and intervertebral disc, *FEBS Lett.,* 123, 195, 1981.

58. **Ayad, S., Abedin, M. Z., Weiss, J. B., and Grundy, S. M.,** Characterization of another short-chain disulphide-bonded collagen from cartilage, vitreous and intervertebral disc, *FEBS Lett.,* 139, 300, 1982.

59. **Ayad, S. and Weiss, J. B.,** Biochemistry of the intervertebral disc, in *The Lumbar Spine and Back Pain,* 3rd ed., Jayson, M. I. V., Ed., Pitman Publ., London, 1986.

60. **Wu, J. J. and Eyre, D. R.,** unpublished results.

61. **Linsenmayer, T. F., Fitch, J. M., Gross, J., and Mayne, R.,** Are collagen fibrils in the developing avian cornea composed of two different collagen types? Evidence from monoclonal antibody studies, *Ann. N.Y. Acad. Sci.,* 460, 232, 1985.

62. **Smith, G. N., Jr., Williams, J. M., and Brandt, K. D.,** Interaction of proteoglycans with the pericellular ($1\alpha2\alpha3\alpha$) collagens of cartilage, *J. Biol. Chem.,* 260, 10761, 1985.

63. **Cornah, M. S., Maechim, G., and Parry, E. W.,** Banded structures in the matrix of human and rabbit nucleus pulposus, *J. Anat.,* 107, 351, 1970.

64. **Smith, J. W. and Serafini-Fracassini, A.,** The distribution of the protein-polysaccharide complex in the nucleus pulposus matrix in young rabbits, *J. Cell Sci.,* 33, 33, 1968.

65. **Wu, J. J., Apone, S., Eyre, D. R., and Slayter, H. S.,** Type VI collagen of the intervertebral disc. Biochemical and electronmicroscope characterization of the native protein, *Biochem. J.,* 248(2), 373, 1987.

66. **Zimmerman, D. R., Treub, B., Winterhalter, K. H., Witmer, R., and Fischer, R. W.,** Type VI collagen is a major component of the human cornea, *FEBS Lett.,* 197, 55, 1986.

67. **Bruns, R. R., Press, W., Engvall, E., Timpl, R., and Gross, J.,** Type VI collagen in extracellular, 100 nm periodic filaments and fibrils: identification by immunoelectron microscopy, *J. Cell Biol.,* in press.

68. **Duance, V. C., Shimokomaki, M., and Bailey, A. J.,** Immunofluorescence localization of type-M collagen in articular cartilage, *Biosci. Rep.,* 2, 223, 1982.

69. **Hartmann, D. J., Magloire, H., Ricard-Blum, S., Joffre, A., Couble, M., Ville, G., and Herbage, D.,** Light and electron immunoperoxidase localization of minor disulfide-bonded collagens in fetal calf epiphyseal cartilage, *Collagen Relat. Res.,* 3, 349, 1982.

70. **Irwin, M. H., Silvers, S. H., and Mayne, R.,** Monoclonal antibody against chicken type IX collagen: preparation, characterization, and recognition of the intact form of type IX collagen secreted by chondrocytes, *J. Cell Biol.,* 101, 814, 1985.

71. **Muller-Glauser, W., Humbel, B., Glatt, M., Stranli, P., Winterhalter, K. H., and Bruckner, P.,** On the role of type IX collagen in the extracellular matrix of cartilage: type IX collagen is localized to intersections of collagen fibrils, *J. Cell Biol.,* 102, 1931, 1986.

72. **Wu, J. J. and Eyre, D. R.,** Cartilage type IX collagen is cross-linked by hydroxypyridinium residues, *Biochem. Biophys. Res. Commun.,* 123, 1033, 1984.

73. **Eyre, D. R., Paz, M. A., and Gallop, P. M.,** Cross-linking in collagen and elastin, *Annu. Rev. Biochem.,* 53, 717, 1984.

74. **Eyre, D. R.,** Collagen stability through covalent cross-linking, *Advances in Meat Research,* Vol. 4, *Collagen as a Food,* Pearson, A. M., Dutson, T. R., and Bailey, A. J., Eds., Van Nostrand Reinhold, New York, 1987, 69.

75. **Bailey, A. J. and Peach, C. M.,** The chemistry of the collagen cross-links. The absence of reduction of dehydrolysinonorleucine and dehydrohydroxylysinonorleucine in vivo., *Biochem. J.,* 121, 257, 1971.

76. **Herbert, C. M., Lindberg, K. A., Jayson, M. I. V., and Bailey, A. J.,** Changes in the collagen of human intervertebral discs during ageing and degenerate disc disease, *J. Mol. Med.,* 1, 79, 1975.

77. **Eyre, D. R., Koob, T. J., and Van Ness, K.,** Quantitation of hydroxypyridinium cross-links in collagen by high performance liquid chromatography, *Anal. Biochem.,* 137, 380, 1984.

78. **Eyre, D. R.,** Collagen cross-linking in normal and diseased skeletal connective tissues, in *Pathogenesis of Idiopathic Scoliosis,* Jacobs, R. R., Ed., Scoliosis Research Society, Chicago, 1984, 107.

79. **Hukins, D. W. L. and Aspden, R. M.,** Composition and properties of connective tissues, *Trends Biochem. Sci.,* 10, 260, 1985.

80. **Eyre, D. R.,** unpublished results.

81. **Harding, J. J.,** Non-enzymatic covalent posttranslational modification of proteins, *in vivo, Adv. Protein Chem.,* 37,. 247, 1985.

82. **Tanzer, M. L., Fairweather, R., and Gallop, P. M.,** Collagen cross-links: isolation of reduced N^c-Hexosylhydroxylysine from borohydride-reduced calf skin insoluble collagen, *Arch. Biochem. Biophys.,* 151, 137, 1972.

83. **Robins, S. P. and Bailey, A. J.,** Age-related changes in collagen: the identification of reducible lysine-carbohydrate condensation products, *Biochem. Biophys. Res. Commun.,* 48, 76, 1972.

84. **Monnier, V. M., Vishwanath, V., Frank, K. E., Elmets, C. A., Dauchot, P., and Kohn, R. R.,** Relation between complications of type I diabetes mellitus and collagen-linked fluorescence, *N. Engl. J. Med.,* 314, 403, 1986.

85. **Monnier, V. M. and Cerami, A.,** Nonenzymatic browning in vivo: possible process for aging of long-lived proteins, *Science,* 211, 491, 1981.

86. **Eble, A. S., Thorpe, S. R., and Baynes, J. W.,** Nonenzymatic glucosylation and glucose-dependent cross-linking of protein, *J. Biol. Chem.,* 258, 9406, 1983.

87. **Pongor, S., Ulrich, P. C., Bencsath, F. A., and Cerami, A.,** Aging of proteins: isolation and identification of a fluorescent chromophore from the reaction of polypeptides with glucose, *Proc. Natl. Acad. Sci. U.S.A.,* 81, 2684, 1984.

88. **Banga, I.,** Investigations of fluorescent peptides and lipofuscins of human intervertebral discs relating to atherosclerosis, *Atherosclerosis,* 22, 533, 1975.

89. **Berthet, C., Hulmes, D. J. S., Miller, A., and Timmins, P. A.,** Structure of collagen in cartilage of intervertebral disk, *Science,* 199, 547, 1978.

90. **Berthet-Colominas, C., Miller, A., Herbage, D., Ronziere, M., and Tocchetti, D.,** Structural studies of collagen fibres from intervertebral disc, *Biochim. Biophys. Acta,* 706, 50, 1982.

91. **Grynpas, M. D., Eyre, D. R., and Kirschner, D. A.,** Collagen type II differs from type I in native molecular packing, *Biochim. Biophys. Acta,* 626, 346, 1980.

92. **Hickey, D. S. and Hukins, D. W. L.,** X-ray diffraction studies of the arrangement of collagenous fibres in human fetal intervertebral disc, *J. Anat.,* 131, 81, 1980.

93. **Klein, J. A. and Hukins, D. W. L.,** Collagen fibre orientation in the annulus fibrosus of intervertebral disc during bending and torsion measured by x-ray diffraction, *Biochim. Biophys. Acta,* 719, 98, 1982.

94. **Klein, J. A. and Hukins, D. W. L.,** X-ray diffraction demonstrates reorientation of collagen fibres in the annulus fibrosus during compression of the intervertebral disc, *Biochim. Biophys. Acta,* 717, 61, 1982.

95. **Klein, J. A., Hickey, D. S., and Hukins, D. W. L.,** Radial bulging of the annulus fibrosus during compression of the intervertebral disc, *J. Biomech.,* 16, 211, 1983.

96. **Hickey, D. S. and Hukins, D. W. L.,** Relation between the structure of the annulus fibrosus and the function and failure of the intervertebral disc, *Spine,* 5, 106, 1980.

97. **Hickey, D. S. and Hukins, D. W. L.,** Collagen fibril diameters and elastic fibres in the annulus fibrosus of human fetal intervertebral discs, *J. Anat.,* 133, 351, 1981.

98. **Hickey, D. S. and Hukins, D. W. L.,** Aging changes in the macromolecular organization of the intervertebral disc, *Spine,* 7, 234, 1982.

99. **Buckwalter, J. A., Maynard, J. A. and Cooper, R. R.,** Sheathing of collagen fibrils in human intervertebral discs, *J. Anat.,* 125, 614, 1978.

100. **Butler, W. F. and Heaps, P.,** An ultrastructural study of glycosaminoglycans associated with collagen and other constituents of the cat annulus fibrosus, *Histochem. J.,* 14, 113, 1982.

101. **Inoue, H. and Takeda, T.,** Three-dimensional observation of collagen framework of lumbar intervertebral discs, *Acta Orthop. Scand.,* 46, 949, 1975.

102. **Inoue, H.,** Three-dimensional architecture of lumbar intervertebral discs, *Spine,* 6, 139, 1981.

103. **Maroudas, A.,** Nutrition and metabolism of the intervertebral disc, in *Symp. Idiopathic Low Back Pain,* White, A. A. and Gordon, S. L., Eds., C. V. Mosby, St. Louis, 1982, 370.

104. **Buckwalter, J. A.,** The fine structure of human intervertebral disc, in *Symp. Idiopathic Low Back Pain,* White, A. A. and Gordon, S. L., Eds., C. V. Mosby, St. Louis, 1982, 108.

105. **Trout, J. J., Buckwalter, J. A., and Moore, K. C.,** Ultrastructure of the human intervertebral disc. II. Cells of the nucleus pulposus, *Anat. Record,* 204, 307, 1982.

106. **Sedowofia, K. A., Tomlinson, I. W., Weiss, J. B., Hilton, R. C., and Jayson, M. I. V.,** Collagenolytic enzyme stystems in human intervertebral disc: their control, mechanism and their possible role in the initiation of biomechanical failure, *Spine,* 7, 213, 1982.

107. **Brickley-Parsons, D. and Glimcher, M. J.,** Is the chemistry of collagen in intervertebral discs an expression of Wolff's Law? A study of the human lumbar spine, *Spine,* 9, 148, 1984.

108. **Bushell, G. R., Ghosh, P., Taylor, T. K. F., and Sutherland, J. M.,** The collagen of the intervertebral disc in adolescent idiopathic scoliosis, *J. Bone Jt. Surg.,* 61B, 501, 1979.

109. **Roberts, S., Beard, H. K., and O'Brien, J. P.,** Biochemical changes of intervertebral discs in patients with spondylolisthesis or with tears of the posterior annulus fibrosus, *Ann. Rheum. Dis.,* 41, 78, 1982.

110. **Artigas, J., Brock, M., and Mayer, H.,** Complications following chemonucleolysis with collagenase, *J. Neurosurg.,* 61, 679, 1984.

111. **Brock, M., Roggendorf, W., Gorge, H. H., and Curio, G.,** Severe local tissue lesions after chemonucleolysis with collagenase, *Surg. Neurol.,* 22, 124, 1984.

112. **Fisher, R. G., Bromley, J. W., Becker, G. L., Brown, M., and Mooney, V.,** Surgical experience following intervertebral discolysis with collagenase, *J. Neurosurg.,* 64, 613, 1986.

113. **Urban, J. P. G. and Maroudas, A.,** Swelling of the intervertebral disc *in vitro, Connect. Tissue Res.,* 9, 1, 1981.

114. **Urban, J. P. G. and McMullin, J. F.,** Swelling pressure of the intervertebral disc: influence of proteoglycan and collagen contents, *Biorheology,* 22, 145, 1985.

115. **Wu, J. J. and Eyre, D. R.,** unpublished results.

Chapter 8

THE NONCOLLAGENOUS PROTEINS OF THE INTERVERTEBRAL DISC*

James Melrose and Peter Ghosh

TABLE OF CONTENTS

---

* Abbreviations for this chapter are as follows: AA, amyloid A protein; AF, annulus fibrosus; α_1-PI, α_1-proteinase inhibitor; CHAPS, 3-[(3-cholamidopropyl)-dimethylammonio]-1-propane sulfonate; DEAE, diethyl amino ethyl-; ELISA, enzyme-linked immunosorbent assay; GAG, glycosaminoglycan; HA, hyaluronic acid; HLE, human leukocyte elastase; IVD, intervertebral disc; JRA, juvenile rheumatoid arthritis; KS, keratan sulfate; NCP, noncollagenous protein; NP, nucleus pulposus; PG, proteoglycan; SAA, serum amyloid A protein; SAP, serum amyloid P component; SDS, sodium dodecyl sulfate.

I. INTRODUCTION

The term noncollagenous proteins is a generalized term encompassing all other proteins present within the disc other than collagen. For the purposes of this review, PGs have been omitted since they are covered extensively elsewhere in this volume (Chapter 6) and type VI collagen will be considered as an NCP since it contains an NCP component, although it is also discussed in Chapter 7. The disc NCPs, therefore, include structural glycoproteins, cell membrane bound receptors and intercalated membrane glycoproteins which are strongly implicated in the interaction of the disc cell with the extracellular matrix. Amyloid and amyloid-related proteins, extravascular plasma proteins, and endogenous proteinases and proteinase inhibitors are also present and would appear to be involved in the aging and degenerative processes.

Despite the fact that the noncollagenous proteins of the human IVD collectively may constitute up to 45% of the dry weight of the NP and 25% of the AF and increase with age,[1-7] it is remarkable that so little is known of their composition and properties. This paucity of data has necessitated, for the purpose of this review, analogies with other connective tissues, particularly hyaline cartilage, where more extensive investigations have been reported. Since the majority of cells resident within the disc may be considered to be fibrochondrocytes,[8,9] synthesizing types I and II collagen as well as PG aggregates with similar characteristics to those of hyaline cartilage, we consider that such analogies are valid.

The intervertebral disc is a heterogenous structure containing regions morphologically identifiable as hyaline and fibro-cartilage. Nevertheless, each is characterized by an abundant extracellular matrix containing relatively few cells which are responsible for the synthesis and degradation of the matrix components.

The morphology of the various cartilages varies with their origin and specialized function. This is reflected by the types and proportions of the noncollagenous proteins present within these tissues (see Table 1).

Fibrocartilage is the most abundant tissue of the disc and is characterized morphologically by an abundance of highly oriented collagen fibers. These bestow high tensile strength to the AF and, in conjunction with PGs and water, also provide resistance to compression which is a prerequisite for disc function (see Chapter 1 and 10). Furthermore, the normal adult disc, like other connective tissues, is largely avascular and is therefore dependent on diffusive processes, which are in turn a function of matrix composition (see Chapter 9). However, these diffusion processes may be augmented by the movement of solutes in and out of the disc during compression and relaxation.[10,11] The cartilage cell is enclosed in a lacunae which, in the intact tissue, is occupied by the chondrocyte and its pericellular matrix. Lacunae may contain one or more cells in the form of clones.[12] Early work suggested that the lacunae, complete with chondrocyte clones and their surrounding territorial matrix, represented specialized regions within the matrix which could be regarded as functional subunits or chondrons. This concept has, however, been challenged by Clarke.[13] While similar studies have not been described for the fibrocartilage of the AF, this tissue is particularly well organized, and recent studies (see Chapter 7) have identified subtleties in the assembly and orientation of the collagens within this tissue, which leads us to conclude that the microenvironment of the disc cell is also highly structured. There is every reason to expect that the matrix noncollagenous proteins occupy a prominent role in such cell-matrix interrelationships.

II. STRUCTURAL GLYCOPROTEINS

A. Solubilization of Extracellular Matrix Glycoproteins

The isolation of structural noncollagenous proteins from connective tissues has been

Table 1
EXTRACELLULAR MATRIX NONCOLLAGENOUS PROTEINS OF THE DISC AND RELATED CONNECTIVE TISSUES

Protein	Known physicochemical characteristics	Tissue distribution/ localization	Functional characteristics	Ref.
Link Proteins				
Human AC link proteins	Link proteins 1,2,3, of 41,44, and 48 kdalton mol wt by SDS PAGE pI 6—7; 9 subcomponents	Widespread throughout cartilaginous tissues, e.g., hyaline cartilage fibrocartilage also present in synovium	Stabilizes proteoglycan aggregates; possible link protein collagen association suggesting a structural role also[407,408]	406
Bovine nasal cartilage link protein	41, 44 and 48 kdalton mol wt by SDS PAGE pI 6—7; subcomponents; 42 kdaltons enzymic breakdown product also evident	Widespread throughout cartilaginous tissues, e.g., hyaline cartilage fibrocartilage also present in synovium	Stabilizes proteoglycan aggregates; possible link protein collagen association suggesting a structural role also[407,408]	409
Human intervertebral disc link proteins	38.9, 44.2, and 50.1 kdaltons mol wt by SDS PAGE on reduction gave 14, 20, and 43-kdalton mol wt species	Found in both NP, AF, and cartilaginous end-plate	Appear to stabilize proteoglycan aggregates less well than the bovine nasal link protein	285
Human intervertebral disc link proteins	Link proteins 1, 2, 3, all evident; however, small mol wt fragments evident also	NP, AF, and cartilaginous end-plate	Link protein from humans aged 3 weeks to 27 years displayed similarities to link proteins from old articular cartilage	410
Hyaluronate Binding Proteins				
Hyaluronic acid-binding protein/ link protein?	70-kdalton molecule reacts with antiarticular cartilage link proteins and has an identical peptide map also; however, does not interact with proteoglycans	Canine articular cartilage and synovial cells	Not known	411
Hyaluronic acid-binding protein from human articular cartilage	60 kdalton mol wt by gel filtration on Sepharose® CL 6B; 75 kdaltons by SDS PAGE possibly derived from proteoglycans	Only identified in human AC so far but probably widespread distribution in cartilages, especially in the IVD	Not known	412, 413

Table 1 (continued)

EXTRACELLULAR MATRIX NONCOLLAGENOUS PROTEINS OF THE DISC AND RELATED CONNECTIVE TISSUES

Protein	Known physicochemical characteristics	Tissue distribution/ localization	Functional characteristics	Ref.
Hyaluronic acid-binding protein from human costal cartilage	50—70 kdalton mol wt mixture of noncollagenous proteins, incompletely characterized; however, HA-binding protein evident	human costal cartilage		414
Hyaluronic acid-binding protein	28-kdalton protein from cell-free cartilage mRNA translation system	Articular cartilage	Not known, possibly matrix stabilization	415
Chondronectin	Intact molecule 180 kdaltons, which on reduction yields 80-kdalton subunit (both estimations by SDS PAGE)	Has only been purified from serum, but chondrocytes in culture synthesize a similar protein which still awaits purification	Chondrocyte adhesion molecule which enables binding to type II collagen	
Calcium-Binding Proteins				
Calcium-binding protein S100	An acidic 21—24-kdalton protein	Found in normal human chondrocytes and cartilage tumors; localized in cytoplasm of cell in osteochondroma, chondromatosis, chondrosarcoma, chondromyxoid-fibroma, enchondroma, clear cell chondrosarcoma.	Implicated in matrix calcification	160, 162, 163, 416
Chondrocalcin, calf epiphyseal cartilage matrix protein	69-kdalton molecule shows strong affinity for hydroxyappatite; composed of 35-kdalton subunits; 4% carbohydrate which is high in mannose oligosaccharides	Fetal and also some adult cartilage, enriched in regions of epiphyseal cartilage where early mineralization is evident	Mineralization of cartilage and endochondral ossification	161, 417
Trimeric IVD NCP possibly related to chondracalcin	105 and 110 kdalton mol wt which on reduction with DTT	Abundant in growing young tissues, e.g., AC and NP	Unclear, possibly related to chondrocalcin (but is trimeric) or a	418

Matrix Glycoproteins

	yields 35- and 37-kdalton subunits resistant to bacterial collagenase but susceptible to pepsin; firmly attached to PG-HA link protein complex		collagen propeptide; structural role in extracellular matrix maturation	
36-kdalton matrix protein	36 kdaltons mol wt not link protein high Leu content	Widespread distribution in mammalian cartilages including AF, articular, epiphyseal, auricular, xiphosternal, nasal, and tracheal cartilages	Not known	419—421
Chondrocyte plasma membrane glycoprotein anchorin CII	31-kdaltons mol wt high glycine content; 183.5 res/1000 res; contains hydroxylysine but no hydroxy protein 30% carbohydrate of which 60% is fucose by GLC; poorly soluble in aq. soln — requires detergents for solubilization. Interacts with collagen	Chondrocyte plasma cell membrane	Links chondrocyte to type II collagen in pericellular matrix; specific receptor for type II collagen	97, 98, 422, 423
Rabbit AC marker protein for OA lesion	160 kdaltons heavily glycosylated; suggested as a marker for OA lesions	Present, localized in fibrillated regions of AC but not in normal AC	Unclear; possibly structural, repair of OA lesions;	424
Rabbit and human AC NCP	Incompletely characterized; 2 glycoproteins present in super PG aggregates but absent in smaller OA PG aggregates		stabilization of PG super aggregates	425
Bovine proximal humeral AC	2.7S NCP extracted by 4 M GuHCl, but not present in 70S PG aggregate by sedimentation velocity ultracentrifugation	Not known	Binding of PG to collagen	426

Table 1 (continued)

EXTRACELLULAR MATRIX NONCOLLAGENOUS PROTEINS OF THE DISC AND RELATED CONNECTIVE TISSUES

Matrix Glycoproteins

Protein	Known physicochemical characteristics	Tissue distribution/localization	Functional characteristics	Ref.
Puppy rib cartilage glycoproteins A and G	Acidic proteins, high Asp and Glu contents; low hydroxy-pro normally present as insoluble complex with collagen — extraction with urea/NaOH/DTT; 87K, 30K, 27.5L subunit has affinity for collagen, fibrinogen, and heparin and reacts with an antibody to fibronectin; highly aggregative	Puppy rib cartilage	Structural, interaction with collagen and other extracellular matrix components	59, 427
Calf rib cartilage glycoproteins	8 Glycoproteins (not link proteins), isolated by SDS PAGE, of mol wt 105, 77, 59, 49, 41, 35, 30, and 22 kdaltons, all relatively rich in Gly and Ala, poorly characterized	Calf rib cartilage	Structural glycoproteins	428
Human costal cartilage glycoprotein	7 PG-associated glycoproteins of mol wt (by SDS PAGE) of 90, 69, 60, 57, 50, 40, and 30 kdaltons, poorly characterized	Human costal cartilage	Structural glycoproteins associated with PG-role in matrix stabilization	414
Human and primate AC NCP	Very poorly and simplistically characterized despite multiple publication; mol wt 87, 64, 56, 46, 41, and 27 kdaltons quoted by SDS PAGE (includes 2 link proteins)	Apparently wide distribution in young and old baboon AC; found in degenerate joints also	Not known	429, 430
Cartilage matrix proteins	Intact mol wt of 148 kdaltons by sedimentation equilibrium ultra-	Widespread in mammalian, rabbit, rat, human, bovine cartilages	Matrix stabilization	419, 420, 431

	Description	Distribution	Function	Ref.
	centrifugation; composed of subunits of 52 kdaltons on reduction; low content aromatic amino acids; no hypro, 3.9% carbohydrate mainly N-linked oligosaccharides of mannose insoluble in 0.1 M GuHCl; interacts with PG	(xiphisternal, auricular, epiphyseal); however, apparently not present in AC or IVD		433
Matrix protein	550-kdalton glycoprotein composed of 116-kdalton subunit; appears not to interact with PG but interacts with type II collagen	Widespread distribution in mammalian hyaline and fibrocartilages, synovium, and aorta; present in IVD, NP and AF; localized in the pericellular region around the chondrocyte.	Structural, matrix stabilization	434—438
Type VI collagen	Heavily disulfide bonded: upon reduction 250—170 kdalton bands obtained; when digested with pepsin yields 40—50 kdalton fragments; technically not NCP, but was originally considered to be one	A prominent matrix component in the IVD also present in meniscus and tendon	Structural	22, 91, 439
Elastin	Highly insoluble macromolecular fibrous protein, rich in hydrophobic amino acids and contains few polar groups; cross-linked by the unique amino acids desmosine and also other cross-links based on lysine; synthesized as a soluble precursor tropoelastin (72,000 mol wt)	Minor component in NP and AF of IVD widely distributed in elastic cartilages from mammals; a component of the hip joint capsule; elastin is synthesized by mesenchymal cells including fibroblasts, chondroblasts, smooth muscle cells, and endothelial cells; a major component of elastic cartilages	Convey dynamic elasticity and resiliency, particularly important in low strain deformation in IVD	69, 70, 72, 92, 440—442

Note: Abbreviations used: DTT, dithiothreitol; SDS PAGE, sodium dodecyl sulfate polyacrylamide gel electorphoresis; NP, nucleus pulposus; AF, annulus fibrosus; AC, articular cartilage; OA, osteoarthritic; HA, hyaluronic acid; PG, proteoglycan; GuHCl, guanidine hydrochloride; NCP, non collagenous protein; and IVD, intervertebral disc.

hampered by their strong interactions with collagen and other insoluble proteins.[1,14-16] Several approaches have been taken to achieve solubilization and these are briefly described.

Dissociative extraction using chaotropic salts or protein denaturants, such as high molarity solutions of NaCl, LiCl, $MgCl_2$, $LaCl_3$, $CaCl_2$, urea, GuHCl, or sodium thiocyanate has been commonly employed.[17-20] Unfortunately, however, after removal of these denaturing salts, there is no guarantee that the native interactive properties of the extracted components will be restored. The relatively insoluble and self-aggregative nature of many of the structural glycoproteins may necessitate that a certain level of salt be present to maintain their solubility. This may impose limitations on the subsequent fractionation steps to be used.

Extraction methods employing specific enzymes under mild conditions represent a gentle, yet effective, method of solubilization of structural proteins in their native state. Selective removal of insoluble collagen has been accomplished using purified collagenase, leaving the structural NCP of interest intact and more readily solubilized by other methods.[21] Glycosidases, such as hyaluronidase or chondroitinase, either singly or in combination, have been used to isolate structural proteins from the IVD after selective removal of PGs and HA from the sample.[22]

Reducing agents such as dithiothreitol, *N*-acetylcysteine, or mercaptoethanol, often used in conjunction with the aforementioned dissociative solvents,[23] have been employed in the extraction of highly disulfide cross-linked glycoproteins. However, the peptide chains so isolated may differ in molecular weight and physicochemical properties from the parent molecule, and this limits the application of this method. It is considered advisable to carry out reduction and alkylation under strongly denaturing conditions to ensure complete modification of sulfhydryl groups. Unless this is done, there is a danger that the addition of thiol-reducing agents under nondenaturing conditions may lead to activation of endogenous proteases with subsequent unwanted modification of the glycoproteins of interest.

Membrane-bound glycoproteins have been solubilized with detergents.[24,25] Three main categories have been used: (1) ionic surfactants, e.g., SDS; (2) nonionic surfactants, e.g., Triton® X-100; and (3) bile salts, e.g., sodium deoxycholate. Each type has particular properties which govern its interaction with lipids and proteins and determines its applicability to the solubilization of membrane glycoproteins. The efficiency of extraction of membrane glycoproteins by nonionic detergents depends on several experimental variables, besides the choice of detergent. These include the ratio of detergent to membrane, temperature, time, number of extractions, ionic strength, and the nature of the ionic species and pH.[26]

Nonionic detergents have little tendency to denature proteins or to influence protein-protein interactions. They are, therefore, of great value in solubilizing membrane glycoproteins, where it is important to maintain protein functionality. Similarly, bile salts are considerably less prone to denature proteins than is SDS.

B. Fractionation of Solubilized Noncollagenous Proteins

Once the glycoprotein of interest has been solubilized, it becomes possible to apply techniques singularly or in combination for its purification and/or fractionation based on solubility, size and shape, charge, density, absorption characteristics, or affinity properties. The fractionation procedure employed may be limited by the extractive conditions used, e.g., strong chaotropic salts, denaturing agents, or ionic detergents, such as SDS. These may result in a loss of native protein conformation and, thus, an inability to fractionate these proteins on the basis of their biological activities. Similarly, nonionic detergents may bind to membrane glycoproteins in such a way as to interfere in subsequent gel filtration or rate zonal centrifugation studies.

1. Fractionation Based on Solubility

This method is related to the variable solubility properties of the noncollagenous proteins. Sequential extractions with dissociative solvents of increasing concentration often may prove suitable as an initial step in the isolation of a particular glycoprotein.[20] Glycoproteins with high carbohydrate contents may be resistant to precipitation by common protein precipitants, such as trichloracetic acid or perchloric acid, and this characteristic may be used to advantage in an isolation procedure. Although the interaction of cetyl trimethyl ammonium and cetyl pyridinium salts with acidic polysaccharides is well known, highly charged glycoproteins may also be precipitated by this procedure.[27,28]

2. Fractionation Based on Size and Shape

Gel filtration techniques employing beads of polymerized dextran (Sephadex®), polyacrylamide (Bio-gel®), or agarose (Sepharose®, Bio-gel®) have found wide application in the purification of glycoproteins and are described extensively in the literature.[29,30] Gel filtration of membrane glycoproteins has been successfully conducted in the presence of ionic detergents such as SDS[31] or deoxycholate, which minimize nonspecific interactions and limit zone broadening.[26] Rate zonal sucrose density gradient centrifugation has also been used to fractionate glycoproteins in which the sedimentation rate depends on molecular size and asymmetry. However, abnormalities in sedimentation rates may be evident if the original extractive method employed detergent. Rate zonal centrifugation may allow separation of proteins with differing sedimentation rates, which may have similar isopycnic densities and are, thus, not separable using conventional equilibrium density gradient ultracentrifugation.

3. Fractionation Based on Charge

Ion-exchange chromatography has been applied extensively in glycoprotein separations following similar methodologies to those utilized for general protein separations.[29] Many structural noncollagenous proteins carry a negative charge at neutral pH and, thus, will bind to DEAE ion-exchange resins.[32] Glycoproteins with high sialic acid content or those which are sulfated are usually bound strongly and require strong salt elution conditions. Peak broadening due to charge interaction of different glycoprotein species can be eliminated by conducting ion-exchange chromatography in the presence of urea or nonionic detergent. Additionally, inclusion of zwitterionic detergents such as CHAPS in buffers may improve recoveries of small quantities of glycoproteins.[33] Isoelectric focusing in polyacrylamide slab gels and chromatography columns has also been utilized in the purification of glycoproteins.[17]

4. Fractionation Based on Density Differences

Ultracentrifugation in density gradients of cesium chloride, cesium sulfate, or cesium bromide allows molecules to be separated on the basis of differences in their buoyant densities. The strong salt solutions used may also prevent ionic interactions during these separations. In addition, the inclusion of protein denaturants such as GuHCl can effect separation of high buoyant density PG from other disc proteins of lower buoyant densities.[34]

Buoyant density is inversely related to partial specific volume. Proteins have values between 0.7 to 0.75 mℓ/g, while values for nonsulfated polysaccharides are between 0.6 to 0.65 mℓ/g. Sulfated glycosaminoglycans have even lower partial specific volumes; thus, chondroitin sulfate has a value of 0.53 mℓ/g. Proteins have isopycnic values in cesium density gradients of about 1.3 g/mℓ, while glycosaminoglycans are isodense between 1.6 to 2.0 g/mℓ. Therefore, depending on carbohydrate content and composition, glycoproteins may have isopycnic densities intermediate to these values. Ultracentrifugation is widely used for the isolation of various cartilage PGs, but may also be employed for the separation of their noncollagenous proteins.

5. Affinity Chromatography

This technique is widely applicable to proteins of differing function and utilizes an interaction via specific antibodies[35] or lectins.[36] The method, however, may be limited by the extractive conditions used, since ionic detergent and chaotropic salts are not compatible with this technique. Concanavalin A[36,37] and wheat germ agglutinin[38,39] have both found application in the isolation of noncollagenous proteins.

C. Glycoproteins of the Disc

The disc noncollagenous proteins exhibit UV fluorescence[40] as do aqueous extracts of disc tissue,[41] which presumably reflects their high tyrosine content.[2,15,16] Structural noncollagenous glycoproteins containing significant amounts of mannose, fucose, and sialic acid have been noted to accumulate in the nucleus pulposus with age.[1,16] At least three noncollagenous proteins (presumably structural glycoproteins) have been distinguished from each other on the basis of their X-ray fiber diffraction patterns and electron microscopic appearances.[15,42] Their X-ray fiber diffraction patterns apparently indicate that these proteins are all in the unoriented β-configuration,[15,42,43] although recently, this has been questioned.[44] The levels of these β-proteins in the disc are reported to increase with age.[2,42,43] The variation of these proteins with aging and degeneration has been reviewed by Taylor and Akeson.[45] As to whether the aforementioned X-ray diffraction patterns are due to a native insoluble protein in the β-form or a denatured globular protein remains to be established. Several authors consider that the apparent increase in β-proteins in the NP with aging (which is suggested by the observed increase in intensity of certain bands of X-ray diffraction patterns) is in actual fact due to an increased contribution by collagen.[46,47] With aging, there is a marked increase in the mean diameter of the collagen fibrils present in the human annulus.[44]

It would appear that the disc β-proteins have properties in common with the collagen degradation product, pseudoelastin.[48] They also resemble the amyloid deposited in primary amyloidosis.[49] Timpl et al.[50] have observed that calf joint-capsule acidic structural glycoproteins resemble amyloid fibril proteins in terms of their solubility, distribution, carbohydrate content, and amino acid composition. (Amyloid is discussed more fully later in this chapter.)

Solubilization of some disc glycoproteins is difficult due to their intimate association with collagen.[51] Thus, they appear similar to structural acidic glycoproteins derived from a variety of other connective tissues.[28,50,52-56] These normally nonextractable glycoproteins would appear to have functional roles (together with the proteoglycans[57]) within the extracellular matrix by providing a structural framework for the assembly of correctly oriented collagen fibrils during fibrillogenesis. However, the nature of the attachment of noncollagenous protein to collagen awaits clarification. It is possible, but unlikely, that the insoluble noncollagenous proteins and collagen are "associated" due to their mutual exclusion from the aqueous phase of the IVD. It has also been suggested that procollagen at certain strategic points may not be fully converted to collagen. For example, the amino terminal portion of procollagen which contains cysteine could be linked to other matrix components via disulfide bonds or the helical section of the procollagen molecule could be cross-linked via lysine- and hydroxylysine-derived aldehydes. Olsen et al.[58] have demonstrated, as has been shown in other connective tissues,[56,59,60] attachment of a globular protein component to collagen by disulfide linkages in lens capsule basement membrane.

Recent investigations[22] have established that type VI collagen is a major constituent of the disc matrix. Type VI collagen is a highly disulfide-linked protein consisting of a short collagenous triple helix bound by relatively large noncollagenous globular domains[61-65] (see Chapter 7). It has only relatively recently been classified as a distinct collagen type and was previously known as short-chain or intima collagen.[62] Type VI collagen has a widespread distribution in connective tissues. It is a major constituent of the human cornea[66] and is also present in the aorta, uterus,[65] and placenta[62,63] as well as in the liver, kidney, ligament, and the skeletal muscle extracellular matrix.[67,68]

Table 1 summarizes the known literature on the matrix noncollagenous proteins of the IVD and related connective tissues. Link proteins of the PG aggregate have received the most attention. However, other disc components such as the NCPs which in vitro bind HA, calcium, PG, and collagen have recently attracted interest. These NCPs are undoubtedly important in the organization of the disc extracellular matrix and have been considered as possible markers for tissue degeneration.

D. Disc Elastin

Although the presence of elastic fibers in the intervertebral disc was originally considered a somewhat controversial finding, their presence has now been clearly established by light[69,70] and electron microscopy.[44,71-74] Elastin is, however, a relatively minor matrix component. It occupies approximately 10% of the disc matrix with its content diminishing slightly with age and declining in the lumbar disc from 12.6% at age 26 to 8.2% at age 62 years, as estimated by manual planimetry.[70] Elastin, nevertheless, is an important structural component which is believed to confer elasticity to the AF.[44,71,75-77]

Elastin is a highly insoluble protein rich in hydrophobic amino acids and contains few polar functional groups. It is synthesized as a soluble precursor molecule, tropoelastin (mol wt 72,000), of similar amino acid composition to insoluble elastin, but contains additional lysine residues which are subsequently involved in cross-link formation. These convert the tyopoelastin to insoluble elastin. Cross-linking is achieved via aldehyde (allysine) formation derived from lysine residues by the enzyme lysyloxidase. The cross-links of elastin contain the unique amino acids desmosine and isodesmosine.[78,79] Other cross-links have recently been described,[80-83] some of which are identical to those present in collagen.[84] However, all of the known cross links of elastin are derived from lysine, whereas hydroxylysine is also utilized in collagen cross-link formation. In mature elastin, dihydrodesmosine and dihydroisodesmosine are more prevalent than the desmosine and isodesmosine ring structures. Problems, however, are encountered in the unequivocal demonstration of cross-linking structures in mature elastin, since the harsh extractive conditions required for its solubilization partially destroy desmosine/isodesmosine and intermediate cross-link structures.[85,86]

Elastic fibers are composed of two distinct morphologic components.[18,87-90] a central amorphic and a microfibrillar outer region. These two components may be distinguished on the basis of their differential staining characteristics with uranyl acetate and lead salts, which stain the microfibrillar structures, but not the dense amorphous central component.[18] The amorphous and microfibrillar components are chemically unrelated, which is apparent by their differential staining characteristics. The former is rich in hydrophobic amino acids such as glycine, alanine, proline, and valine, while the microfibrillar component is much more acidic and apparently has a high content of cysteine and a high glycoprotein content.[23,87,88] Collagen fibrils which occur associated with elastin fibrils in AF tissue may be distinguished from microfibrillar components by their specific staining with uranyl acetate or phosphotungstic acid and the lack of staining with lead salts.

During the early stages of fibrillogenesis, the microfibrillar structures are major components of the elastin fibril and have a characteristic fibrous appearance by light microscopy.[87] These are easily discernible from other fibrillar structures present in the intervertebral disc,[91] as has been clearly demonstrated in micrographs of human fetal annulus.[71] In later stages of fibrillogenesis, the amorphous central component assumes a major proportion of the elastin fibril.[18,87,92]

It has been suggested that elastic fibers impart resilience to annular tissue, where they are present as a composite mixture with collagen fibrils.[75,93] It has also been observed by Johnson et al.[69] that elastic fibers in the annulus occur in close proximity to annular attachment points with the vertebral end-plate. Annular collagen fibers under light microscopy assume a characteristic crimped appearance, suggesting that when a fiber is stretched, it may not transmit a force until it is fully extended.[75,76,94] Elastic fibers may help to maintain the collagen crimping and, thus, provide a means of protecting annular collagen against rupture during sudden impact loading.

III. CELL SURFACE GLYCOPROTEINS IMPLICATED IN THE CONTROL OF DISC METABOLISM

A. Cell Membrane Glycoprotein Receptors and Cell Adhesion Glycoproteins

It has been suggested that intricate attachment of the chondrocyte via specific cell membrane receptors and intercalated transmembrane glycoproteins[95-98] to constituents of its extracellular matrix may enable it to respond subtly to any changes in its matrix and permits coordination of any growth and repair processes.[99] Growth is a fundamental characteristic of all living organisms and is predominantly associated with the early stages of embryonic and postnatal development. However, it remains a dormant feature in most human tissues throughout adult life. While the metabolism of the normal disc is slow,[100-102] it is clear that the disc cells are capable of rapidly responding to changes in their environment during immobilization[103] and chemonucleolysis (see Chapter 13). These studies indicate that disc cells may produce an extracellular matrix more appropriate to counteracting the new stress or nutritional status to which they have been subjected.[34,103] During remodeling, changes are most noticeable in the major structural matrix components of the IVD, such as collagen and proteoglycan, and have been investigated in some detail.[34,103,104] The extensive remodeling of the IVD matrix due to changes in phenotypic expression of the chondrocyte during progression of the scoliotic curve[105,106] is further evidence that the disc cell may readily respond to alterations in its environment.

Cellular morphogenesis, adhesion, motility, proliferation, and cyto-differentiation have all been shown to be modified by certain extracellular matrix components.[107-111] Specific cell-surface receptors or intermediate linking molecules, such as fibronectin or laminin, are undoubtedly involved in these processes. Thus, treatment of oncogenically transformed fibronectin-deficient fibroblastic cells with purified cellular fibronectin has been shown to restore normal cell shape, adhesiveness, cell surface morphology, and actin filament organization.[112,113] Moreover, isolated epithelial cells cease "blobbing" and reorganize cortical microfilaments after treatment with purified fibronectin, laminin, or collagen.[114] Cartilage chondrocytes, when treated with purified cellular fibronectin, have also been shown to alter their morphology and patterns of biosynthesis, thus causing reversion from chondrocyte-specific synthesis of type II collagen and proteoglycans to a mesenchymal cell pattern.[115,116]

Some of the individual matrix components which have been shown to have important roles in the regulation of cell behavior and matrix assembly include HA binding proteins.[117-119] HA is found to accumulate in the extracellular matrix of the IVD with aging. However, the possible influence of HA on disc cellular metabolism is largely unexplored. HA also interacts with other proteins besides proteoglycans.[117-120] These so called hyaluronic acid binding proteins (HABP) have been shown in vitro to greatly influence formation of HA fibrils[117,121] and dramatically increase the binding of HA to collagen. This has also been noted in embryonic extracellular matrices,[120] suggesting a possible matrix stabilization role for the HABP. Neither fibronectin nor chondroitin sulfate (which both bind to HA) increase binding of HA to collagen.[108,117,118] Both cellular and plasma fibronectin also bind to HA,[121,122] although the latter does so only to a small extent. Cell adhesion proteins, believed to play roles in the adhesion, migration, and/or anchorage of cells to the extracellular matrix, include fibronectin,[123-130] chondronectin,[95,131] laminin,[132] and laminin-associated glycoproteins, such as entactin,[133] nidogen,[19] GP-2,[134] and the novel basement membrane protein BM40.[135] Other adhesion molecules, including N-CAM, L1, J1, NILE, and ovomarulin, have recently been described.[136]

Type VII collagen has recently been shown to form a network of anchoring fibrils[137] between epithelial cells and the basal lamina. The intervertebral disc extracellular matrix has also recently been shown to contain several of the so-called minor collagens, (see Chapter 7) and it is also emerging that the disc extracellular matrix is highly ordered. It is therefore highly probable that similar structural roles are played by these minor collagens in the anchoring of the intervertebral disc fibrochondrocyte in its matrix.

Anchorin CII is a chondrocyte transmembrane glycoprotein of mol wt 31,000,[96-98] whose function is attachment of the chondrocyte to type II collagen in the extracellular matrix. Alternative mechanisms for the adhesion of chondrocytes to collagen would appear to exist involving chondronectin, a soluble extracellular matrix adhesion molecule, rather than an integral component of the chondrocyte surface.[95] Other adhesion proteins may resemble intercalated cell surface proteoglycans, such as a heparin sulfate proteoglycan described by Kjellen et al. in 1981,[138] although this component has not been identified in the chondrocyte. Similar intercalated membrane matrix receptors for laminin are present on tumor cells and skeletal muscle cells.[139-142] A 140-kdalton cell membrane-associated probable fibronectin receptor has also been described.[143] A transmembrane connection between pericellular fibronectin and intracellular microfilament bundles in fibroblasts, termed fibronexus, has been reported.[144] Three different systems of intracellular filaments and microtubules have also been described which can function independently. It has been suggested that these may provide cell surface modulating assemblies which affect intracellular organelles involved in maintenance of the extracellular matrix homeostasis.[145]

Another possible means of communication between the chondrocyte and its extracellular matrix is via cilia.[146,147] It has been proposed that these may carry a variety of extrinsic stimuli to intracellular organelles responsible for homeostatic feedback responses to changes in the extracellular matrix microenvironment.

The aforementioned examples illustrate the importance of transmembrane proteins in the interactive relationship between the connective tissue cell and its extracellular matrix, including the extent of its hydration.[148] It has recently been found that polyethylene glycol may be used to control the hydration of disc tissue in culture.[149,150] By this means, it has been possible to culture dog and rabbit disc tissues and determine the metabolic activity of disc cells. These latest developments of in vitro culture methods, which can preserve disc cell integrity for several weeks,[150] may permit more detailed investigations of disc cell surface proteins and interactions with matrix components to be undertaken.

The nature of extracellular materials interacting with the cell surface has important regulatory and structural consequences, and an extensive literature now exists on this subject. Most of this work, however, is beyond the scope of this review and the interested reader is referred to excellent reviews[55,108,109,122,151-154] on this subject for supplementary reading.

B. Miscellaneous Factors Involved in Maintaining the Integrity of the Intervertebral Disc Extracellular Matrix

The normal healthy disc is characterized by its avascularity and presumably contains antiangiogenesis factors[155,156] to maintain this state. Following prolapse and/or degeneration, blood vessels and granulation tissue may enter the disc. However, as to whether this situation arises primarily from a decline in levels of antiangiogenesis factors with senescence or as a secondary reaction to acute inflammation remains to be determined.

Mineralization of the IVD has been noted to increase after surgery, and it has been suggested that this may not be as infrequent as previously throught.[160] Regulation of bone mineralization is a complicated process controlled by many factors including serum calcium and phosphate concentrations, hormones, enzymes, and the structural components of the extracellular matrix. Mineralization of the bone matrix has also been shown to be inhibited by specific noncollagenous proteins, such as bone Gla protein (BGP), osteonectin, and prothrombin.[158] Bone Gla protein has been shown to be the seventh most abundant protein in vertebrates.[159] Since IVD calcification may be considered as a sequelae of degeneration (see Chapter 12), it would seem logical *vide infra* that proteins similar or identical to BGP are present within the healthy disc. However, experimental studies have not been undertaken to examine this proposition as far as we are aware. Calcium binding NCPs have been isolated from various cartilage types,[160-163] including fibrocartilage (see Table 1), and as mentioned above, these play an important role in the mineralization of the matrix in bone. However, it again remains to be established whether such proteins are functional during mineralization of disc tissues.

IV. AMYLOID DEPOSITION

The term amyloidosis relates to a group of diseases (rather than a single disease entity) characterized by the extracellular deposition of proteinaceous material — amyloid in various tissues and organs. Amyloid has been shown to occur in the disc with aging.[164-169] With development of the amyloid deposit, displacement of normal tissue structures may give rise to progressive, often fatal, functional disturbances and may induce mechanical abnormalities due to organ or tissue enlargement.

A. Characterization of Amyloid and Its Constituent Proteins

The name amyloid was suggested by Virchow[170] who considered it "starch-like" (GK *amylon,* starch), since it stained with iodine. This is a misnomer since the proteinaceous nature of amyloid was suggested by Friedreich and Kekule[171] more than a century earlier. Today, it is recognized that the carbohydrates which stain positively with periodate, Schiff's reagent, or metachromatically with toluidine or Alcian blue[172,173] are part of the PG matrix in which the amyloid protein filament is embedded. Apparently, completely unrelated proteins can constitute the subunit from which amyloid is constructed. However, despite the significant chemical variations possible (Table 2), all amyloids have certain characteristics in common, namely:

1. All show positive Congo red staining and display greenish birefringence (dichroism) under polarized light.
2. Amyloid fibrils are characterized by electron microscopy as being straight, nonbranching, nonanastomosed filaments 6 to 10 nm in diameter. There are no periodical cross bands as in collagen fibrils. In the amyloid mass, filaments run in various random directions and, therefore, lack the orderly formations found in collagen fibril bundles. Medium electron-dense material between filaments, probably representing proteoglycan, is also evident.[174]
3. Amyloid filaments are composed of aggregates of polypeptide chains of overall small molecular weight (4.5 to 31 kdaltons). These proteins are of such a size that entry into the IVD by normal diffusive processes is possible; X-ray crystallographic analysis indicates that the protein subunits are assembled in antiparallel, β-pleated sheet arrangements.[174]

Amyloid deposition in the intervertebral disc, in common with other articulating structures, is an age-dependent phenomenon.[164-169,175-182] It has also been recognized that aging of the intervertebral disc is accompanied by an increase in noncollagenous proteins, as determined by an increase in β-pleated sheet structures, as identified by X-ray diffraction methods.[42,43,183] The appearance of a 4.65 Å diffuse X-ray diffraction ring from degenerate and prolapsed discs supports the proposition that amyloid and proteins giving rise to this 4.65 Å diffraction pattern are related. A protein having a similar diffraction pattern has been obtained from rheumatoid tissues, where it was considered to be derived from immunoglobulins.[184]

Glenner[185] has suggested fibrillosis as an alternative, possibly more appropriate term to replace amyloidosis. Fibrillosis would emphasize the structural assembly of the amyloid proteins as a unifying characteristic of this family of diseases.

Table 2
CLASSIFICATION OF THE AMYLOIDOSES ON THE BASIS OF THEIR CONSTITUENT FIBRIL PROTEINS

Type of amyloidosis[a]	Chemical designation	Fibril protein(s)[b]	Putative precursor(s)
Primary systemic myeloma associated[443]	AL	Immunoglobulin Variable kappa and lambda L chain N terminal fragments AL protein	Ig L chain Kappa Lambda regions
Reactive (secondary) and some familial types (e.g., FMF)[192,444]	AA	AA protein	SAA
Localized, organ specific, and some familial types:			
Medullary thryoid carcinoma		Thyrocalcitonin	Precalcitonin
Pancreatic insulinoma[445]		Insulin B	(Pre-) proinsulin
Danish familial cardiomyopathy[446]		Variant pre-albumin	Variant prealbumin
Chronic hemodialysis[447]		β_2-Microglobulin	β_2-Microglobulin
Familial polyneuropathy[448-453]		Variant pre-albumin	Variant prealbumin

Note: Abbreviations: FMF = familial Mediterranean fever; SAA = serum amyloid A protein; AL, AA = amyloid A, L proteins, respectively.

[a] As yet, the particular form of amyloid present in aged intervertebral discs awaits detailed characterization. However, the green dichroism in polarized light shown by Congo red-stained disc specimens after treatment with potassium permaganate indicates the absence of amyloid A protein in such disc amyloid deposits. The amyloid is therefore nonsecondary.[164] Disc amyloids so far are identified as the primary or myeloma associated form.[167,168]

[b] In addition, most amyloid deposits also contain another amyloid-specific protein, AP, the amyloid P component, whose putative precursor is SAP, serum amyloid protein, a normal plasma glycoprotein. However, in cerebral plaques, such as are found in Alzheimers' disease,[240,454] SAP is often absent, probably due to its inability to penetrate the blood-brain barrier.

During the last 15 years, it has become apparent that amyloid fibrils may be composed of apparently completely unrelated protein subunits. However, the recognition and characterization of these low molecular weight amyloid protein subunits have enabled a chemical and immunological classification system to emerge which correlates to some extent with the clinical descriptions of amyloidosis.[186-189] Over ten subtypes of amyloidosis are known,[185] however, only three main forms may be identified on the basis of their constituent fibril proteins (Table 2). Recommendations of the 3rd International Symposium on Amyloidosis suggested a classification based on three major clinical designations. These were (1) familial, (2) associated with (or reactive to) an underlying disease, and (3) idiopathic. These clinical descriptions are discussed more fully elsewhere.[189]

B. Formation and Deposition of Amyloid

While much knowledge has accumulated regarding the chemical composition of amyloid, very little is known about its formation and deposition in tissues. Formation of amyloid fibrils appears to result from overproduction and/or decreased clearance of amyloid precursor proteins, particularly in localized organ-specific forms of amyloid.

It has been established[190,191] that individuals prone to develop secondary amyloidosis have an enzymatic defect characterized by incomplete breakdown of SAA. This results in an increased concentration of AA and eventually in the formation of amyloid.[192,193] Normally, however, SAA is degraded to much smaller fragments which are more readily removed by the reticuloendothelial system leaving no excess of protein AA for subsequent amyloid formation. It is likely that similar principles are operative during formation of other amyloid types. It is of interest to note that SAP, another amyloid-specific protein, which is deposited on amyloid AA fibrils,[192,194-196] has also been reported to be an elastase inhibitor.[197] This may be of particular relevance, since it has been suggested that the major source of amyloid degrading activity in serum is due to leukocyte elastase.[191,198-200] In amyloidosis associated with rheumatoid arthritis[187,201] and familial Mediterranean fever,[200] a reduced amyloid degrading activity in serum has also been noted. In these two cases, this was considered to be largely due to elevated serum α-PI levels, rather than deposition of a specific amyloid bound elastase inhibitor.

Purified α_1-PI has been shown to effectively inhibit degradation of SAA by human leukocyte elastase.[199,201] As already indicated, it appears that the amyloid degrading activity of serum is due largely to human leukocyte elastase (HLE), since an antibody to HLE and a specific chloromethyl ketone elastase inhibitor effectively abolished the amyloid degrading activity of serum.[198] Human leukocyte elastase has been found intimately associated with AA fibrils.[198,202] Therefore, deposition of SAP, an elastase inhibitor on SAA fibrils, would presumably prevent breakdown of these fibrils in vivo, although this has as yet to be proven.

It has been shown that the amyloid degrading activity of serum, as determined by clearing of turbid agarose-AA gels, is at least partly a nonspecific calcium-mediated effect[203-207] which correlates well with the serum albumin content. This process apparently does not involve degradation of amyloid fibrils. Ethylenediaminetetra acetic acid has also been shown (as have other specific chelators of calcium) to mimic "amyloid degrading activity" by causing clearing zones in agarose-AA gels.[206,207] While the above-mentioned clearing phenomena are of doubtful physiological significance and cast doubts on unequivocal demonstration of enzymic degradation of SAA by this technique, these data, nevertheless, serve to illustrate the involvement of calcium in amyloid assembly.

Serum amyloid A protein, the high density lipoprotein associated amyloid-related serum component,[208,209] is an acute phase reactant in man. Its serum concentration is elevated in a number of inflammatory, infectious, and neoplastic disorders. In the acute phase state, SAA can reach levels that are 100- to 1000-fold higher than found normally. In this respect, it resembles C-reactive protein (CRP), but contrasts with other liver-produced acute phase proteins such as α_1-PI, α_1-antichymotrypsin, fibrinogen, hapto-globulin, and α-1-acid-glycoprotein which only increase two to four times in an acute-phase reaction. This has led to the suggestion that SAA is a more sensitive marker for certain pathological conditions than CRP.[208-215]

Chronic inflammatory diseases such as adult and juvenile rheumatoid arthritis are important underlying disorders which increase the likelihood for the development of secondary amyloidosis. In the majority of such patients, there is a continuous overproduction of SAA which appears to be a prerequisite for AA amyloidosis. Only a small proportion of patients with elevated SAA levels, however, subsequently develop secondary amyloidosis, implicating the involvement of other factors.[215]

As already mentioned, the normal production and subsequent serum concentration of SAA is very low, but increases several hundredfold within 24 hr of inflammatory stimuli known to induce an acute phase response.[215] The signal for SAA induction is mediated by a monokine, interleukin-1 released by activated mononuclear phagocytes, e.g., monocytes and macrophages.[216]

Although the mechanism by which interleukin-1 stimulates the liver to produce SAA is unknown,[217] activation of mononuclear phagocytes appears to be a key step for the production and release into the serum of SAA. In this regard, it is relevant to note that the activated macrophage (and thus interleukin-1) are a characteristic feature of synovial inflammation in rheumatoid arthritis and may partly explain the incidence of amyloid deposits in the tissues of such patients.[177-182,218]

Human amyloid enhancing factor (AEF) has also been shown to induce amyloid deposition in mice[219] and is transferable from one mouse to another without loss of effect. Such mediators[219-223] may therefore represent control mechanisms for amyloid production and deposition and may explain why the many individuals with elevated SAA levels, as a consequence of an underlying inflammatory condition, do not necessarily progress to clinically identifiable amyloidosis.

Human SAA is heterogeneous. Six forms have been identified,[190,208,212,216,224] and it has been speculated[190,212,224] that only certain molecular species of SAA are precursors of AA. Thus, individuals who produce these particular isotypes of SAA may be more prone to develop amyloidosis. Such a situation may be further exacerbated by defective catabolism of the SAA isotypes.[190,191] Moreover, the SAA isotypes appear to be synthesized at varying rates in vivo and are products of different genes.[190]

C. Amyloid Deposition and Inflammatory Conditions

In the last 100 years, several reports of deposition of amyloid in articular structures have appeared, primarily as case reports of severe arthropathy in association with myelomatosis,[225-228] primary amyloidosis,[167,229] and rheumatoid arthritis.[230-233] In 1972, Christensen and Sorensen[181] described the presence of amyloid in the capsular lining of hip joints obtained at total joint replacement. However, it has only been during the last 5 years that amyloid in joint connective tissues, including the disc, has been studied systematically.[164-169,175-182]

Amyloid deposits, formerly regarded as infrequent and of little pathological significance in osteoarthritic joint tissues, are, in fact, fairly common. Ten of eighteen consecutive patients who underwent knee or hip arthroplasty as a consequence of progressive osteoarthritis had significant amyloid deposits present in articular tissues removed at surgery.[218] Amyloid deposits have also been reported in 33% of osteoarthritic hip joints removed during reconstructive surgery[181,178] and also in a follow-up study in 43% of hip capsular tissues from unselected autopsy cases.[180] Goffin et al.[233] have identified amyloid in 56% of unselected autopsy specimens of hip and sternoclavicular joints. In all of the aforementioned cases the presence of amyloid was strongly age dependent with little deposition evident in patients below the age of 40. More severe deposition was evident in individuals aged 60 and above.

Amyloid deposits in intervertebral discs were first described by Bywaters and Dorling in 1970[167] in a patient with myelomatosis. Amyloid in disc tissue has also been described in association with severe primary amyloidosis.[168] More recently, amyloid has been described in tissue from surgically removed herniated intervertebral discs.[166,175] Contrary to previous opinions, deposits of this material in the disc are fairly common. It has been reported that 41% of surgically removed disc specimens contained amyloid.[164] Ladefoged[165] reported that 93% of spines from 30 nonselected autopsies contained significant deposits of amyloid.

An age-dependent deposition of amyloid in the human intervertebral disc is indicated from the positive identification of this protein in discs of an age group greater than 65 years, but not in specimens of a group of less than 25 years.[166] A similar situation has been reported for discs of young and senescent mice.[169]

A close relationship between pyrophosphate and amyloid deposits has been reported in autopsy material and surgical specimens from hip joints[176,177,182,234,235] as well as in surgical[164] and autopsy disc specimens.[165] The incidence of these deposits was found to be higher than that reported by Andres and Trainer,[157] who considered calcification (pyrophosphate deposition) in disc tissue a rare finding.

Amyloid deposition, herniation, and chondrocalcinosis are all age-related phenomena in the human IVD. However, any possible pathogenetic link between these events has as yet to be established.

The prognosis of reactive AA amyloidosis is more favorable than for idiopathic or myeloma associated amyloidosis. The reported survival rates are about 2 years[236] for the former and 4 months for the latter.[237] Amyloidosis has been estimated to be the cause of 43 to 47% of deaths among European patients with JRA,[238] while the lower incidence of this condition in the U.S. reflects the lower death rate there from JRA.[215] The proportion of deaths caused by amyloidosis in adult onset rheumatoid arthritis is variable, but generally much lower than for JRA. Koota et al.[239] reported that amyloidosis was the cause of deaths in 8% of rheumatoid arthritis patients examined at autopsy.

D. Serum Amyloid P Component (SAP)

Serum amyloid P Component (SAP) is a normal plasma glycoprotein[195] with an apparent morphological and immunochemical identity to the P component found in most types of amyloid deposits.[194] It is, however, absent in cerebral amyloid plaques due to its inability to penetrate the blood-brain barrier.[240] Serum amyloid P component is composed of 10 covalently linked globular subunits each of 25,500 daltons arranged "face to face" as cyclic pentameric rings. This is a characteristic of the so-called pentraxins, of which C-reactive protein is also a member.[241] The molecular configuration of SAP is influenced by Ca^{++} (as well as Cu^{++} and Zn^{++}) in certain circumstances[242] which, in an ill-defined manner, contributes to the self-aggregation of this protein[196] and its binding to certain ligands,[243-246] including amyloid fibrils.[194] Serum amyloid P component shows strong amino acid sequence homology (60%) and ultrastructural similarity to C reactive protein (CRP).[241,247-249] However, in man, SAP (unlike SAA or CRP) is not an acute phase protein. It has been postulated that both SAA and CRP have evolved from a common ancestral protein which has been conserved throughout evolution.[250] All vertebrate species so far identified contain both SAP and CRP in their serum. Strict preservation of the Ca^{++}-dependent ligand-binding specificity of SAP implies an important underlying function which has as yet to be ascertained. Amyloid P component has never been demonstrated in any extra or intracellular deposit other than amyloid, even in longstanding calcified lesions. It, therefore, has a more discerning specificity than Ca^{++} itself.

In addition to its deposition in amyloid, which may or may not be of physiological significance, SAP has also been found to be associated with normal vascular basement membrane.[251,252] It is also found in peripheral microfibrillar elastic fibers[253,254] where, in degenerative conditions, it may be a constituent of the "amyloid-like" protein called colloid.[254] This may explain the intimate structural association of amyloid and elastic fibers in systemic and cutaneous amyloidosis.[255]

In the presence of calcium, SAP binds to various ligands, including zymosan,[242,245] agarose (and other polysaccharides), amyloid fibers,[194] heparin, fibronectin,[246] C4 binding protein,[246] and modified C3b. Binding of SAP to ligands was recently found to be proportional to their pyruvate acetal content,[256] although, it is unlikely that this reflects the physiological specificity of SAP. However, the chemically analogous β-turn structures present in some SAP proteinaceous ligands[256] have exposed carbonyl groups at their "hair pin bends" which coordinate Ca^{++}, and thus may also represent physiological SAP binding centers. Binding of SAP to some of these ligands has been shown in the presence of Ca^{++}, Zn^{++}, and Cd^{++}. Binding with Cu^{++} is enhanced at an acid pH (5.0), while binding with Zn^{++} is unaffected at this pH, and binding is diminished with Ca^{++} under these conditions.[242]

During inflammatory processes both Cu^{++} and Zn^{++} are rapidly sequestered into hepatic and extracellular tissues where these ions contribute to biosynthetic and oxidative pathways known to be operative during the immune response. The observed SAP binding reactivities in the presence of Cu^{++} and Zn^{++} may be of particular importance during inflammatory or necrotic processes, since inflammatory foci can become acidic and Cu^{++} and Zn^{++} are rapidly mobilized during inflammatory reactions. Serum Cu^{++} levels increase in association with elevation in ceruloplasmin. This is a copper transport protein donating Cu^{++} to enzymes, such as cytochrome oxidase and lysyl oxidase, which are active during processes of basic cellular metabolism and tissue remodeling. Exchange of Cu^{++} from ceruloplasmin is favored by an acid pH. Therefore, such an exchange may potentially represent a means of altering the biochemical reactivities of these proteins during an acute inflammatory episode and may suggest a physiological role for SAP.

It is not clear how these biological processes relate to the IVD, since it is generally assumed that its avascularity restricts entry of many inflammatory proteins. The work of Fricke,[257] and Fricke and Hadding[258] reported the presence of serum albumin, transferrin, and α_1-acid glycoprotein in the human NP and AF. Yet preliminary work by Urban and Maroudas[100] has suggested that albumin does not gain access to the IVD by passive diffusion, although serum amyloid P component and SAA would appear to be small enough to gain entry.

The liver is probably the main site of synthesis of SAP, as it is for C-reactive protein (CRP).[259] Serum levels of SAP tend to be subnormal in patients with hepatocellular insufficiency irrespective of the cause. Staining of hepatocytes with anti-SAP, after administration of colchicine (which inhibits hepatic release of SAP), results in more intense intracellular staining suggesting again the liver as the site of SAP synthesis. Using immunolocalization, SAP has also been identified in normal human fibroblasts.[260]

E. Physiological Function of SAP

The suggestions that SAP participated in complement activation[261] or was involved in the coagulation cascade have now been discounted. SAP is not a special type of collagen[262] despite its possible fibrillar structure. Nor is it a subunit of the first component of complement,[263,264] despite the fact that CRP shows strong homology with complement subcomponent Clt[265] and does interact in the complement system.[265-267]

However, SAP has been found at physiological concentrations to have an immunosuppressive effect on human peripheral blood mononuclear cells, inhibiting the normal proliferative responses of such cells to Phytohemagglutinin, Concanavalin A, and Staphylococcal protein A.[268,269] This characteristic, together with the aforementioned ligand specificities of SAP, suggests, therefore, that it could be regarded as a circulating mammalian lectin with the functional ability to modulate the immune response. Such an important role may explain

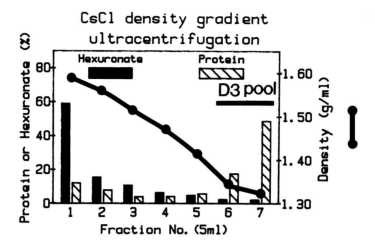

FIGURE 1. CsCl density gradient ultracentrifugation under dissociative conditions of a 4 *M* GuHCl extract, of normal lumbar disc tissue from a 53-year-old male. The extract was brought to a starting density of 1.5 g/mℓ with solid CsCl, centrifuged at 100,000 × *g*. Tubes were manually fractionated into 7 × 5.0 mℓ fractions, which were monitored for hexuronate and protein by specified methods. The density of the samples was measured by weighing aliquots of known volume. The D3 protein pool was pooled as indicated by the bar.

the conservation of SAP (and CRP) throughout vertebrate evolution.[250] Recent in vitro studies have also suggested a regulatory effect of CRP on the complement system[266] as well as on platelets[270,271] and an inhibitory effect on T-lymphocytes.[270,272-275] It is of interest to note that abnormal platelet function has been observed in patients with adolescent idiopathic scoliosis,[276-279] but the significance of this finding has yet to be determined.

V. EXTRAVASCULAR PLASMA PROTEINS

Although there is very little information available concerning the permeability properties of the healthy IVD to plasma proteins, it is widely regarded that this structure excludes these proteins. Fricke[257] and Fricke and Hadding[258] reported the presence of albumin, α_1-acid glycoprotein, transferrin, and γ-globulin in the nucleus pulposus and albumin, transferrin, and γ-globulin in the annulus fibrosus of the human intervertebral disc. These results have been questioned by Naylor et al.[184] who were unable to detect plasma components in normal and prolapsed intervertebral discs. However, these authors did concede that loss of immunogenicity of such proteins may have occurred during their fractionation procedures or that they became bound to other matrix components which prevented their detection. A preliminary study conducted in our laboratories has shown that normal disc tissues contain a wide variety of soluble proteins, some of which appear to be identical with serum proteins. These proteins were isolated by dissociative CsCl density gradient ultracentifugation of 4.0 *M* GuHCl disc extracts (as shown in Figure 1). The low buoyant density proteins were obtained from the top of the gradient and fractionated by Sephadex® G75F chromatography (Figure 2) into void volume (sample a) and included proteins (sample b). Each pool was then examined by SDS PAGE (Figure 3). The molecular weight distribution of extractable disc proteins was found to be between 10 to 67 kdaltons with intense staining of bands at 67 kdaltons, 50 to 56 kdaltons, 30 kdaltons, and 15 kdaltons (Figure 3). The low molecular weight proteins were readily separated from the larger species by gel filtration chromatography on Sephadex® G75F (Figure 2). Sulfated polymeric GAGs representing the KS-rich regions of degraded PGs were also evident in the void volume of these Sephadex® G75F

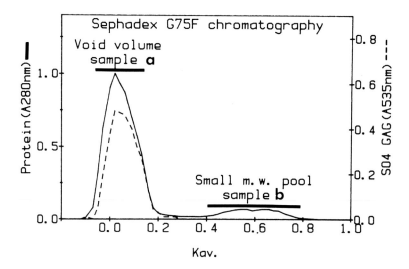

FIGURE 2. Sephadex® G75F gel permeation chromatography of concentrated D3 protein pool from Figure 1. The sample (5.0 mℓ) was applied to a column of Sephadex® G75F and eluted with 0.05 *M* Tris-HCl pH 7.5 containing 1.0 *M* NaCl and 0.01 *M* CaCl$_2$. Eluant fractions were monitored for protein (A280 nm) and sulfated GAG. Void volume protein pool a and included protein pool b were collected as indicated by the bars.

separations (Figure 2). As is evident from Figure 3, (track b) at least nine low molecular weight proteins appear to be present. Two of these minor bands correspond to the disc serine proteinase inhibitors[280,281] which are discussed in more detail later in this chapter. The major contribution to the low molecular weight species in the disc was two cationic proteins (pI ≥ 10.0) which were active on lysozyme substrates[282] (*Micrococcus lysodekticus*). Since the disc is rich in sulfated proteoglycans, it is not unreasonable to assume that the cationic proteins detected arose from the circulation and accumulated in the disc as a function of time by binding to these polyanions. Furthermore, human plasma has been shown to contain proteins, including lysozyme, with molecular weights within the range of those found in the disc.[283,284] On the other hand, it is possible that the disc cells may also be a source of lysozyme, and studies need to be undertaken to resolve this point. The 67-kdalton protein identified in the void volume fractions of the Sephadex® G75F column (Figure 3, track a) was shown by isoelectric focusing and immunodiffusion techniques to be identical to serum albumin. Using the same techniques, a band corresponding to molecular weight of 39 to 42 kdaltons (Figure 3, track a) was identified as α$_1$-acid glycoprotein. These data confirm the original observations of Fricke[257] and Fricke and Hadding[258] that plasma proteins are indeed present within the disc.

Although the protein bands within the molecular weight range 48 to 55 kdaltons undoubtedly contain link proteins,[28] isoelectric focusing also demonstrated a protein with multiple pI species between 4.6 to 4.9, suggesting the presence of α$_1$-proteinase inhibitor. As the physiological role of this protein could be to attenuate the action of the serine proteinase previously identified by us in disc tissue,[281,286] it was considered important to isolate and quantitate the amounts present.

A. Isolation of α$_1$-Proteinase Inhibitor

The α$_1$-proteinase inhibitor was isolated and purified[286] from normal disc tissues using the scheme shown in Figure 4. The initial purification step involved ion-exchange chromatography of DEAE Sephadex® A50 in the presence of 6.0 *M* urea (Figure 5). This facilitated the separation of the disc PGs from the neutral and cationic proteins. As is evident

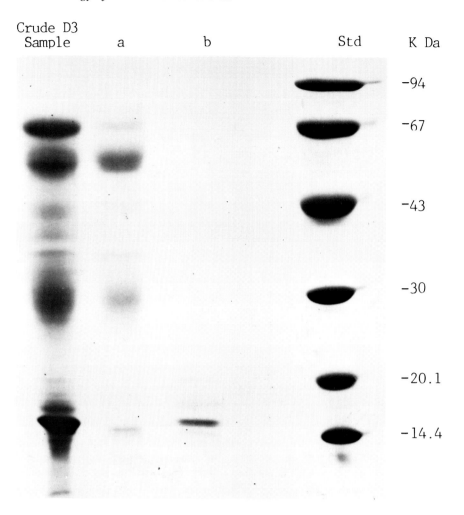

FIGURE 3. Disc proteins (isolated as in Figures 1 and 2) were subjected to 0.1% SDS PAGE employing the Laemlli discontinuous buffer system under reducing and denaturing conditions. Samples were fixed and stained overnight in 0.02% Coomassie R250 dissolved in methanol:acetic acid:H_2O (30:10:60) and destained in the same solvent mixture. The samples electrophoresed were as follows: crude — D3, protein sample (35 µg); a. Sephadex® G75F void volume, protein sample a (15 µg); b. Sephadex® G75F small molecular weight pool, protein sample b (10 µg); standard — molecular weight protein standards, phosphorylase b (94,000), bovine serum albumin (67,000), ovalbumin (43,000), carbonic anhydrase (30,000), soyabean trypsin inhibitor (20,100), and α-lactalbumin (14,400).

from Figure 5, fractions containing α_1-proteinase inhibitor activity were considerably less abundant than the cationic proteinase inhibitors present in pools 1 and 2. α_1-Proteinase inhibitor does, however, represent the majority (78%) of the large molecular weight trypsin inhibitory activity present in disc extracts. It was not possible to detect any other high molecular weight plasma proteinase inhibitors by immunological methods in these samples. The purity of the α_1-proteinase inhibitor purified to step 5 (Figure 4) was established by isoelectric focusing (in the pH range 3.5 to 9.5) as well as by crossed immunoelectrophoresis.[286]

VI. THE ENDOGENOUS PROTEINASE INHIBITORY PROTEINS

A. Comparison with Related Proteins from Similar Connective Tissues

Several mammalian connective tissues have been shown to contain low molecular weight

Step 1. 4 *M* GuHCl extract of pooled lumbar disc tissue, mixed NP/AF from male 19 and female 18

> Dialyzed extract equilibrated in 6.0 *M* urea
> ↓ 0.1 *M* Tris pH 6.8

Step 2. DEAE Sephadex® A50 ion exchange chromatography in 6.0 *M* urea 0.1 Tris pH 6.8

> α-1-Proteinase inhibitor pooled and dialyzed
> ↓ in Sephadex® G75F equilibration buffer

Step 3. Sephadex® G75F gel permeation chromatography in 0.05 *M* Tris pH 7.5, containing 1.0 *M* NaCl 0.01 *M* CaCl$_2$

> Void volume α-1-proteinase inhibitor pool
> dialyzed against dist H$_2$O, then equilibrated
> ↓ in 0.05 *M* phosphate buffer pH 6.7

Step 4. Cibacron blue affinity chromatography

> Nonbound α-1-proteinase inhibitor pooled
> and dialyzed against 0.025 *M* phosphate
> ↓ buffer pH 6.5

Step 5. DEAE Sepharose® CL 6B ion-exchange chromatography in 0.025 *M* phosphate buffer pH 6.5; column eluted with a linear 0 to 0.2 *M* NaCl gradient in the aforementioned buffer

FIGURE 4.   Scheme for the purification of α$_1$-proteinase inhibitor from the intervertebral disc.

proteinase inhibitors. It has been suggested that these inhibitors bestow on cartilage resistance against neoplastic and capillary cell invasion.[155,156,287-293] It has also been proposed that they provide protection to matrix components against degradation by some of the enzymes involved in bone resorption[294-296] or cartilage degradation by endogenous or exogenous enzymes in osteoarthritis.[297-305] Collagenase has been suggested as a mediator of tumor spread either directly[306-310] or by facilitating the growth of capillaries in tumor-induced neovascularization.[287,289,291] It is, therefore, significant that connective tissues contain specific inhibitors of this enzyme.[288,311-314]

Such inhibitors have been detected in the IVD,[314] which may explain the avascularity of this tissue and its resistance to tumor invasion. A similar explanation has been suggested for other avascular connective tissues.[155,156,287,289,291,308] The low molecular weight proteinase inhibitors of bovine hyaline cartilage[287,289,290,311,315-317] have been extensively studied, while those of human hyaline cartilage[298,312,313,318] have attracted less attention. Low molecular weight proteinase inhibitors have also been reported in human costal cartilage[319] as well as aorta[311] and cornea.[320] Kuettner et al.[315] have reported that articular cartilage, aorta, cornea, and the pulmonary vein, are the richest sources of these proteins in the canine. Fibrocartilage, including the human meniscus[321] and the annulus fibrosus of the intervertebral discs,[322] also contains appreciable quantities of low molecular weight inhibitors of serine proteinases. In the human intervertebral disc, these low molecular weight inhibitors which were active against trypsin, chymotrypsin, human leukocyte elastase, and cathepsin G were localized in the nucleus pulposus with a decreasing concentration gradient towards the periphery of the annulus fibrosus.[322] Although collagenase inhibitors have been detected in the human intervertebral disc[314] and articular cartilage,[312,313] they have not been purified to homogeneity. Collagenase inhibitors are widely distributed in other human tissues which presumably reflects their physiological importance. Collagenase inhibitors may be particularly significant for the integrity of the intervertebral disc, since collagen is a major structural component of its extracellular matrix. During growth and repair, collagen is relatively rapidly turned over, and it would seem logical that there must be subtle cellular mechanisms to control these

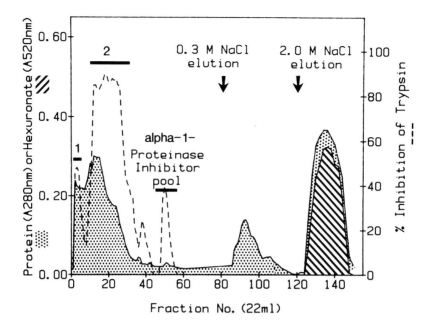

FIGURE 5.   DEAE Sephadex® A50 ion-exchange chromatography of pooled 4.0 *M* GuHCl extract of macroscopically normal female 18 and male 19 lumbar disc specimens. The 4 *M* GuHCl extract was dialyzed and equilibrated in starting buffer (6.0 *M* urea 0.1 *M* Tris pH 6.8) and applied to a column of DEAE Sephadex® A50. The column was washed step-wise with starting buffer, 0.3 *M* NaCl and 2.0 *M* NaCl (the latter two washes both in starting buffer). Column eluates were monitored for protein (A280 nm) and hexuronate (A520 nm). Aliquots (2.0 mℓ) of the fractions were dialyzed exhaustively against 0.01 *M* Tris-HCl pH 7.4, then freeze-dried and redissolved in dist H$_2$O (0.5 mℓ) and their trypsin inhibitory activity determined as previously specified.[286] Earlier experiments with specific antisera had established the identity of the α_1-proteinase inhibitor, which was pooled as indicated.

processes. The local biosynthesis of inhibitors of the collagenolytic enzymes would be one way of achieving such control. Immunologically and functionally identical (by Ouchterlony, ELISA, and inhibition studies) collagenase inhibitors have been detected in human skin, corneal, gingival, and lung fibroblasts, human fetal osteoblasts, uterine smooth muscle cells, fibrosarcoma cells, and explants of human tendon[323] and articular cartilage.[324,325] Human amniotic fluid,[300,326] rheumatoid synovial fluid,[327] and human plasma[328-330] also contain potent collagenase inhibitors. Collagenase inhibitors are also elaborated into culture media from human skin fibroblasts,[331,332] human polymorphonuclear leukocytes,[333] and human platelets.[334] Rabbit and chick bone collagenase inhibitors[335-337] have been obtained by similar methods. The collagenase inhibitors of bovine aorta,[338] rabbit skin, and uterus[339] appear to be similar. Subsequent studies have established that the aforementioned collagenase inhibitors are indeed closely related and collectively have been named TIMP (tissue inhibitor of metalloproteases). This was first purified from human amniotic fluid.[300,326] It is a glycoprotein of 28,000 mol wt and combines irreversibly with tissue metalloproteinases. Apart from TIMP, the serum proteinase inhibitor α_2-macroglobulin is the only other major collagenase inhibitor of relevance to the disc. However, due to its large size (780 kdaltons), α_2-macroglobulin is probably confined to sites close to blood vessels and is very unlikely to gain access to the disc except perhaps following its rupture. The endogenous disc collagenase inhibitor described[314] is likely to bear a close resemblance to TIMP, but this has yet to be confirmed.

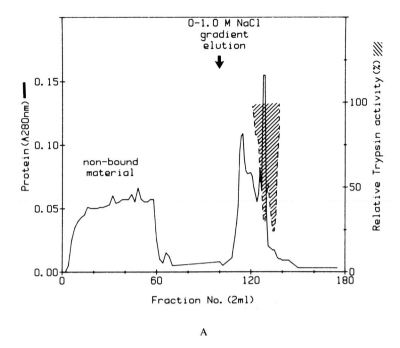

A

FIGURE 6. (A) CM Sepharose® CL 6B ion exchange chromatography of pooled inhibitor 1 from DEAE Sephadex® A50 ion exchange chromatography (Figure 5) of an extract from pooled normal lumbar disc specimens. Samples (100 mℓ) were equilibrated in 0.5 M Tris-HCl pH 7.5, then applied to CM Sepharose® CL 6B in the same buffer and washed with the same buffer (100 mℓ) to remove nonbinding material. The column was then washed with a gradient (150 mℓ) of 0—1.0 M NaCl in the above buffer. Eluant fractions were monitored for protein A280 nm, lysozyme, and trypsin inhibitory activities as specified.[340] To aid interpretation, fractions 110 to 140 are shown enlarged (B). Gradient-elution was started at fraction 100. Therefore, the trypsin-inhibitory fractions illustrated eluted from the column at between 0.4 to 0.6 M NaCl. Inhibitory activities 1a and 1b were pooled as indicated by the bars.

B. Serine Proteinase Inhibitors of the Intervertebral Disc

Early studies by Knight et al.[280,322] suggested the presence of multiple serine proteinase inhibitory activities in human disc tissues, but it was not until recently that these were investigated in any detail.[281] As already discussed in the section on the isolation of α_1-proteinase inhibitor from the disc, the major trypsin inhibitory activities present in 4.0 M GuHCl disc extracts could be resolved from proteoglycan and noncationic inhibitors by DEAE Sephadex® A50 chromatography run in the presence of 6.0 M urea (Figure 5). Application of pool 1 or 2 (Figure 5) to a CM Sepharose® CL-6B column (Figure 6A) removed a large proportion of extraneous proteins, but also demonstrated that those fractions with trypsin inhibitory activity contained high lysozyme activity (Figure 6B). However, it was possible to separate the lysozyme activity from the trypsin inhibitory proteins using trypsin affinity chromatography (Figure 7). More detailed investigation of the cationic trypsin inhibitors present in pools 1 and 2 obtained from the DEAE column (Figure 5) revealed at least three independent species.[340] All the endogenous disc trypsin inhibitory proteins were of low molecular weight (7 to 16 kdaltons) and were highly cationic (pI 10.0), but differed in ionic properties which facilitated their subsequent separation. Such characteristics are also displayed by bovine pancreatic trypsin inhibitor (BPTI) which has been more fully characterized. Originally isolated from bovine pancreas by Kunitz and Northrop in 1936,[341] BPTI is of low molecular weight (6500), is highly cationic (pI 10 to 11), and also displays molecular heterogeneity. Fioretti et al.[342] have shown that four isoinhibitor forms are evident during

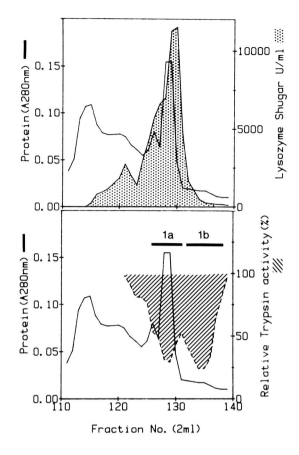

FIGURE 6B.

ion-exchange chromatography of affinity purified pancreatic inhibitor. The bovine kunitz inhibitor (identical to BPTI) shows widespread distribution in various bovine organs including lung, spleen, thyroid, salivary glands, calf thymus, and pancreas.[341-344] It has been suggested that this ubiquitous distribution is due to localization of the inhibitor in tissue mast cells. Trypsin inhibitors similar to those identified in disc tissues would appear to be present in human articular cartilage.[298,318,345] While the origin of these human disc and articular cartilage trypsin inhibitors remains uncertain, it seems likely that some are synthesized by disc cells or articular chondrocytes as a means of controlling matrix turnover. In this regard, they work in conjunction with the collagenase inhibitors[312-314] which have already been discussed.

The major endogenous serine proteinase inhibitors in the human intervertebral disc exist as enzyme-inhibitor complexes as well as in the free form.[281,346] Trypsin affinity chromatography provided a convenient and reproducible means of separating these inhibitors from endogenous neutral proteinase and lysozyme (a protein, which because of its similar size and charge, copurifies with these proteins).

The endogenous disc proteinase inhibitors were shown to have potent activity against several serine proteinases including trypsin, chymotrypsin, plasmin, urokinase, kallikrein, and human leukocyte elastase. They also effectively prevented degradation of disc proteoglycans and synthetic substrates by a number of endogenous disc neutral proteinases. Provided that the levels of the disc serine proteinase inhibitors are in excess, degradation of matrix components by serine proteinases cannot readily occur. Furthermore, these inhibitors have the potential to abrogate activation of latent enzyme systems such as collagenase by plasmin,[347-349] kallikrein,[350,351] or other serine proteinases.[301,352,353]

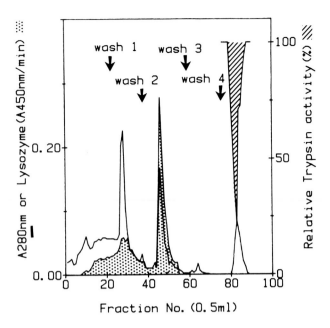

FIGURE 7. Trypsin affinity chromatography of disc inhibitor pool 1a from CM Sepharose® CL 6B ion exchange chromatography (Figure 6). Inhibitor sample (10 mℓ) was equilibrated and applied in starting buffer (0.02 *M* Tris-HCl pH 7.5) to a column of TPCK treated trypsin immobilized on beaded agarose (0.5 mℓ). The column was washed sequentially with 20 bed volumes of: (1) starting buffer; (2) 1*M* NaCl in starting buffer; (3) 2 *M* NaCl in starting buffer; and (4) pH 2.0 glycine HCl 0.05 *M* containing 1 *M* NaCl. Washing steps are indicated in the diagram by arrows. Eluant fractions (0.5 mℓ) were monitored for protein (A280 nm), lysozyme, and trypsin inhibitory activity as specified.[340]

As discussed in Chapter 11, it is not uncommon at autopsy to find prolapse of the annulus and entry of blood vessels into discs of elderly subjects. Such conditions could provide access to the disc of plasma components normally excluded. An important role of the endogenous serine proteinase inhibitors might be to prevent initiation of the complement and fibrinolytic cascades within these tissues.

Preliminary experiments in this laboratory have also established the presence of cysteine-proteinase inhibitors in the greyhound disc[455] These inhibitors may have important regulatory roles to play over pericellular proteolysis by cysteine proteinases as suggested by Dingle and co-workers.[354-356]

VII. THE ENDOGENOUS PROTEINASES

Although there has been considerable interest in the variation with aging and degeneration of the matrix components of the IVD, there is relatively little known about the enzyme systems which might be responsible for their catabolism. Whether this reflects a disinterest towards a tissue which has been regarded as metabolically "inert" or arises from the technical problems associated with the separation of these proteinases from the endogenous inhibitors is difficult to assess. Certainly, under normal circumstances the turnover of proteoglycans within the disc is reported to be relatively slow.[100-102] It is only recently that methods have been developed to permit experiments to be undertaken with disc tissues in which the normal extent of hydration has been preserved in vitro. The availability of such methods may, as was the case for hyaline cartilage, generate data which up to the present have been lacking.[34,101,149] With aging and degeneration[34,101] or immobilization[103] of the disc, proteoglycan catabolism is markedly increased. Using a group of mature beagles, which is a chondrodystrophoid breed,[357] it was found that half of the newly synthesized ^{35}S-labeled disc PGs had lost their ability to aggregate within 60 days.[34] This finding was assumed to arise from cleavage of the hyaluronate binding regions of the disc PGs by endogenous proteinases, since this was known to be a region frequently attacked.[358,359]

Work on disc proteinases, prior to 1975, was concerned mainly with the autolytic changes which occurred most readily at an acid pH.[184,360,361] Dziewiatowski et al.[362] reported significant degradation of denatured hemoglobin at pH 3.6 by extracts of disc autopsy specimens. Since hemoglobin was the most sensitive protein substrate known for cathepsin D (which has a pH optimum between 2.8 and 5), it seems likely that this was the proteinase responsible.[363] Using prolapsed disc material obtained at the time of surgery, Naylor et al.[184] also demonstrated that autolysis of disc tissues could occur at an acid pH. The enzymes responsible were not studied in detail, but these authors did confirm the presence of cathepsin D in these preparations by using specific antibodies. Additional studies by this group showed that enzyme activity at pH 4 to 5 was enhanced by EDTA and DTT. Under these conditions, degradation of PG and the synthetic substrates, benzoyl arginine nitroanilide and naphthylamide, readily occurred. As this latter substrate was particularly sensitive for cathepsin B,[364] it suggested the presence of thiol proteinases with cathepsin B-like specificity within disc tissues.

However, cathepsin B and D have little, if any, enzymic activity against PGs at physiological pH.[365,366] The pericellular localization of these cathepsins in normal and pathological articular cartilage has been described.[367,368] It has been suggested that the pericellular regions around chondrocytes in articular cartilage may be maintained at an acidic pH[354,355] due to lactic acid production under anaerobic glycolysis. A pH environment of 6 has been suggested, and there is some recent evidence using fluorescent diphosphitidyl ethanolamine[355] that this could be achieved at or near the chondrocyte surface. Holm et al.[11] have demonstrated using dogs that a gradient of lactic acid exists across the disc due to anaerobic metabolism even at elevated oxygen tensions. It has been calculated that a lactic acid content of 10 μmol/g wet weight tissue could exist in the disc which would result in a pH 1 unit lower than in plasma (see Chapter 9). Thus, the central part of the NP may assume a pH of around 6.1. In this environment, proteinases such as cathepsins B and D could quite readily degrade proteoglycans.

More recent investigations on the enzymes of the disc have been concerned with proteinases active within a neutral pH range.[314,346,369,370] Sedowofia et al.[314,369] reported the presence in human disc tissues of a collagenase and of at least two other neutral proteinases. These neutral proteinases were active against gelatin and were considered to be present as zymogens rather than as enzyme-inhibitor complexes. The zymogens were activated with APMA, a finding which was in agreement with recent studies from these laboratories.[346] Apart from collagenase, an elastase-like proteinase activity was also identified in human disc tissues by Sedowofia et al.[314] but these enzymes were not characterized nor their specificities determined in any detail. A preliminary report of collagenase and gelatinase activities from immature pig intervertebral discs[370] suggested that, unlike normal mammalian collagenases, these disc enzymes were not inhibited by EDTA, but were activated by this treatment.

A. Isolation and Charaterization of Disc Neutral Proteinases

Proteinases may be isolated from lumbar disc tissue using ultracentrifugation and gel filtration chromatography as outlined in Figures 1 and 8. However, trypsin-affinity chromatography subsequent to Sephadex® G75 gel filtration (Figure 7) provided the crucial step for the separation of the proteinases from their endogenous inhibitors. Since some proteinase

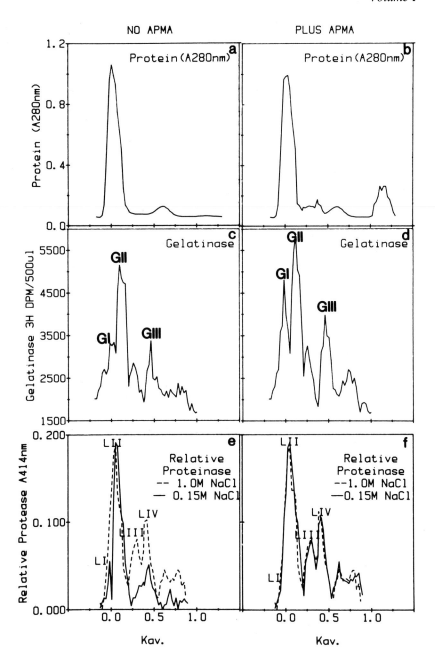

FIGURE 8.   Aliquots (4 mℓ) of crude D3 protein sample (isolated as depicted in Figure 4) were chromatographed with (b,d,f) and without (a,c,e) pretreatment with APMA (1 mM). Relative gelatinase (c,d) and esterolytic activities (e,f), using N-α-CBZ-L-lysine thiobenzyl ester as substrate (with NaCl digest concentrations of 0.15 and 1.0 M), were monitored. Samples were pooled, on the basis of esterolytic activity (enzyme pools LI to LIV) and purified further by trypsin affinity chromatography. (From Melrose, J., Ghosh, P., and Taylor, T. K. F., *Biochim. Biophys. Acta.*, 923, 483, 1987. With permission.)

activity was demonstrable prior to application to the affinity column (Figure 8), partial activation of the disc zymogen in the presence of the chaotropic extractant (4.0 M GuHCl)

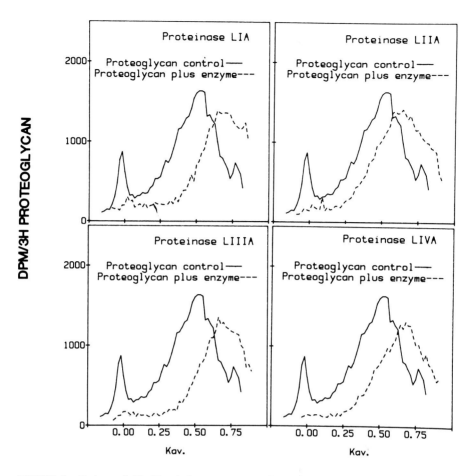

FIGURE 9. Sepharose® CL 2B gel chromatography of ³H-proteoglycan samples preincubated with (----) and without (——) trypsin affinity-purified enzyme pools LIA-LIVA. Aliquots (0.5 mℓ) of eluant fractions were monitored for ³H by liquid scintillation spectrometry. (From Melrose, J., Ghosh, P., and Taylor, T. K. F., *Biochim. Biophys. Acta.*, 923, 483, 1987. With permission.)

may have occurred. As shown in Figure 8 c and d, at least three pools (GI, GII, and GIII) of neutral proteinase activities were present in extracts of human discs and could be separated by Sephadex® G75F chromatography. These activities were increased on exposure to APMA, a result which could be interpreted to indicate their similarity to the cartilage-latent metal-loproteoglycanases.[299,371-375] However, more detailed studies showed that the APMA was activated by removal or modification of endogenous proteinase inhibitors which co-eluted in fractions GI, GII, and GIII. Application of LI, LII, LIII, and LIV enzyme pools (Figure 8 e) to the trypsin affinity column provided efficient resolution of the inhibitors from proteinases, but, surprisingly, also resulted in a very significant increase in enzymic-specific activity. The most significant increase was evident in the void-volume protease pool LI. These data were interpreted to indicate that, apart from removal of endogenous inhibitors, disc zymogens were also activated as a consequence of exposure to the immobilized trypsin. Thus, zymogen activation as well as suppression by specific endogenous inhibitors both appear to be important mechanisms for controlling disc-proteolytic activity.[281]

Characterization of the disc zymogen-active proteinase system[346] indicated many similarities to the plasminogen-plasmin-miniplasmin system. For this reason we have proposed the names, discinogen and discin for the disc zymogens and their active forms. As is shown in Figure 9, the discins can degrade proteoglycans, but, like plasmin,[376,377] the degradation products generated by their action are still quite large.

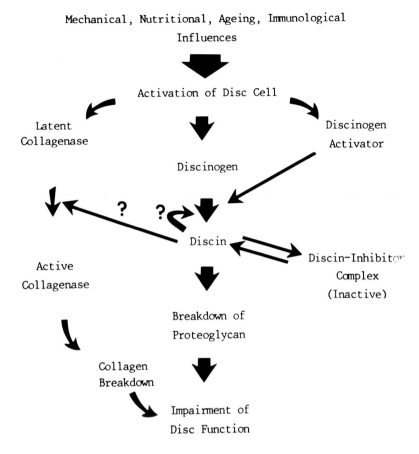

FIGURE 10. Pathways considered by the authors to be implicated in the pathogenesis of disc degeneration.

The question of how discinogen can be converted to discin in vivo has not yet been answered, but is clearly important to our understanding of the pathogenesis of disc degeneration. A specific activator could be involved which was released by the disc cell in response to trauma, intercellular messenger (e.g., IL-1), or nutritional deficiency (see Figure 10). It has been noted that various normal and neoplastic human tissues cultured in vitro secrete plasminogen activators[348,378,379] which, via plasmin, can activate latent collagenase.[347,348,380] Plasminogen activators have recently been shown to be secreted by chondrocytes.[381] Thus, it remains a possibility that disc cells may produce similar activators whose function is to convert discinogen into an active form. As it is most likely that extracellular proteolysis is a largely pericellular event,[354,355] we consider that these discinogen activators may be membrane bound since such enzymes are known to exist in other cellular systems.[347,379,381-384]

The turnover of the extracellular matrix at sites remote from disc cells may also be mediated by enzymes bound to their respective substrates which could be components of the extracellular matrix. Immunolocalization studies have demonstrated that mammalian collagenases are localized on stromal elements, particularly collagen fibers. Moreover, it has been suggested that the tissue-bound collagenase was present in an inactive form.[336,385-387] However, this proposition has been disputed,[388,389] since it is known that human skin collagenase is

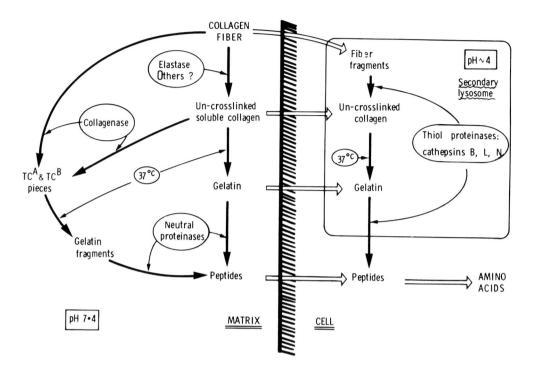

FIGURE 11.   Pathways of collagen degradation. (From Barrett, A. J. and Saklatvala, J., Proteinases in joint disease, in *Textbook of Rheumatology,* Vol. 1, Kelly, W. N., Harris, E. D., Ruddy, S., and Sledge, C. B., Eds., W. B. Saunders, Philadelphia, 1981. With permisssion.)

secreted by cells in an inactive proenzyme form[390] which does not bind to collagen fibrils.[391,392] In addition, the latent form of synovial fluid collagenase shows less binding to collagen than the active form.[393] Recent immunolocalization studies[394] have also established that only active collagenase binds to collagen fibrils. A major unresolved problem, however, is the mechanism by which latent collagenase and related metalloproteinases are activated in vivo. This has recently been reviewed by Murphy and Reynolds[395] and Harris et al.[396] and is summarized in Figure 11.

Immobilized fibronectin and its 120-kdalton fragment and laminin have been shown to specifically bind plasminogen and its activator.[397] A novel oligomeric plasminogen-binding protein from plasma, tetranectin, has also recently been described.[398] Although the biological role of tetranectin has yet to be determined, it was suggested by the authors that it might be involved in the binding of plasminogen and plasminogen-activator to cell surfaces. Thus, laminin and fibronectin (and perhaps tetranectin) may represent possible binding sites for plasminogen and plasminogen activator in vivo[379] as well as discinogens. However, as in the case with collagenase, the key step of activation in vivo of disc zymogens has yet to be resolved. Elastases have also been noted to bind specifically to their native substrate elastin. Therefore, it may be a general principle that the extracellular matrix is laid down with components which can result in its ultimate destruction.

Disc matrix destruction in common with other connective tissue is likely to involve the synergistic action of a number of proteolytic enzymes similar to those depicted in Figure 11.[347,348,378,380,399-405] The two major structural components of the disc extracellular matrix are collagen and proteoglycan, and while degradation of the latter is readily achieved by a variety of proteolytic enzymes,[358,359] native helical collagen requires the synergistic action of collagenase and other neutral proteinases such as those indicated in Figure 11.[347,378,395,399-401,405] Furthermore, the products of matrix breakdown are further processed intracellularly[355,400,401,405] (Figure 11) and provide a feedback mechanism for a variety of events, including the biosynthesis and export of matrix components and enzymes. Such cellular processes have yet to be established for disc cells.

REFERENCES

1. **Pearson, C. H., Happey, F., Naylor, A., Turner, R. L., Palframan, J., and Shentall, R. D.,** Collagens and associated glycoproteins in the human IVD. Variations in sugar and amino acid composition in relation to location and age, *Ann. Rheum. Dis.,* 31, 45, 1972.
2. **Dickson, I. R., Happey, F., Pearson, C. H., Naylor, A., and Turner, R. L.,** Variations in the protein components of human intervetebral disc with age, *Nature (London),* 215, 52, 1967.
3. **Ghosh, P., Taylor, T. K. F., Braund, K. G., and Larsen, L. H.,** The collagenous and non-collagenous protein of the canine intervertebral disc and their variation with age, spinal level and breed, *Gerontology,* 22, 124, 1976.
4. **Happey, F., Pearson, C. H., Naylor, A., and Turner, R. L.,** The ageing of the human intervertebral disc, *Gerontologia,* 15, 174, 1969.
5. **Pearson, C. H., Happey, F., Shentall, R. D., Naylor, A., and Turner, R. L.,** The non-collagenous proteins of the human intervertebral disc, *Gerontologia,* 15, 189, 1969.
6. **Happey, F.,** A study of the changes in collagen and allied polysaccharides and proteins in ageing of the human intervertebral disc, *J. Polym. Sci., Polym. Symp.,* 42, 1481, 1973.
7. **Naylor, A. and Shentall, R.,** Biochemical aspects of the intervertebral discs in ageing and disease, in *The Lumbar Spine and Backpain,* Jayson, M., Ed., Sector Publ., London, 1976, 317.
8. **Trout, J. J., Buckwalter, J. A., Moore, K. C., and Landas, S. K.,** Ultrastructure of the human intervertebral disc. I. Changes in notochordal cells with age, *Tissue Cell,* 14, 359, 1982.
9. **Trout, J. J., Buckwalter, J. A., and Moore, K. C.,** Ultrastructure of the human intervertebral disc. II. Cells of the nucleus pulposus, *Anat. Rec.,* 204, 307, 1982.
10. **Urban, J., Holm, S., and Maroudas, A.,** Diffusion of small solutes in the intervertebral disc: an in vivo study, *Biorheology,* 15, 203, 1978.
11. **Holm, S., Maroudas, A., Urban, J. P. G., Selstam, G., and Nachemson, A.,** Nutrition of the intervertebral disc: solute transport and metabolism, *Connect. Tissue Res.,* 8, 101, 1981.
12. **Stockwell, R. A.,** *Biology of Cartilage Cells,* Cambridge University Press, London, 1979.
13. **Clarke, I. C.,** Articular cartilage: a review and scanning electron microscope study. II. The territorial fibrillar architecture, *J. Anat.,* 118, 261, 1974.
14. **Steven, F. S., Jackson, D. S., and Broady, K.,** Proteins of the human intervertebral disc: the association of collagen with a protein fraction having an unusual amino acid composition, *Biochim. Biophys. Acta,* 160, 435, 1968.
15. **Pearson, C. H., Dickson, I. R., Happey, F., Naylor, A., and Turner, R. L.,** The protein and carbohydrate constituents of the human intervertebral disc, in *Biochimie et Physiologie du Tissu Conjective,* Comte, P., Ed., Lyon, 1966, 327.
16. **Ghosh, P., Taylor, T. K. F., and Horsburgh, B. A.,** The composition and protein metabolism in the immature rabbit IVD, *Cell Tissue Res.,* 163, 223, 1975.
17. **Lafuma, C., Moczar, M., and Robert, L.,** Isolation and characterisation of lung connective tissue glycoproteins, *Biochem. J.,* 203, 593, 1982.
18. **Greenlee, T. K., Jr., Ross, R., and Hartman, J. L.,** The fine structure of elastic fibres, *J. Cell Biol.,* 30, 59, 1966.
19. **Timpl, R., Dziadek, M., Fujiwara, S., Nowack, H., and Wick, G.,** Nidogen: a new, self-aggregating basement membrane protein, *Eur. J. Biochem.,* 137, 455, 1983.
20. **Orkin, R. W., Gehron, P., McGoodwin, E. B., Martin, G. R., Valentine, T., and Swarm, R.,** A murine tumor producing a matrix of basement membrane, *J. Exp. Med.,* 145, 204, 1977.
21. **Freytag, J. W., Dalrymple, P. N., Maguire, M. H., Strickland, D. K., Carraway, K. L., and Hudson, B. G.,** Glomerular basement membrane, *J. Biol. Chem.,* 253, 9069, 1978.
22. **Wu, J. J., Apone, S., and Eyre, D. R.,** Type VI collagen: a prominent matrix component of the intervertebral disc, *Trans. Orthop. Res. Soc.,* 11, 416, 1986.
23. **Robert, B., Szigeti, M., Derouette, J. C., and Robert, L.,** Studies on the nature of the microfibrillar component of elastic fibres, *Eur. J. Biochem.,* 21, 507, 1971.
24. **Helenius, A. and Simons, K.,** Solubilisation of membranes by detergents, *Biochim. Biophys. Acta,* 415, 29, 1975.

25. **Tanford, C. and Reynolds, J. A.,** Characterisation of membrane proteins in detergent solution, *Biochim. Biophys. Acta,* 457, 133, 1976.
26. **Letarte-Muirhead, M., Barclay, A. N., and Williams, A. F.,** Purification of the Thy-1 molecule, and major cell surface glycoprotein of rat thymocytes, *Biochem. J.,* 151, 685, 1975.
27. **Scott, J. E.,** Alphatic ammonium salts in the assay of acidic polysacchirides from tissues, *Methods Biochem. Anal.,* 8, 145, 1963.
28. **Anderson, J. C.,** Glycoproteins of the connective tissue matrix, *Int. Rev. Connect. Tissue Res.,* 7, 251, 1976.
29. **Scopes, R.,** *Protein Purification,* Springer-Verlag, New York, 1982.
30. **Fischer, L.,** Laboratory techniques, in *Biochemistry and Molecular Biology,* Vol. 1, Work, T. S. and Work, E., Eds., North-Holland, Amsterdam, 157, 1969.
31. **Hamaguchi, H. and Cleve, H.,** Solubilisation of human erthyrocyte membrane glycoproteins and separation of the MN glycoprotein with 1,5 and A activity, *Biochim. Biophys. Acta,* 278, 271, 1972.
32. **Muir, L. W., Bornstein, P., and Ross, R.,** A presumptive subunit of elastic fibre microfibrils secreted by arterial smooth muscle cells in culture, *Eur. J. Biochem.,* 64, 105, 1976.
33. **Yanagishita, M. and Hascall, V. C.,** Characterisation of low buoyant density dermatan sulfate proteoglycans synthesised by rat ovarian granulosa cells in culture, *J. Biol. Chem.,* 258, 12847, 1983.
34. **Cole, T.-C., Ghosh, P., and Taylor, T. K. F.,** Variations of the proteoglycans of the canine intervertebral disc with ageing, *Biochim. Biophys. Acta,* 880, 209, 1986.
35. **Sakashita, S. and Ruoslahti, E.,** Laminin like glycoproteins in the extracellular matrix of endodermal cells, *Arch. Biochem. Biophys.,* 205, 283, 1980.
36. **Anderson, J. C.,** Isolation of a glycoprotein and proteodermatan sulphate from bovine achilles tendon by affinity chromatography on concanavalin A-sepharose, *Biochim. Biophys. Acta,* 379, 444, 1975.
37. **Glant, T. T.,** Concanavalin A binding link protein in the proteoglycan aggregate of hyaline cartilage, *Biochem. Biophys. Res. Commun.,* 106, 158, 1982.
38. **Carlsson, H. E., Lonngren, J., Goldstein, I. J., Christner, J. E., and Jourdian, G. W.,** The interaction of wheat-germ agglutinin with keratan from cornea and nasal cartilage, *FEBS Lett.,* 62, 38, 1976.
39. **Choi, H. U., Tang, L. H., Johnson, T. L., and Rosenberg, L.,** Proteoglycans from bovine nasal and articular cartilages — fractionation of the link proteins by wheat germ agglutinin, *J. Biol. Chem.,* 260, 3370, 1985.
40. **Moschi, A. and Little, K.,** Fluorescent properties of the non-collagenous components of the intervertebral disc, *Nature (London),* 212, 722, 1966.
41. **Peereboom, J. W. C.,** Age dependent changes in the human intervertebral disc. Fluorescent substances and amino acids in the annulus fibrosus, *Gerontologia,* 16, 352, 1970.
42. **Taylor, T. K. F. and Little, K.,** Intercellular matrix of the intervertebral disc in ageing and in prolapse, *Nature (London),* 208, 384, 1965.
43. **Blakely, P. R., Happey, F., Naylor, A., and Turner, R. L.,** Protein in the nucleus pulposus of the intervertebral disc, *Nature (London),* 195, 73, 1962.
44. **Hickey, D. S. and Hukins, D. W. L.,** Ageing changes in the macromolecular organisation of the intervertebral disc: an x-ray diffraction and electron microscope study, *Spine,* 7, 234, 1982.
45. **Taylor, T. K. F. and Akeson, W. H.,** A review of morphological and biochemical knowledge concerning the nature of prolapse, *Clin. Orthop. Relat. Res.,* 76, 54, 1971.
46. **Davidson, E. A. and Woodall, B.,** Biochemical alterations in herniated intervertebral discs, *J. Biol. Chem.,* 234, 2951, 1959.
47. **Mallen, A.,** The collagen and ground substance of human intervertebral discs at different ages, *Acta Chem. Scand.,* 16, 705, 1962.
48. **Hall, D. A. and Reed, F. B.,** Protein-polysacharide relationships in tissue subjected to repeated stress throughout life. II. The intervertebral disc, *Age Ageing,* 2, 218, 1973.
49. **Cohen, A. S.,** Preliminary chemical analysis of partially purified amyloid fibrils, *Lab. Invest.,* 15, 66, 1966.
50. **Timpl, R., Wolff, I., and Weiser, M.,** A new class of structural proteins from connective tissue, *Biochim. Biophys. Acta,* 168, 168, 1968.
51. **Steven, F. S., Knott, J., Jackson, D. S., and Podrazky, V.,** Collagen-protein polysaccharide interactions in human IVD, *Biochim. Biophys. Acta,* 188, 307, 1969.
52. **Honda, A., Kanke, Y., and Mori, Y.,** Biochemical study of cardiac valvular tissue. The isolation of glycoproteins and proteoglycans from salt insoluble materials of bovine heart valve, *J. Mol. Cell. Cardiol.,* 7, 715, 1975.
53. **Robert, A. M., Robert, B., and Robert, L.,** Chemical and physical properties of structural glycoproteins, in *Chemistry and Molecular Biology of the Intercellular Matrix,* Balazs, E. A., Ed., Academic Press, New York, 1970, 237.
54. **Robert, L. and Dische, Z.,** Analysis of a sialofucoglucosaminogalactomannosidoglycan from corneal stroma, *Biochem. Biophys. Res. Commun.,* 10, 209, 1963.

55. **Timpl, R. and Martin, G. R.,** Immunochemistry of the Extracellular Matrix, Furthmayr, H., Ed., CRC Press, Boca Raton, Fla., Vol. 2, 1982, 119.

56. **Wolf, I., Fuchswans, W., Weiser, M., Furthmayr, H., and Timpl, R.,** Acidic structural proteins of connective tissue. Characterisation of their heterogeneous nature, *Eur. J. Biochem.,* 20, 426, 1971.

57. **Junqueira, L. C. U. and Montes, G. S.,** Biology of collagen — proteoglycan interaction, *Arch. Histol. Jpn.,* 46, 589, 1983.

58. **Olsen, B. R., Alpen, R., and Kefalides, N. A.,** Structural characterisation of a soluble fraction from lens-capsule basement membrane, *Eur. J. Biochem.,* 38, 220, 1973.

59. **Shipp, D. W. and Bowness, J. M.,** Insoluble non-collagenous cartilage glycoproteins with aggregating subunits, *Biochim. Biophys. Acta,* 379, 282, 1975.

60. **Furthmayr, H. and Timpl, R.,** Acidic structural proteins of connective tissue II. Evidence for disulphide cross links, *Biochim. Biophys. Acta,* 221, 396, 1970.

61. **Furuto, D. K. and Miller, E. J.,** Isolation of a unique collagenous fraction from limited pepsin digest of human placental tissue, *J. Biol. Chem.,* 225, 290, 1980.

62. **Jander, R., Rauterberg, J., and Glanville, R. W.,** Further characterisation of the three polypeptide chains of bovine and human short-chain collagen (intima collagen), *Eur. J. Biochem.,* 133, 39, 1983.

63. **Odermatt, E., Risteli, J., Van Delden, V., and Timpl, R.,** Structural diversity and domain composition of a unique collagenous fragment (intima collagen) obtained from human placenta, *Biochem. J.,* 211, 295, 1983.

64. **Furthmayr, H., Wiedemann, H., Timpl, R., and Odermatt, E.,** Electron microscopical approach to a structural model of intima collagen, *Biochem. J.,* 211, 303, 1983.

65. **Trueb, B. and Bornstein, P.,** Characterisation of a precursor form of type VI collagen, *J. Biol. Chem.,* 259, 8597, 1984.

66. **Zimmerman, D. R., Truels, B., Winterhatter, K. H., Witmewr, R., and Fischer, R. W.,** Type VI collagen is a major component of the human cornea, *FEBS Lett.,* 197, 55, 1986.

67. **Von Der Mark, H., Aumailley, M., Wick, G., Fleischmajer, R., and Timpl, R.,** Immunochemistry, genuine size and tissue localisation of type VI collagen, *Eur. J. Biochem.,* 142, 493, 1984.

68. **Hessle, H. and Engvall, E.,** Type VI collagen. Studies on its localisation, structure and biosynthetic form with monoclonal antibodies, *J. Biol. Chem.,* 259, 3955, 1984.

69. **Johnson, E. F., Chetty, K., Moore, I. M., Stewart, A., and Jones, W.,** The distribution and arrangement of elastic fibres in the IVD of the adult human, *J. Anat.,* 135, 301, 1982.

70. **Johnson, E. F., Caldwell, R. W., Berryman, H. E., Miller, A., Chetty, K.,** Elastic fibres in the annulus fibrosus of the dog intervertebral disc, *Acta Anat.,* 118, 238, 1984.

71. **Hickey, D. S. and Hukins, D. W. L.,** Collagen fibril diameters and elastic fibres in the annulus fibrosus of human fetal intervertebral disc, *J. Anat.,* 133, 351, 1981.

72. **Buckwalter, J. A., Cooper, R. R., and Maynard, J. A.,** Elastic fibers in human intervertebral discs, *J. Bone Jt. Surg.,* 58A, 73, 1976.

73. **Sylvest, J., Bent, H., and Kobayashi, T.,** Ultrastructure of prolapsed disc, *Acta Orthop. Scand.,* 48, 32, 1977.

74. **Postacchini, F., Bellocci, M., Ricciards-Pollins, P. T., and Modesti, A.,** An ultrastructural study of recurrent disc herniation, *Spine,* 7, 492, 1982.

75. **Minns, R. J., Soden, P. D., and Jackson, D. S.,** The role of the fibrous components and ground substance in the mechanical properties of biological tissues: a preliminary investigation, *J. Biomech.,* 6, 153, 1973.

76. **Hukins, D. W. L. and Aspden, R. M.,** Composition and properties of connective tissues, *Trends Biol. Sci.,* 10, 260, 1985.

77. **Hickey, D. S. and Hukins, D. W. L.,** Relation between the structure of the annulus fibrosus and the function and failure of the intervertebral disc, *Spine,* 5, 106, 1980.

78. **Partridge, S. M., Elsden, D. F., and Thomas, J.,** Constitution of the cross-linkages in elastin, *Nature (London),* 197, 1297, 1963.

79. **Thomas, J., Elsden, D. F., and Partridge, S. M.,** Degradation products from elastin, partial structure of two major degradation products from the cross linkages in elastin, *Nature,* 200, 651, 1963.

80. **Franzblau, C., Sinex, F. M., Faris, B., and Lampidis, R.,** Identification of a new cross linking amino acid in elastin, *Biochem. Biophys. Res. Commun.,* 21, 575, 1965

81. **Starcher, B. C., Partridge, S. M., and Elsden, D. F.,** Isolation and partial characterisation of a new amino acid from reduced elastin, *Biochemistry,* 6, 2425, 1967.

82. **Lent, R. W. and Franzblau, C.,** Studies on the reduction of bovine elastin: evidence for the presence of 6,7 dehydrolysinonorleucine, *Biochem. Biophys. Res. Commun.,* 26, 43, 1967.

83. **Paz, M. A., Pereyra, B., Gallop, P. M., and Seifter, S.,** Isomers of desmosine and isodesmosine and related reduced compounds in elastin, *J. Mechanochem. Cell Motil.,* 2, 231, 1974.

84. **Eyre, D. R.,** Cross linking in collagen and elastin, *Annu. Rev. Biochem.,* 53, 717, 1984.

85. **Paz, M. A., Keith, D. A., and Gallop, P. M.,** Elastin isolation and cross-linking, *Methods Enzymol.,* 82A, 571, 1982.

86. **Paz, M. A., Keith, D. A., and Traverso, H. P.,** Isolation, purification and cross-linking profiles of elastin from lung and aorta, *Biochemistry,* 15, 4912, 1976.

87. **Ross, R.,** The elastic fibre: a review, *J. Histochem. Cytochem.,* 21, 199, 1973.

88. **Ross, R. and Bornstein, P.,** The elastic fibre. I. The separation and partial characterisation of its macromolecular components, *J. Cell Biol.,* 40, 366, 1969.

89. **Sandberg, L. B., Soskel, N. T., and Leslie, J. G.,** Elastin structure, biosynthesis and relation to disease states, *N. Engl. J. Med.,* 304, 566, 1981.

90. **Rosenbloom, J.,** Elastin: biosynthesis, structure, degradation and role in disease processes, *Connect. Tissue Res.,* 10, 73, 1982.

91. **Buckwalter, J. A., Maynard, J. A., and Cooper, R. R.,** Banded structures in human nucleus pulposus in the intervertebral disc, *Clin. Orthop. Relat. Res.,* 139, 259, 1979.

92. **Quintarelli, G., Starcher, B. C., Bocaturo, A., Gianfillippo, F., Gotte, L., and Mecham, R. P.,** Fibrillogenesis and biosynthesis of elastin in cartilage, *Connect. Tissue Res.,* 7, 1, 1979.

93. **Hukins, D. W. L.,** Properties of spinal materials, in *The Lumbar Spine and Back Pain,* 3rd ed. Jayson, M. I. V., Ed., Pitman, Tunbridge Wells, England, Chap. 6, in press.

94. **Hukins, D. W. L., Knight, D. P., and Woodhead-Galloway, J.,** Orientation of normal collagen fibrils during ageing, *Science,* 194, 622, 1976.

95. **Hewitt, A. T., Kleinmann, H. K., Pennypacker, J. P., and Martin, G. R.,** Identification of an adhesion factor for chondrocytes, *Proc. Natl. Acad. Sci. U.S.A.,* 77, 385, 1980.

96. **Mollenhauer, J., Bee, J. A., Lizarbe, A., and Van Der Marl, K.,** Role of anchorin CII, a 31,000 mol wt membrane protein in the interaction of chondrocytes with type II collagen, *J. Cell Biol.,* 98, 1572, 1984.

97. **Mollenhauer, J. and Von Der Mark, K.,** Isolation and characterisation of a collagen binding glycoprotein from chondrocyte membranes, *Eur. Mol. Biol. Organ J.,* 2, 45, 1983.

98. **Von Der Mark, K., Mollenhauer, J., Kuhl, U., Bee, J., and Lesot, H.,** Anchorins, a new class of membrane proteins involved in cell matrix interactions, Trelstad, R., Ed., *42nd Ann. Meet. Am. Soc. Dev. Biol.,* 1983.

99. **Huang, D.,** Extracellular matrix cell interactions and chondrogenesis, *Clin. Orthop. Rel. Res.,* 123, 169, 1977.

100. **Urban, J. and Maroudas, A.,** The chemistry of the intervertebral disc in relation to its physiological function and requirement, *Clin. Rheum. Dis.,* 6, 51, 1980.

101. **Lyons, G., Eisenstein, S. A., and Sweet, M. B. E.,** Biochemical changes in intervertebral disc degeneration, *Biochim. Biophys. Acta,* 673, 443, 1981.

102. **Lohmander, S., Antonopoulos, C. A., and Friberg, U.,** Chemical and metabolic heterogeneity of chondroitin sulphate and keratan sulphate in guinea pig cartilage and nucleus pulposus, *Biochim. Biophys. Acta,* 304, 430, 1973.

103. **Cole, T.-C., Burkhardt, D., Ghosh, P., Ryan, M., and Taylor, T. K. F.,** Effects of spinal fusion on the proteoglycans of the canine intervertebral disc, *J. Orthop. Res.,* 3-3, 277, 1985.

104. **Cole, T. -K., Ghosh, P., Hannan, N., Taylor, T. K. F., and Bellenger, C.,** The response of the intervertebral disc to immobilization is dependent on constitutional factors, *J. Orthop. Res.,* 5, 337, 1987.

105. **Parsons, D. B., Brennan, M. B., Glisscher, M. J., and Hall, J.,** Scoliosis: collagen defect in the intervertebral disc, *Trans. Orthop. Res. Soc.,* 7, 52, 1982.

106. **Pedrini-Mille, A., Pedrini, V. A., Tudisco, C., Ponseti, I. V., Weinstein, S. L., and Maynard, J. A.,** Proteoglycans of human scoliotic intervertebral disc, *J. Bone Jt. Surg.,* 65A, 815, 1983.

107. **Hay, E. D.,** Extracellular matrix, *J. Cell Biol.,* 91, 2055, 1981.

108. **Yamada, K. M.,** Cell surface interactions with extracellular materials, *Annu. Rev. Biochem.,* 52, 761, 1983.

109. **Kimata, K., Okayama, M., Oohira, A., and Suzuki, S.,** Cytodifferentiation and proteoglycan biosynthesis, *Mol. Cell. Biochem.,* 1, 211, 1973.

110. **Hughes, R. C., Pena, S. D. J., and Fischer, P.,** *Cell Adhesion and Motility,* Curtis, A. S. G. and Pitts, J. D., Eds., Cambridge University Press, New York, 329, 1980.

111. **Edelman, G. M.,** Surface modulation in cell recognition and cell growth: some new hypotheses on phenotypic alteration and transmembrane control of cell surface receptors, *Science,* 192, 218, 1976.

112. **Yamada, K. M., Yamada, S. S., and Pastan, I.,** Cell surface protein partially restores morphology adhesiveness, and contact inhibition of movement to transformed fibroblasts, *Proc. Natl. Acad. Sci. U.S.A.,* 73, 1217, 1976.

113. **Ali, I. U., Mautner, V., Lanza, R., and Hynes, R. O.,** Restoration of normal morphology, adhesion and cytoskeleton in transformed cells by addition of a transformation sensitive surface protein, *Cell,* 11, 115, 1977.

114. **Surgue, S. P. and Hay, E. D.,** Response of basal epithelial cell surface and cytoskeleton to solubilized extracellular matrix molecules, *J. Cell Biol.,* 91, 45, 1981.

115. **Pennypacker, J. P., Hassell, J. R., Yamada, K. M., and Pratt, R. M.,** The influence of an adhesive cell surface protein on chondrogenic expression *in vitro, Exp. Cell Res.,* 121, 411, 1979.

116. **West, C. M., Lanza, R., Rosenbloom, J., Lowe, M., Holtzer, H., and Avdalovic, N.,** Fibronectin alters the phenotypic properties of cultured chick embryo chondroblasts, *Cell,* 17, 491, 1979.

117. **Turley, E. A.,** Purification of a hyaluronate binding protein fraction that modifies cell social behaviour, *Biochem. Biophys. Res. Commun.,* 108, 1016, 1982.

118. **Turley, E. A. and Moore, D.,** Hyaluronate binding proteins also bind to fibronectin laminin and collagen, *Biochem. Biophys. Res. Commun.,* 121, 808, 1984.

119. **Delpech, A. and Delpech, B.,** Expression of hyaluronic acid binding glycoprotein, hyaluronectin, in the developing rat embryo, *Dev. Biol.,* 101, 391, 1984.

120. **Delpech, B. and Halavent, C.,** Characterization and purification from human brain of a hyaluronic acid binding glycoprotein, hyaluronectin, *J. Neurochem.,* 36, 855, 1981.

121. **Turley, E. A., Erickson, C. A., and Tucker, R. P.,** The retention and ultra structural appearances of various extracellular matrix molecules incorporated into three dimensional hydrated collagen lattices, *Dev. Biol.,* 109, 347, 1985.

122. **Yamada, K. M., Ed.,** *Cell Interactions and Development: Molecular Mechanisms,* John Wiley & Sons, New York, 1983, 287.

123. **Miller, D. R., Mankin, H. J., Shoji, H., and D'Aambosia, R. D.,** Identification of fibronectin in preparation of osteoarthritic human cartilage, *Connect. Tissue Res.,* 12, 267, 1984.

124. **Haas, R. and Culp, L. A.,** Binding of fibronectin to gelatin and heparin: effect of surface denaturation and detergents, *FEBS Lett.,* 174, 279, 1984.

125. **Mazurier, C., Lefevre, A., Henon, M. P. and Goudemand, M.,** Gross immunoelectrophoretic analysis of heparin and gelatin binding capacity of fibronectin, *Clin. Lab. Haematol.,* 6, 193, 1984.

126. **Engvall, E. and Ruoslahti, E.,** Binding of soluble form of fibroblast surface protein fibronectin to collagen, *Int. J. Cancer,* 20, 1, 1977.

127. **Wurster, N. B. and Lust, G.,** Synthesis of fibronectin in normal and osteoarthritic articular cartilage, *Biochim. Biophys. Acta,* 800, 52, 1984.

128. **Scott, D. L. and Walton, K. W.,** The significance of fibronectin in rheumatoid arthritis, *Semin. Arthritis Rheum.,* 13, 244, 1984.

129. **Vartio, T. and Vaheri, A.,** Fibronectin: chains of domains with diversified functions, *Trends Biol. Sci.,* 442, 1983.

130. **Martin, D. E., Reece, M., and Reese, A. C.,** Effect of plasma fibronectin, macrophages and glycosaminoglycans on tumor cell growth, *Cancer Invest.,* 2, 339, 1984.

131. **Hewitt, A. T., Varner, H. H., Silver, W., Dessau, W. I., Wilkes, C. M., and Martin, G. R.,** The isolation and partial characterisation of chondronectin, an attachment factor for chondrocytes, *J. Biol. Chem.,* 257, 2330, 1982.

132. **Timpl, R., Engel, J., and Martin, G. R.,** Laminin — a multifunctional protein of basement membranes, *Trends Biol. Sci.,* 207, 1983.

133. **Carlin, B., Jaffe, R., Bender, B., and Chung, A. E.,** Entactin, a novel Basal lamina associated sulphated glycoprotein, *J. Biol. Chem.,* 256, 5209, 1981.

134. **Chung, A. E., Jaffe, R., Freeman, I. L., Vergnes, J. P., Braginslis, J. E., and Carlin, B.,** Properties of a basement membrane related glycoprotein synthesised in culture by a mouse embryonal carcinoma derived cell line, *Cell,* 16, 277, 1979.

135. **Dziadek, M., Paulsson, M., and Timpl, R.,** Characterisation of a new small basement membrane protein BM 40, 5th Ann. Meet. Aust. and N.Z. Soc. Cell Biol., *Regulatory Mechanisms of the Cell,* Sydney, 1986.

136. **Sames, J. R., Schachner, M., and Covault, J.,** Expression of several adhesive macromolecules (N-CAM, LI, JI, NILE, uvomorulin, laminin, fibronectin and a heparan sulphate proteoglycan) in embryonic, adult and denervated adult skeletal muscle, *J. Cell Biol.,* 102, 420, 1986.

137. **Keene, D. R., Sakai, L. Y., Lunstrom, G. P., Morris, N. P., and Burgeson, R. E.,** Type VII collagen forms an extended network of anchoring fibrils, *J. Cell Biol.,* 104, 611, 1987.

138. **Kjellen, L., Petterson, I., and Hook, M.,** Cell surface heparin sulphate an intercalated membrane proteoglycan, *Proc. Natl. Acad. Sci. U.S.A.,* 78, 5371, 1981.

139. **Rao, N. C., Barsky, S. H., Terranova, V. P., and Liotta, A.,** Isolation of a tumor cell laminin receptor, *Biochem. Biophys. Res. Commun.,* 111, 804, 1983.

140. **Malinoff, H. L. and Wicha, M. S.,** Isolation of a cell surface receptor protein for laminin from murine fibrosarcoma cells, *J. Cell Biol.,* 96, 1475, 1983.

141. **Lesot, H., Kuhl, U., and Von Der Mark, K.,** Isolation of a laminin binding protein from muscle cell membranes, *Eur. Mol. Biol. Organ J.,* 2, 861, 1983.

142. **Terranova, V. P., Rao, C. N., Kalebic, T., Margulies, I. M., and Liotta, L. A.,** Laminin receptor on human breast carcinoma cells, *Proc. Natl. Acad. Sci. U.S.A.,* 80, 444, 1983.

143. **Akiyama, S. A., Yamda, S. Y., and Yamada, K. M.,** Characteristics of a 140kD cell surface antigen as a fibronectin binding molecule, *J. Cell Biol.,* 102, 442, 1986.

144. **Singer, I. I.,** The fibronexus: a transmembrane association of fibronectin containing fibres and 5nm microfilaments in hamster and human fibroblasts, *Cell,* 16, 675, 1979.

145. **Pollard, T. D.,** Cytoskeletal functions of cytoplasmic contractile proteins, *J. Supramol. Struct.,* 5, 317, 1976.

146. **Poole, C. A., Flint, M. H., and Beaument, B. W.,** Analysis of the morphology and function of primary cilia in connective tissues: a cellular cybernetic probe?, *Cell Motility,* 5, 175, 1985.

147. **Poole, C. A., Flint, M. H., and Beaument, B. W.,** A role for primary cilia in connective tissues: the cellular cybernetic probe? 5th Ann. Meet., Aust. N.Z. Soc. Cell Biol., *Regulatory Mechanisms of the Cell,* Australia and New Zealand Society for Cell Biology, Sydney, 1986.

148. **Broom, N. D. and Myers, D. B.,** A study of the structural response of wet hyaline cartilage to various loading situations, *Connect. Tissue Res.,* 7, 227, 1980.

149. **Urban, J. P. G. and McMullin, J. F.,** Swelling pressure of the intervertebral disc: influence of proteoglycan and collagen contents, *Biorheology,* 22, 145, 1985.

150. **Bayliss, M. T., Urban, J. P. G., Johnstone, B., and Holm, S.,** In vitro method for measuring synthesis rates in the intervertebral-disk, *J. Orthop. Res.,* 4, 10, 1986.

151. **Hay, E., Ed.,** *Cell Biology of the Extracellular Matrix,* Plenum Press, New York, 1981, 417.

152. **Grinnell, F.,** Cellular adhesiveness and extracellular substrata, *Int. Rev. Cytol.,* 53, 65, 1978.

153. **Kleinman, H. K., Klebe, R. J., and Martin, G. R.,** Role of collagenous matrices in the adhesion and growth of cells, *J. Cell Biol.,* 88, 473, 1981.

154. **Hay, E. D.,** *Spatial Organisation of Eukaryotic Cells,* McIntosh, J. R., Ed., Alan R. Liss, New York, 1982.

155. **Jacobsen, B., Dorfman, T., Basu, K., and Hasang, S. M.,** Inhibition of vascular endothelial cell growth and trypsin activity by vitreous, *Exp. Eye Res.,* 41, 581, 1985.

156. **Taylor, C. M. and Weiss, J. B.,** Partial-purification of a 5.7K glycoprotein from bovine vitreous which inhibits both angiogenesis and collagenase activity, *Biochem. Biophys. Res. Commun.,* 133, 911, 1985.

157. **Andres, T. L. and Trainer, T. D.,** Intervertebral chondrocalcinosis. A coincidental finding possibly related to previous surgery, *Arch. Pathol. Lab. Med.,* 104, 269, 1980.

158. **Haunschka, P. V., Lian, J. B., and Gallop, P. M.,** Direct identification of the calcium binding amino acid — carboxyglutamate in mineralised tissue, *Proc. Natl. Acad. Sci., U.S.A.,* 72, 3925, 1975.

159. **Price, P. A., Otsuka, A. S., Poser, J. P., Kristanponis, J. A., and Raman, N.,** Characterisation of a γ-carboxyglutamic acid containing protein from bone, *Proc. Natl. Acad. Sci. U.S.A.,* 73, 1447, 1976.

160a. **Romberg, R. W., Werness, P. G., Riggs, B. L., and Mann, K. G.,** Inhibition of hydroxy apatite crystal growth by bone specific and other calcium binding proteins, *Biochemistry,* 25, 1176, 1986.

160. **Weiss, A. P. C. and Dorfmann, H. D.,** S-100 protein in human cartilage lesions, *J. Bone Jt. Surg., Am. Am. Vol.,* 68A, 521, 1986.

161. **Poole, A. R., Pidoux, I., Reiner, A., Choi, H., and Rosenberg, L. C.,** Association of an extracellular protein (chondrocalcin) with the calcification of cartilage in endochondral bone formation, *J. Cell Biol.,* 98, 54, 1984.

162. **Stefanson, K., Woolmann, R. L., Moore, B. W., and Arnason, B. G. W.,** S-100 protein in human chondrocytes, *Nature (London),* 295, 63, 1982.

163. **Nakamura, Y., Becker, L. E., and Marks, A.,** S-100 protein in tumors of cartilage and bone, *Cancer,* 52, 1820, 1983.

164. **Ladefoged, C. H. R., Fedders, O., and Peterson, O. F.,** Amyloid in intervertebral discs: a histopathological investigation of surgical material from 100 consecutive operations on herniated discs, *Ann. Rheum. Dis.,* 45, 239, 1986.

165. **Ladefoged, C.,** Amyloid in intervertebral discs (a histopathological investigation of intervertebral discs from 30 randomly selected autopsies), *Appl. Pathol.,* 3, 96, 1985.

166. **Wagner, T. and Mohr, W.,** Age distribution of amyloid in the intervertebral disc, *Ann. Rheum. Dis.,* 43, 663, 1984.

167. **Bywaters, E. G. L. and Dorling, J.,** Amyloid deposits in articular cartilage, *Ann. Rheum. Dis.,* 29, 294, 1970.

168. **Ballou, S. P., Kahn, M. A., and Kushner, I.,** Diffuse intervertebral disc calcification in primary amyloidosis, *Ann. Intern. Med.,* 85, 616, 1976.

169. **Shimuzu, K., Ishii, M., Yamamuro, T., Takeshita, S., Hosokawa, M., and Takeda, T.,** Amyloid deposition in intervertebral discs of senescence accelerated mouse, *Arthritis Rheum.,* 25, 710, 1982.

170. **Virchow, R.,** *Cellular Pathology,* Dover Publ., New York, 1971, 415.

171. **Friedreich, N. and Kekule, A.,** Zur Amyloidfrage, *Virchows Arch. (Pathol. Anat.),* 16, 50, 1859.

172. **Pennock, C. A.,** Association of acid mucopolysaccharides with isolated amyloid fibrils, *Nature (London),* 217, 753, 1968.

173. **Stiller, D. and Katenkamp, D.,** Demonstration of orderly arranged acidic groups in amyloid by Alcian blue, *Histochemistry,* 39, 163, 1974.

174. **Eanes, E. D. and Glenner, G. G.,** X-ray diffraction studies on amyloid fibrils, *J. Histochem. Cytochem.,* 16, 673, 1968.

175. **Takeda, T., Sanada, H., Ishii, M., Matsushita, M., Yamamuro, T., Shimizu, K., and Hosokawa, M.,** Age associated amyloid deposition in surgically removed herniated intervertebral discs, *Arthritis Rheum.,* 27, 1063, 1984.

176. **Ladefoged, C.,** Amyloid deposits in human hip joints, *Acta Pathol. Microbiol. Scand. Sect. A,* 90, 2, 1982.

177. **Ladefoged, C.,** Amyloid in osteoarthritic hip joints, *Acta Orthop. Scand.,* 53, 581, 1982.

178. **Sorensen, K. H. and Christensen, H. E.,** Local amyloid formation in the hip capsule in osteoarthritis, *Acta Orthop. Scand.,* 44, 460, 1973.

179. **Ladefoged, C., Christensen, H. E., and Sorensen, K. H.,** Amyloid in osteoarthritic hip joints, *Acta Orthop. Scand.,* 53, 587, 1982.

180. **Ladefoged, C. and Christensen, H. E.,** Congophilic substance with green dichroism in hip joints in autopsy material, *Acta Pathol. Microbiol. Scand. Sect. A,* 88, 55, 1980.

181. **Christensen, H. E. and Sorensen, K. H.,** Local amyloid formation of capsule fibrosa in arthritis coxae, *Acta Pathol. Microbiol. Scand. Sect. A,* 233, 128, 1972.

182. **Ladefoged, C.,** Amyloid in osteoarthritic hip joints: deposits in relation to chondromatosis, pyrophosphate and inflammatory cell infiltrate in the synovial membrane and fibrous capsule, *Ann. Rheum. Dis.,* 42, 659, 1983.

183. **Happey, F.,** A biophysical study of the human intervertebral disc, the lumbar spine and back pain, Jayson, M., Ed., Sector Publ., London, 1976, 293.

184. **Naylor, A., Shentall, R. D., and West, D. C.,** Current investigations on the biochemical aspects of intervertebral disc degeneration and herniation, in *Biopolymere ind Biomechanik von Brindegewebssystemen,* Hartmann, F., Ed., Springer-Verlag, Berlin, 1974, 77.

185. **Glenner, G. G.,** A retrospective and prospective overview of the investigations on amyloid and amyloidosis: the B-fibrilloses, in *Amyloid and Amyloidosis,* Glenner, G. G., Costa, P. P., and Freitas, F., Eds., Excerpta Medica, Amsterdam, 1980, 3.

186. **Husby, G.,** A chemical classification of amyloid, *Scand. J. Rheumatol.,* 9, 60, 1980.

187. **Husby, G.,** Amyloisosis and rheumatoid arthritis, *Clin. Exp. Rheumatol.,* 3, 173, 1985.

188. **Kimamoto, T., Tateishi, J., Hikita, K., Nagara, H., and Takeshita, I.,** A new method to classify amyloid fibril proteins, *Acta Neuropathol. (Berlin),* 67, 272, 1985.

189. **Glenner, G. G. and Osserman, E. F., Eds.,** *Amyloidosis,* Plenum Press, New York, 1984.

190. **Bausserman, L. L., Bernier, D. N., McAdam, K. P. W. J., and Herbert, P. N.,** Immunochemical and metabolic studies of human serum amyloid A polymorphism, *Clin. Res.,* 33, 504A, 1985.

191. **Lavie, G., Zucker-Franklin, D., and Franklin, E. C.,** Degradation of serum amyloid A protein by surface associated enzymes of human blood monocytes, *J. Exp. Med.,* 148, 1020, 1978.

192. **Husebekk, A., Skogen, B., Husby, G., and Marhaug, G.,** Transformation of amyloid precursor SAA to protein AA and incorporation into amyloid fibrils in vivo, *Scand. J. Immunol.,* 21, 283, 1985.

193. **Thoenes, W. and Schneider, H.-M.,** Human glomerular amyloidosis — with special regard to proteinuria and amyloidogenesis, *Klin. Wochenschr.,* 58, 667, 1980.

194. **Pepys, M. B., Dyck, R. F., De Beer, F. C., Skinner, M., and Cohen, A. S.,** Binding of serum amyloid P-components (SAP) by amyloid fibrils, *Clin. Exp. Immunol.,* 38, 284, 1979.

195. **Pepys, M. B., Dash, A. C., Munn, E. A., Feinstein, A., Skinner, M., Cohen, A. S., Gewutz, H., Osmand, A. P., and Painter, R. H.,** Isolation of amyloid P component (Protein AP) from normal serum as a calcium-dependent binding protein, *Lancet,* 1, 1029, 1977.

196. **Baltz, M. L., De Beer, F. C., Feinstein, A., and Pepys, M. B.,** Calcium dependent aggregation of human serum amyloid P components, *Biochim. Biophys. Acta,* 701, 229, 1982.

197. **Li, J. J. and McAdam, K. P. W. J.,** Human amyloid P component: an elastase inhibitor, *Scand. J. Immunol.,* 20, 219, 1984.

198. **Skinner, M., Schneller, S. I., Connors, L. H., Kagan, H. M., Stone, P. J., Shirahama, T., Sipe, J. D., O'Connor, C., Calore, J. D., Franzblau, C., and Cohen, A. S.,** Observations on the amyloid degrading activity of serum and its relationship to human neutrophil elastase, *Trans. Am. Assoc. Physicians,* 437, 1984.

199. **Silverman, S. L., Cathcart, E. S., Skinner, M., Cohen, A. S., and Burnett, L.,** A pathogenetic role for polymorphonuclear leukocytes in the synthesis and degradation of SAA protein, *Amyloid and Amyloidosis,* Glenner, G. G., Costa, P. P., and Freitas, F., Eds., Excerpta Medica, Amsterdam, 1980, 420.

200. **Kedar, I., Ravid, M., and Sohar, E.,** Amyloid degrading activity in human serum, in *Amyloid and Amyloidosis,* Glenner, G. G., Costa, P. P., and Freitas, F., Eds., Excerpta Medica, Amsterdam, 1980.

201. **Wegelius, O., Teppo, A.-M., and Maury, C. P. J.,** Reduced amyloid A degrading activity in serum in amyloidosis associated with rheumatoid arthritis, *Br. Med. J.,* 284, 617, 1982.

202. **Skinner, M., Stone, P., Shiraham, T., Connors, L. H., Calore, J., and Cohen, A. S.,** The association of an elastase with amyloid fibrils, *Proc. Soc. Exp. Med.,* 181, 211, 1986.

203. **Scott, D. L., Bracken, P., Bacon, P. A., and Husby, G.,** Amyloid degrading factor activity — a nonspecific calcium mediated effect, *Clin. Res.,* 68, 333, 1985.

204. **Caspi, D., Baltz, M. L., Feinstein, A., Munn, E. A., and Pepys, M. B.,** Amyloid degrading activity of human serum an in vitro clearing effect which does not involve degradation of amyloid fibrils, *Clin. Exp. Immunol.,* 57, 647, 1984.

205. **Caspi, D., Baltz, M. L., and Pepys, M. B.,** Serum amyloid degrading activity, *Clin. Sci.,* 65, 16P, 1983.

206. **Kedar, I., Sohar, E., and Ravid, M.,** Degradation of amyloid by a serum component and inhibition of degradation, *J. Lab. Clin. Med.,* 99, 693, 1982.

207. **Teppo, A. M., Maury, C. P. J., and Wegelius, O.,** Characteristics of the amyloid A fibril degrading activity of human serum, *Scand. J. Immunol.,* 16, 309, 1982.

208. **Marhaug, G., Sletten, K., and Husby, G.,** Characteristics of amyloid related protein SAA complexed with serum lipoproteins (apo SAA), *Clin. Exp. Immunol.,* 50, 382, 1982.

209. **Parks, J. S. and Rudel, L. L.,** Alteration of high density lipoprotein subfraction distribution with induction of serum amyloid A protein (SAA) in the human and primate, *J. Lipid Res.,* 26, 82, 1985.

210. **Laurent, P.,** The clinical usefulness of C-reactive protein measurement, in *Marker Proteins in Inflammation,* Allen, R. C., Bienvenu, J., Laurent, P., and Suskind, R. M., Eds., Walter de Gruyter, New York, 1982, 69.

211. **Maury, C. P. J. and Wegelius, O.,** Clinical value of serum amyloid A and C-reactive protein measurements in secondary amyloidosis, *Int. J. Tissue React.,* VII, 405, 1985.

212. **Maury, C. P. J., Ehnholm, C., and Lukka, M.,** Serum amyloid A protein (SAA) subtypes in acute and chronic inflammatory conditions, *Ann. Rheum. Dis.,* 44, 711, 1985.

213. **Grindulis, K. A., Scott, D. L., Robinson, M. W., Bacon, P. A., and McConkey, B.,** Serum amyloid A protein during the treatment of rheumatoid arthritis with second line drugs, *Br. J. Rheumatol.,* 24, 158, 1985.

214. **Maury, C. P. J.,** Comparative study of serum amyloid A protein and C reactive protein in disease, *Clin. Sci.,* 68, 233, 1985.

215. **Filipowicz-Sosnowska, A. M., Rostropowicz-Denisiewicz, K., Rosenthal, C. J., and Baum, J.,** The amyloidosis of juvenile rheumatoid arthritis — comparative studies in Polish and American children. I. Levels of serum SAA protein, *Arthritis Rheum.,* 21, 699, 1978.

216. **McAdam, K. P. W. J., LI, J., Knowles, J., Foss, N. T., Dinarello, C. A., Rosenwasser, L. T., Selinger, M. J., Kaplan, M. M., and Goodman, R.,** The biology of SAA: identification of the inducer, in vitro synthesis, and heterogeneity demonstrated with monoclonal antibodies, *Ann. N.Y. Acad. Sci.,* 389, 126, 1982.

217. **Takahashi, M., Yokota, T., Yamashita, Y., Ishihara, T., and Uchino, F.,** Ultrastructural evidence for the synthesis of serum amyloid A protein by murine hepatocytes, *Lab. Invest.,* 52, 220, 1985.

218. **Egan, M. S., Goldenberg, D. L., Cohen, A. S., and Segal, D.,** The association of amyloid deposits and osteoarthritis, *Arthritis Rheum.,* 25, 204, 1982.

219. **Varga, J., Shirahama, T., and Cohen, A. S.,** Accelerated induction of amyloid in mice with human amyloid enhancing factor, *Fed. Proc. Fed. Am. Soc. Exp. Biol.,* 44, 747, 1985.

220. **Axelrad, M. A. and Kisilevski, R.,** Biological characterisation of amyloid enhancing factor, in *Amyloid and Amyloidosis,* Glenner, G. G., Costa, P. P., and Freitas, F., Eds., Excerpta Medica, Amsterdam, 1980, 527.

221. **Axelrad, M. A., Kisilevski, R., Willmer, J., Chen, S. J., and Skinner, M.,** Further characterisation of amyloid enhancing factor, *Lab. Invest.,* 47, 139, 1982.

222. **Cathcart, E. S., Rodgers, O. G., and Cohen, A. S.,** Amyloid-inducing factor and immunological unresponsiveness, *Ann. Rheum. Dis.,* 1, 303, 1972.

223. **Hol, P. R., Van Andel, A. C., Vanedere, A. M., Draayer, J., and Gruys, E.,** Amyloid enhancing factor in hamster, *Br. J. Exp. Pathol.,* 66, 689, 1985.

224. **Bausserman, L. L., Herbert, P. N., and McAdam, K. P. W. J.,** Heterogeneity of human serum amyloid A proteins, *J. Exp. Med.,* 152, 641, 1980.

225. **Kruse, P.,** Amyloid artropati, *Ugeskr. Laeg.,* 133, 1777, 1971.

226. **Wiernick, P. H.,** Amyloid joint disease, *Medicine (Baltimore),* 51, 465, 1972.

227. **Kavanaugh, J. H.,** Multiple myeloma, amyloid arthropathy and pathological fractures of the femur, *J. Bone Jt. Surg. Am. Vol.,* 60, 135, 1978.

228. **French, B. T.,** Amyloid arthropathy in myelomatosis — intracytoplasmic synovial deposits, *Histopathology,* 4, 21, 1980.

229. **Gamarski, J. and Netto, M. B.,** Manifestaqaes osteoarticulares na amyloidose primaria — apresentaqao de caso, *Arch. Interam. Rheumatol.,* 2, 651, 1959.

230. **Laine, V., Vainio, K., and Ritana, V. V.,** Occurrence of amyloid in rheumatoid arthritis, *Acta Rheumatol. Scand.,* 1, 43, 1955.

231. **Linke, R. P. and Konig, G.,** Diagnostische signifikanz eines ioslichen, synoviale Proteins mit Immunologisher Kreuzreaktion mit dem Amyloid — Fibrillen Protein A, *Verh. Dtsch. Ges. Rheumatol.,* 5, 330, 1978.

232. **Liard, M. E., Cywiner-Golenzer, C. L., and Leclerc, J. P.,** Les micro depots amyloides en rheumatologie, *Arch. Anat. Cytol. Pathol.,* 27, 343, 1979.

233. **Goffin, Y. A., Thoua, Y., and Potvliege, P. R.,** Micro deposition of amyloid in the joints, *Ann. Rheum. Dis.,* 40, 27, 1981.

234. **Teglebjaerg, P. S., Ladefoged, C., Sorensen, K. H., and Christensen, H. E.,** Local articular amyloid deposition in pyrophosphate arthritis, *Acta Pathol. Microbiol. Scand. Sect. A,* 87, 307, 1979.

235. **Ryan, L. M., Bernhard, G. C., Liang, G., and Kozin, F.,** Amyloid arthropathy in the absence of dysproteinemia: a possible association with chondrocalcinesis, *Arthritis Rheum.,* 21, 587, 1978.

236. **Wright, J. R. and Collins, E.,** Clinico-pathologic differentiation of common amyloid syndromes, *Medicine (Baltimore),* 60, 429, 1981.

237. **Dyle, R. A.,** Amyloidosis, *Clin. Hematol.,* 60, 429, 1982.

238. **Baum, J. and Gutowska, G.,** Death in juvenile rheumatoid arthritis, *Arthritis Rheum.,* 20(s), 245, 1977.

239. **Koota, K., Isomaki, H. A., and Mutru, O.,** Death rate and causes of death in patients with rheumatoid arthritis, *Scand. J. Rheumatol.,* 4, 205, 1975.

240. **Westermark, P., Shirahama, T., Skinner, M., Brun, A., Cameron, R., and Cohen, A. S.,** Immunohistochemical evidence for the lack of amyloid P component in some intra cerebral amyloids, *Lab. Invest.,* 46, 457, 1982.

241. **Pepys, M. B., Baltz, M. L., De Beer, F. A., Dyck, R. F., Holford, S., Breathnach, S. M., Black, M. M., Tribe, C. R., Evans, D. J., and Feinstein, A.,** Biology of serum amyloid P component, *Ann. N.Y. Acad. Sci.,* 389, 286, 1982.

242. **Potempa, L. A., Kubak, B. M., and Gewurz, H.,** Effect of divalent metal ions and pH upon the binding reactivity of human serum amyloid P component, a C-reactive protein homologue for zymosan, *J. Biol. Chem.,* 260, 12142, 1985.

243. **White, A., Fletcher, T. C., Pepys, M. B., and Baldo, B. A.,** The effects of inflammatory agents on C-reactive protein and serum amyloid P-components levels in plaice (Pleuronectes platessa L) serum, *Comp. Biochem. Physiol.,* 69C, 325, 1981.

244. **Pepys, M. B., Dash, A. C., Markham, E., Thomas, H. C., Williams, B. D., and Petrie, A.,** Comparative clinical study of protein SAP (amyloid P component) and C-reactive protein in serum, *Clin. Exp. Immunol.,* 32, 119, 1978.

245. **Kubak, B., Potempa, L. A., Mahklouf, S., Venegas, M., Anderson, B., and Gewurz, H.,** Mannose and anionic polysaccharides as ligands for the serum amyloid P component, *Fed. Proc. Fed. Am. Soc. Exp. Biol.,* 44, 1189, 1985.

246. **De Beer, C. F., Baltz, M., Holford, S., Feinstein, A., and Pepys, M. B.,** Fibronectin and C4-binding protein are selectively bound by aggregated amyloid P component, *J. Exp. Med.,* 154, 1134, 1981.

247. **De Beer, F. C., Baltz, M. L., Munn, E. A., Feinstein, A., Taylor, J., Bruton, C., Clamp, J. R., and Pepys, M. B.,** Isolation and characterisation of C-reactive protein and serum amyloid P component in the rat, *Immunology,* 45, 55, 1982.

248. **Olieveira, E. B., Gotschlich, E. C., and Liu, T.-Y.,** Primary structure of C-reactive protein, *Proc. Natl. Acad. Sci. U.S.A.,* 74, 3148, 1977.

249. **Gotschlich, E. C. and Edelman, G. M.,** Binding properties and specificity of C-reactive protein, *Proc. Natl. Acad. Sci. U.S.A.,* 57, 706, 1967.

250. **Baltz, M. L., De Beer, F. C., Feinstein, A., Munn, E. A., Milstein, C. P., Fletcher, T. C., March, J. F., Taylor, J., Bruton, C., Clamp, J. R., Davies, A. J. S., and Pepys, M. B.,** Phylogenetic aspects of C-reactive protein and related proteins, *Ann. N.Y. Acad. Sci.,* 389, 49, 1982.

251. **Dyck, R. F., Lockwood, C. M., Kershaw, M., McHuch, N., Duance, V. C., Baltz, M. L., and Pepys, M. B.,** Amyloid P-component is a constituent of normal human glomerular basement membrane, *J. Exp. Med.,* 152, 1162, 1980.

252. **Dyck, R. F., Evans, D. J., Lockwood, C. M., Rees, A. J., Turner, D., and Pepys, M. B.,** Amyloid P-component in human glomerular basement membrane, *Lancet,* 2, 606, 1980.

253. **Breathnach, S. M., Melrose, S. M., Bhogal, B., De Beer, F. C., Dyck, R. F., Tennent, G., Black, M. M., and Pepys, M. B.,** Amyloid P-component is located on elastic fibre microfibrils in normal human tissue, *Nature (London),* 293, 652, 1981.

254. **Hashimoto, K.,** Diseases of amyloid, colloid and hyalin, *J. Cutaneous Pathol.,* 12, 322, 1985.

255. **Yanagihara, M., Kato, F., Shikano, Y., Fukushima, N., and Mori, S.,** Intimate structural association of amyloid and elastic fibres in systemic and cutaneous amyloidoses, *J. Cutaneous Pathol.,* 12, 110, 1985.

256. **Hind, C. R. K., Collins, P. M., Baltz, M. L., and Pepys, M. B.,** Human serum amyloid P component, a circulating lectin with specificity for the cyclic 4,6-pyruvate acetal of galactose, *Biochem. J.,* 225, 107, 1985.

257. **Fricke, R.,** Serum proteins in connective tissues, in *Protides of the Biological Fluids,* Peeters, H., Ed., Elsevier, Amsterdam, 1962, 249.

258. **Fricke, R. and Hadding, U.,** Connective tissue proteins, in *Protides of the Biological Fluids,* Peeters, H., Ed., Elsevier, Amsterdam, 1963, 52.

259. **Pepys, M. B.,** C-reactive protein fifty years on, *Lancet,* 1, 653, 1981.

260. **Spark, E. C., Shirahama, T., Skinner, M., and Cohen, A. S.,** The identification of amyloid P-component (protein AP) in normal cultured human fibroblasts, *Lab. Invest.,* 38, 556, 1978.

261. **Baltz, M. L., Holford, S., De Beer, F. C., Whaley, K., and Pepys, M. B.,** The interaction between human serum amyloid P component (SAP) and fixed complement, *Ann. N.Y. Acad. Sci.,* 389, 429, 1982.

262. **Schneider, H.-M. and Loos, M.,** Amyloid P component — a special type of collagen?, *Virchows Arch. Sect. B. Cell Pathol.,* 29, 225, 1978.

263. **Painter, R. H.,** Evidence that C1 (amyloid P component) is not a subcomponent of the first component of complement (C1), *J. Immunol.,* 119, 2203, 1977.

264. **Cooper, N. R. and Ziccardi, R. J.,** Amyloid-P component (Clt) and complement: lack of physical or functional relationship, *Mol. Immunol.,* 16, 821, 1979.

265. **Osmand, A. P., Friedensen, B., Gewurz, H., Painter, R. H., Hofmann, T., and Shelton, E.,** Characterisation of C reactive protein and the complement subcomponent Clt as homologous proteins displaying cyclic pentameric symmetry (pentraxins), *Proc. Natl. Acad. Sci. U.S.A.,* 74, 739, 1977.

266. **Claus, D. R., Siegel, J., Osmand, A. P., and Gewurz, H.,** Interactions of C-reactive protein with the first component of human complement, *J. Immunol.,* 119, 187, 1977.

267. **Siegel, J., Osmand, A. P., Wilson, M. F., and Gewurz, H.,** Interactions of C reactive protein with the complement system, *J. Exp. Med.,* 142, 709, 1974.

268. **Levo, Y. and Wollner, S.,** Effects of serum amyloid P component on human lymphocytes, *Int. Arch. Allergy Appl. Immunol.,* 77, 322, 1985.

269. **Li, J. J., Pereira, M. E. A., De Lellis, R. A., and McAdam, K. P. W. J.,** Human amyloid P component a circulatory lectin that modulates immune responses, *Scand. J. Immunol.,* 19, 227, 1984.

270. **Fiedel, B. A., Simpson, R. M., and Gewurz, H.,** Interaction between C-reactive protein (CRP) and platelets, in *Marker Proteins in Inflammation,* Allen, R. C., Bienvenu, J., Laurent, P., and Suskind, R. M., Eds., Walter de Gruyter, New York, 1982, 111.

271. **Kilpatrick, J. M. and Vinella, G.,** Inhibition of platelet activating factor by C-reactive protein, *Clin. Res.,* 33, A380, 1985.

272. **James, K. K., Mold, C., and Gewurz, H.,** Interactions between CRP and mononuclear cells, in *Marker Proteins in Inflammation,* Allen, R. C., Bienvenu, J., Laurent, P., and Suskind, R. M., Eds., Walter de Gruyter, New York, 1982, 131.

273. **Mortensen, R. F., Osmand, A. P., and Gewurz, H.,** Effects of C reactive protein on the lymphoid system I binding to thymus dependent lymphocytes and alteration of their functions, *J. Exp. Med.,* 141, 821, 1975.

274. **Mortensen, R. F. and Gewurz, H.,** Effects of C reactive protein on the lymphoid system II inhibition of mixed lympocyte reactivity and generation of toxic lymphocytes, *J. Immunol.,* 116, 1244, 1976.

275. **Fiedel, B. A. and Gewirz, H.,** Effects of C reactive protein on platelet function, *J. Immunol.,* 116, 1289, 1976.

276. **Sabato, S., Rotman, A., Robin, G. C., and Floman, Y.,** Platelet aggregation abnormalities in idiopathic scoliosis, *J. Pediatr. Orthop.,* 5, 588, 1985.

277. **Cohen, D. S., Solomans, C. C., and Lowe, T.,** Altered platelet calmodulin activity in idiopathic scoliosis, in Proc. Scoliosis Res. Soc. Meet., Orlando, Florida, 1984.

278. **Floman, Y., Liefergall, M., Robin, G. C., and Elder, A.,** Abnormalities of aggregation, thromboxane A2 synthesis and 14C serotonin release in platelets of patients with idiopathic scoliosis, *Spine,* 8, 236, 1983.

279. **Yarom, R., Myhlrad, A., Hodges, A., and Robin, G. C.,** Platelet pathology in patients with idiopathic scoliosis, *Lab. Invest.,* 43, 208, 1980.

280. **Knight, J. A., Stephens, R. W., Bushell, G. R., Ghosh, P., and Taylor, T. K. F.,** Neutral protease inhibitors from human intervertebral disc and femoral head articular cartilage, *Biochim. Biophys. Acta,* 584, 304, 1979.

281. **Melrose, J. and Ghosh, P.,** Low molecular weight serine proteinase inhibitors of the human intervertebral disc, *Biochem. Int.,* 15, 117, 1987.

282. **Melrose, J., Ghosh, P., and Taylor, T. K. F.,** Multiple forms of lysozyme in the human intervertebral disc, submitted.

283. **Pandey, S. R. and Schmid, K.,** Basic proteins of Cohn fraction III of normal human plasma, *Biochem. Biophys. Res. Commun.,* 43, 1112, 1971.

284. **Iwasaki, T. and Schmid, K.,** Isolation and characterization of a low molecular weight basic protein of human plasma, *J. Biol. Chem.,* 242, 5247, 1967.

285. **Tengblad, A., Pearce, I., Reiner, A., and Rosenberg, L.,** Demonstration of link protein in proteoglycan aggregates from human intervertebral disc, *Biochem. J.,* 222, 85, 1984.

286. **Melrose, J., Ghosh, P., and Taylor, T. K. F.,** Alpha-1-proteinase inhibitor in the human intervertebral disc, submitted.

287. **Eisenstein, R., Kuettner, K. E., Neapolitan, C., Soble, L. W., and Sorgente, N.,** The resistance of certain tissues to invasion. II. Cartilage extracts inhibit the growth of fibroblasts and endothelial cells in culture, *Am. J. Pathol.,* 81, 337, 1975.

288. **Kuettner, K. E., Soble, L., Croxen, R. L., Marczynska, B., Hiti, J., and Harper, E.,** Tumor cell collagenase and its inhibition by a cartilage derived protease inhibitor, *Science,* 196, 653, 1977.

289. **Langer, R., Brem, H., Falterman, K., Klein, M., and Folkman, J.,** Isolation of a cartilage factor that inhibits tumor neovascularisation, *Science,* 193, 70, 1976.

290. **Rifkin, D. B. and Crowe, R. M.,** Isolation of a protease inhibitor from tissue resistant to tumor invasion, *Hoppe Seyler's Z. Physiol. Chem.,* 358, 1525, 1977.

291. **Sorgente, N., Kuettner, K. E., Soble, L. W., and Eisenstein, R.,** The resistance of certain tissues to invasion. II. Evidence for extractable factors in cartilage which inhibit invasion by vascularised mesenchyme, *J. Lab. Invest.,* 32, 217, 1975.

292. **Pauli, B. U., Memoli, V. A., and Kuettner, K. E.,** In vitro determination of tumor invasiveness using extracted hyaline cartilage, *Cancer Res.,* 41, 2084, 1980.

293. **Pauli, B. U., Memoli, V. A., and Kuettner, K. E.,** In vitro determination of tumor invasiveness using extracted hyaline cartilage, *J. Natl. Cancer Inst.,* 67, 65, 1981.

294. **Horton, J. E., Wezeman, F. H., and Kuettner, K. E.,** Inhibition of bone resorption in vitro by a cartilage derived anticollagenase factor, *Science,* 19, 1342, 1978.

295. **Ehrlich, M. G., Armstrong, A. L., and Mankin, H. J.,** Partial purification and characterisation of a proteoglycan degrading neutral protease from bovine epiphyseal cartilage, *J. Orthop. Res.,* 2, 126, 1984.

296. **Horton, J. E., Tarpely, T. M., and Davis, W. F., Eds.,** Mechanisms of localized bone loss, Proc. 1st Scientific Evaluation Workshop on Localized Bone Loss, November 14, 1977, Information Retrieval Inc., Washington, D.C., 1978.

297. **Stephens, R. W., Ghosh, P., and Taylor, T. K. F.,** The pathogenesis of osteoarthritis, *Med. Hypotheses,* 5, 809, 1979.

298. **Walton, E. A., Upfold, L. I., Stephens, R. W., Ghosh, P., and Taylor, T. K. F.,** The role of serine protease inhibitors in normal and osteoarthritic human articular cartilage, *Semin. Arthritis Rheum.,* 11(s), 73, 1981.

299. **Sapolsky, A. I., Malemud, C. J., Norby, D. P., Moskowitz, W., Matsuta, K., and Howell, D. S.,** Neutral proteinases from articular chondrocytes in culture. II. Metal dependent latent proteoglycanase and inhibitory activity, *Biochim. Biophys. Acta,* 658, 138, 1981.

300. **Murphy, G., Cawston, T. E., and Reynolds, J. J.,** An inhibitor of collagenase from human amniotic fluid, *Biochem. J.,* 195, 167, 1981.

301. **Eisenberh, M., Johnson, L., and Moon, K. E.,** Serine proteinase activation of latent human skin collagenase, *Biochem. Biophys. Res. Commun.,* 125, 279, 1984.

302. **Martel-Pelletier, J., Pelletier, J-P., Cloutier, J-M., Howell, D. S., Ghandur-Mnaymneh, L., and Woessner, J. F., Jr.,** Neutral proteases capable of proteoglycan digesting activity in osteoarthritic and normal human articular cartilage, *Arthritis Rheum.,* 27, 305, 1984.

303. **Sandy, J. D., Sriratana, A., Brown, H. L. G., and Lowther, D. A.,** Evidence for polymorphonuclear leukocyte derived proteinases in arthritic cartilage, *Biochem. J.,* 193, 193, 1981.

304. **Lowther, D. A., Sandy, J. D., Srirantana, A., and Brown, H. L. G.,** A neutral serine dependent proteoglycanase from polymorphonuclear leukocytes is present in articular cartilage during joint inflammation, *Semin. Arthritis Rheum.,* 11, 63, 1981.

305. **Lowther, D. A., Sandy, J. D., Cartwright, E. C., and Brown, H. L. G.,** Isolation and secretion of proteolytic enzymes from articular cartilage in organ culture, *Semin. Arthritis Rheum.,* 11, 65, 1981.

306. **Dresden, M. H., Heilman, S. A., and Schmidt, J. D.,** Collagenolytic enzymes in human neoplasms, *Cancer Res.,* 32, 993, 1972.

307. **Harris, E. D., Faulkner, C. S., and Wood, S.,** Collagenase in carcinoma cells, *Biochem. Biophys. Res. Commun.,* 48, 1247, 1972.

308. **Taylor, A. C., Levy, B. M., and Simpson, J. W.,** Collagenolytic activity of sarcoma tissues in culture, *Nature (London),* 228, 366, 1970.

309. **Liotta, L. A., Thorgeirsson, U. P., and Garbisa, S.,** Role of collagenases in tumor cell invasion, *Cancer Metastasis Rev.,* 1, 277, 1982.

310. **Turpeenniemi-Hujanen, T., Thorgeirsson, U. P., and Liotta, L. A.,** Collagenases in tumor cell extravasation, in *Topics in Biology,* Egan, T., Ed., John Wiley, New York, 1984, 231.

311. **Kuettner, K. E., Hiti, J., Eisenstein, R., and Harper, E.,** Collagenase inhibition by cationic proteins derived from cartilage and aorta, *Biochem. Biophys. Res. Commun.,* 72, 40, 1976.

312. **Ehrlich, M. G., Mankin, H. J., Jones, H., Wright, R., Crispen, C., and Vigliani, G.,** Collagenase and collagenase inhibitors in osteoarthritic and normal human cartilage, *J. Clin. Invest.,* 59, 226, 1977.

313. **Killackey, J. J., Roughley, P. J., and Mort, J. S.,** Proteinase inhibitors of human articular cartilage, *Collagen Rel. Res.,* 3, 419, 1983.

314. **Sedowofia, K. A., Tomlinsen, I. W., Weiss, J. B., Hilton, R. C., and Jayson, M. I. V.,** Collagenolytic enzyme systems in human intervertebral disc. Their control, mechanism and their possible role in the initiation of biomechanical failure, *Spine,* 7, 213, 1982.

315. **Kuettner, K. E., Croxen, R. J., Eisenstein, R., and Sorgente, N.,** Proteinase inhibitor activity in connective tissues, *Experimentia,* 30, 595, 1974.

316. **Sorgente, N., Kuettner, K. E., and Eisenstein, R.,** *Proc. 23rd Colloqiuum on Protides of Biological Fluids,* Peeters, H., Ed., Pergamon Press, Oxford, 1976, 227.

317. **Roughley, P. J., Murphy, G., and Barrett, A. J.,** Proteinase inhibitors of bovine nasal cartilage, *Biochem. J.,* 169, 721, 1978.

318. **Lesjak, M. S. and Ghosh, P.,** Polypeptide proteinase inhibitor from human articular cartilage, *Biochim. Biophys. Acta,* 789, 266, 1984.

319. **Kuettner, K. E., Pauli, B. U., and Soble, L. W.,** Morphological studies on the resistance of cartilage to invasion by osteosarcoma cells in vitro and in vivo, *Cancer Res.,* 38, 277, 1978.

320. **Skoza, L., Herp, A., Bloomfield, S. E., and Dunn, M. W.,** Demonstration of a protease inhibitor in cornea, *Invest. Ophthal. Visual Sci.,* 18, 827, 1979.

321. **Nakagawa, T., Ghosh, P., and Nagai, Y.,** Serine proteinase and serine proteinase inhibitors of normal and degenerate knee joint menisci, *Biomed. Res.,* 4, 25, 1983.

322. **Knight, J., Stephens, R. W., Ghosh, P., Bushell, G. R., and Taylor, T. K. F.,** A comparative study of the proteoglycanase inhibitors in intervertebral discs of various mammalian species, *Proc. Aust. Biochem. Soc.,* 12, 27, 1979.

323. **Vater, C. A., Mainardi, C. L., and Harris, E. D., Jr.,** Inhibitor of human collagenase from cultures of human tendon, *J. Biol. Chem.,* 254, 3045, 1979.

324. **Murphy, G., McGuire, M. B., Russell, R. G. G., and Reynolds, J. J.,** Characterisation of collagenase, other metalloproteinase and an ihibitor (TIMP) produced by human synovium and cartilage in culture, *Clin. Sci.,* 61, 711, 1981.

325. **Welgus, H. G. and Stricklin, G. P.,** Human skin fibroblast collagenase inhibitor, *J. Biol. Chem.,* 258, 12252, 1983.

326. **Aggeler, J., Engvall, E., and Werb, Z.,** An irreversible tissue inhibitor of collagenase in human amniotic fluid: characterisation and separation from fibronectin, *Biochem. Biophys. Res. Commun.,* 100, 1195, 1981.

327. **Cawston, T. E., Mercer, E., De Silva, M., and Hazleman, B. L.,** Metalloproteinases and collagenase inhibitors in rheumatoid synovial fluid, *Arthritis Rheum.,* 27, 285, 1984.

328. **Macartney, H. W. and Tschesche, H.,** Characterisation of β1-anticollagenase from human plasma and its reaction with polymorphonuclear leukocyte collagenase by Disulphide/Thiol interchange, *Eur. J. Biochem.,* 130, 85, 1983.

329. **Macartney, H. W. and Tschesche, H.,** Interaction of β1-anticollagenase from human plasma with various tissues and competition with α_2-macroglobulin, *Eur. J. Biochem.,* 130, 93, 1983.

330. **Woolley, D. E., Roberts, D. R., and Evanson, J. M.,** Small molecular weight β1 serum protein which specifically inhibits human collagenases, *Nature (London),* 261, 326, 1976.

331. **Welgus, H. G., Stricklin, G. P., Eisen, A. Z., Bauer, E. A., Cooney, R. V., and Jeffrey, J. J.,** A specific inhibitor of vertebrate collagenase produced by human skin fibroblasts, *J. Biol. Chem.,* 254, 1938, 1978.

332. **Stricklin, G. P. and Welgus, H. G.,** Human skin fibroblast collagenase inhibitor, *J. Biol. Chem.,* 258, 12252, 1983.

333. **Macartney, H. W. and Tschesche, H.,** The collagenase inhibitor from human polymorphonuclear leukocytes, *Eur. J. Biochem.,* 130, 79, 1983.

334. **Cooper, T. W., Stricklin, G. P., Eisen, A. Z., and Welgus, H. G.,** Platelet derived collagenase inhibitor, *Clin. Res.,* 32, 306A, 1984.

335. **Galloway, W. A., Mercer, E., Murphy, G., and Reynolds, J. J.,** Purification of rabbit bone inhibitor of collagenase, *Biochem. J.,* 195, 159, 1981.

336. **Sakamoto, S., Sakamoto, M., Matsumoto, A., Nagayama, M., and Glimcher, M. J.,** Chick bone collagenase inhibitor and latency of collagenase, *Biochem. Biophys. Res. Commun.,* 103, 339, 1981.

337. **Sellers, A., Murphy, G., Meikle, M. C., and Reynolds, J. J.,** Rabbit bone collagenase inhibitor blocks the activity of other neutral metalloproteinases, *Biochem. Biophys. Res. Commun.,* 87, 581, 1979.

338. **Nolan, J. C., Ridge, S. C., Aronsky, A. L., and Kerwar, S. S.,** Purification and properties of a collagenase inhibitor from cultures of bovine aorta, *Atherosclerosis,* 35, 93, 1980.

339. **Murphy, G., Cartwright, E. C., Sellers, A., and Reynolds, J. J.,** The detection and characterisation of collagenase inhibitors from rabbit tissues in culture, *Biochim. Biophys. Acta,* 483, 493, 1977.

340. **Melrose, J., Ghosh, P., and Taylor, T. K. F.,** The serine proteinase inhibitors of the human intervertebral disc, Proc. Connective Tissue Society of Australia and New Zealand, Port Stephens, 1985.

341. **Kunitz, M. and Northrop, J. H.,** Isolation from beef pancreas of crystalline trypsinogen, trypsin, trypsin inhibitor, and inhibitor-trypsin compound, *J. Gen. Physiol.,* 19, 991, 1936.

342. **Fioretti, E., Binotti, I., Barra, D., Citro, G., Ascoli, F., and Antonini, E.,** Heterogeneity of the basic pancreatic inhibitor (Kunitz) in various bovine organs, *Eur. J. Biochem.,* 130, 13, 1983.

343. **Vogel, R., Trantschold, I., and Werle, E.,** *Natural Proteinase Inhibitors,* Academic Press, New York, 1968.

344. **Laskowski, M., Jr., Mars, P. H., and Laskowski, M., Sr.,** Comparison of trypsin inhibitor from colostrum with other crystalline trypsin inhibitors, *J. Biol. Chem.,* 198, 745, 1952.

345. **Ghosh, P., Andrews, J., Lesjak, M., and Osborne, R.,** Variation with ageing and degeneration of the serine and cysteine proteinase inhibitors of human articular cartilage, *Trans. Orthop. Res. Soc.,* 11, 428, 1986.

346. **Melrose, J., Ghosh, P., and Taylor, T. K. F.,** The neutral proteinases of the human intervertebral disc, *Biochim. Biophys. Acta,* 923, 483, 1987.

347. **Werb, Z., Mainardi, C. L., Vater, C. A., and Harris, E. D.,** Endogenous activation of latent collagenase by rheumatoid synovial cells. Evidence for a role of plasminogen activator, *N. Engl. J. Med.,* 296, 1017, 1977.

348. **O'Grady, R. L., Upfold, L. I., and Stephens, R. W.,** Rat mammary carcinoma cells secrete active collagenase and activate latent enzyme in the stroma via plasminogen activator, *Int. J. Cancer,* 28, 509, 1981.

349. **Harris, E. D., Vater, C. A., Mainardi, C. L., and Werb, Z.,** Cellular control of collagen breakdown in rheumatoid arthritis, *Agents Actions,* 8, 36, 1978.

350. **Vaes, G. and Eeckhout, Y.,** Procollagenase and its activation, in *Dynamics of Connective Tissue Macromolecules,* Burleigh, P. M. C. and Poole, A. R., Eds., North-Holland, Amsterdam, 1975, 129.

351. **Stancikova, M., Rybak, M., Trnavsky, K., and Simonianova, E.,** Kallikrein in rheumatoid synovial fluid and its relation to the activation of latent leukocyte collagenase, *Biologia (Bratislava),* 40, 769, 1985.

352. **Armour, P. C., Levi, S., Golds, E., Poole, A. R., Mort, J. S., and Roughley, P. J.,** Activation of latent collagenase by serum proteinases that interact with immobilised immunoglobulin G, *Rheumatol. Int.,* 4, 151, 1984.

353. **Woessner, J. F.,** A latent form of collagenase in the involuting rat uterus and its activation by a serine proteinase, *Biochem. J.,* 161, 535, 1977.

354. **Dingle, J. T.,** The secretion of enzymes into the pericellular environment, *Philos. Trans. R. Soc. London Ser. B:,* 271, 315, 1975.

355. **Dingle, J. T. and Knight, C. G.,** The role of the chondrocyte microenvironment in the degradation of cartilage matrix, in *Degenerative Joints,* Vol. 2, Verbruggen, G. and Veys, E. M., Eds., Excerpta Medica, Amsterdam, 1985, 69.

356. **Dingle, J. T. and Dingle, T. T.,** The site of cartilage matrix degradation, *Biochem. J.,* 190, 431, 1980.

357. **Braund, K. G., Ghosh, P., Taylor, T. K. F., and Larsen, L. H.,** Morphological studies of the canine intervertebral disc. The assignment of the beagle to the achondroplastic classification, *Res. Vet. Sci.,* 19, 167, 1975.

358. **Roughley, P. J.,** The degradation of cartilage proteoglycans by tissue proteinases. Proteoglycan heterogeneity and the pathway of proteolytic degradation, *Biochem. J.,* 167, 639, 1977.

359. **Roughley, P. J. and Barrett, A. J.,** The degradation of cartilage proteoglycans by tissue proteinases. Proteoglycan structure and its susceptibility to proteolysis, *Biochem. J.,* 167, 629, 1977.

360. **Naylor, A., Happey, F., Turner, R. L., Shentall, R. D., West, D. C., and Richardson, C.,** Enzymic and immunological activity in the intervertebral disc, *Orthop. Clin. N. Am.,* 6, 51, 1975.

361. **Happey, F., Osborn, J. M., Pearson, C. H., Naylor, A., and Turner, R. L.,** Proteoglycan degradation in the human intervertebral disc, *Z. Klin. Chem. Klin. Biochem.,* 9, 72, 1971.

362. **Dziewiatowski, D. D., Tourtelotte, C. D., and Campo, R. D.,** *The Chemical Physiology of Mucopolysaccharides,* Quintarelli, G., Ed., J & A Churchill, London, 1968, 63.

363. **Barrett, A. J. and McDonald, J. K., Eds.,** Cathepsin D, in *Mammalian Proteases,* Vol. 1, Academic Press, New York, 1980, 338.

364. **Barrett, A. J.,** An improved color reagent for use in Barretts assay of Cathepsin B, *Anal. Biochem.,* 76, 374, 1976.

365. **Woessner, J. F.,** Purification of Cathepsin D from cartilage and uterus and its action on the protein-polysaccharide complex of cartilage, *J. Biol. Chem.,* 248, 1634, 1973.

366. **Barrett, A. J.,** *Proteases and Biological Control,* Reich, E., Rifkin, D. B., and Shaw, E., Eds., Cold Spring Harbor Laboratory, Cold Spring Harbor, N.Y., 1975, 467.

367. **Mort, J. S., Recklies, A. D., and Poole, A. R.,** Extracellular presence of the lysosomal proteinase Cathepsin B in rheumatoid synovium and its activity at neutral pH, *Arthritis Rheum.,* 27, 509, 1984.

368. **Poole, A. R., Hembry, R. M., and Dingle, J. T.,** Cathepsin D in cartilage: the immunohistochemical demonstration of extracellular enzyme in normal and pathological conditions, *J. Cell Sci.,* 14, 139, 1974.

369. **Sedowofia, S. K. A., Tomlinsen, I., Jayson, M. I. V., and Weiss, J. B.,** Identification of collagenase and other neutral proteinases in human intervertebral discs, *Ann. Rheum. Dis.,* 38, 573, 1979.

370. **Tomlinsen, I., Jayson, M. I. V., and Weiss, J. B.,** Unusual collagenase and gelatinase enzymes in pig intervertebral discs, *Ann. Rheum. Dis.,* 38, 573, 1979.

371. **Woessner, J. F. and Selzer, M. G.,** Two latent metalloproteases of human articular cartilage that digest proteoglycan, *J. Biol. Chem.,* 259, 3633, 1983.

372. **Sapolsky, A. I., Keiser, H., Howell, D. S., and Woessner, J. F.,** Metallo-proteases of human articular cartilage that digest proteoglycan at neutral and acid pH, *J. Clin. Invest.,* 58, 1030, 1976.

373. **Malemud, C. J., Weitzman, G. A., Norby, D. P., Sapolsky, A. I., and Howell, D. S.,** Metal dependent neutral proteoglycanase activity from monolayer cultured lapine articular chondrocytes, *J. Lab. Clin. Med.,* 93, 1018, 1979.

374. **Salopsky, A. I. and Howell, D. S.,** Further characterisation of a neutral metallo-protease isolated from human articular cartilage, *Arthritis Rheum.,* 25, 981, 1982.

375. **Sapolsky, A. I., Matsuta, K., Woessner, J. F., and Howell, D. S.,** Metal dependent neutral proteoglycanase from normal and ulcerated human articular cartilage, *Trans. Orthop. Res. Soc.,* 3, 71, 1978.

376. **Mochan, E. and Keler, T.,** Plasmin degradation of cartilage proteoglycan, *Biochim. Biophys. Acta,* 800, 312, 1984.

377. **Oegema, T. R. and Farnham, B. J.,** Extracellular matrix proteoglycan turnover: a possible role for plasmin, *Trans. Orthop. Res. Soc.,* 11, 256, 1986.

378. **Wilson, E. L. and Dowdle, E.,** Secretion of plasminogen activator by normal, reactive and neoplastic human tissues cultured in vitro, *Int. J. Cancer,* 22, 390, 1978.

379. **Saksela, O.,** Plasminogen activation and regulation of pericellular proteolysis, *Biochim. Biophys. Acta,* 823, 35, 1985.

380. **Zucker, S., Lysik, R. M., Wieman, J., Wilkie, D. P., and Lane, B.,** Diversity of human pancreatic-cancer cell proteinases — role of cell-membrane metalloproteinases in collagenolysis and cytolysis, *Cancer Res.,* 45, 6168, 1985.

381. **Meats, J. E., Elford, P. R., Burning, R. A. D., and Russell, R. G. G.,** Retinoids and synovial factor(s) stimulates the production of plasminogen activator by cultured human chondrocytes. A possible role for plasminogen activator in the resorption of cartilage in vivo, *Biochim. Biophys. Acta,* 838, 161, 1985.

382. **Steven, F. S., Griffin, M. M., Itzhaki, S., and Al-Habib, A.,** A trypsin like neutral protease on Ehrlich ascites cell surfaces: its role in the activation of tumour-cell zymogen of collagenase, *Br. J. Cancer,* 42, 712, 1980.

383. **Dano, K., Andersen, P. A., Grondahl-Hansen, J., Kristensen, P., Nielsen, L. S., and Skriver, L.,** Plasminogen activators, tissue degradation and cancer, *Adv. Cancer Res.,* 44, 139, 1985.

384. **Kenny, A. J.,** Endopeptidase-24.11: an ectoenzyme capable of hydrolysing regulatory peptides at the surface of many different cell types, in *Cellular Biology of Ectoenzymes,* Kreutzberg, G. W., Reddington, M., and Zimmerman, H., Eds., Springer-Verlag, Berlin, 1986, 257.

385. **Montfort, I. and Perez-Tamayo, R.,** The distribution of collagenase in normal rat tissues, *J. Histochem. Cytochem.,* 23, 910, 1975.

386. **Mechanic, G. L., Binderman, I., and Harell, A.,** A novel hypothesis for bone resorption and remodeling, in *Current Advances in Skeletogenesis,* Silbermann, M. and Slavkin, H. C., Eds., Excerpta Medica, Amsterdam, 1982, 322.

387. **Pardo, A., Rosenstein, I., Montfort, I., and Perez-Tamayo, R.,** Immunohistochemical identification of collagenase in carrageenin granuloma, *J. Histochem. Cytochem.,* 31, 641, 1983.

388. **Woessner, J. F.,** Total, latent and active collagenase during the course of post-partum involution of the rat uterus, *Biochem. J.,* 180, 95, 1979.

389. **Woolley, D. E. and Evanson, J. M., Eds.,** *Normal and Pathological Connective Tissues,* John Wiley & Sons, New York, 1980, 105.

390. **Stricklin, G. P., Bauer, E. A., Jeffrey, J. J., and Elsen, A. Z.,** Human skin collagenase isolation of precursor and active forms from both fibroblast and organ cultures, *Biochemistry,* 16, 1607, 1977.

391. **Stricklin, G. P., Bauer, E. A., and Jeffrey, J. J.,** Human skin fibroblast collagenase: chemical properties of precursor and active forms, *Biochemistry,* 17, 2331, 1978.

392. **Welgus, H. G., Jeffrey, J. J., Eisen, A. Z., Roswit, W. T., and Stricklin, G. P.,** Human skin fibroblast collagenase: interaction with substrate and inhibitor, *Collagen Relat. Res.,* 5, 167, 1985.

393. **Vater, C. A., Mainardi, C. L., and Harris, E. D.,** Binding of latent rheumatoid synovial collagenase to collagen fibrils, *Biochim. Biophys. Acta,* 539, 238, 1978.

394. **Hembry, R. M., Murphy, G., Cawston, T. E., Dingle, J. T., and Reynolds, J. J.,** Characterisation of a specific antiserum for mammalian collagenase from several species: immunolocalisation of collagenase in rabbit chondrocytes and uterus, *J. Cell Sci.,* 81, 105, 1980.

395. **Murphy, G. and Reynolds, J. J.,** Current views of collagen degradation. Progress towards understanding the resorption of connective tissues, *Biol. Essays,* 1, 55, 1985.

396. **Harris, E. D., Welgus, H. G., and Krane, S. M.,** Regulation of mammalian collagenases, *Collagen Relat. Res.,* 4, 493, 1984.

397. **Salonen, E.-M., Zitting, A., and Vaheri, A.,** Laminin interacts with plasminogen and its tissue type activator, *FEBS Lett.,* 172, 29, 1984.

398. **Clemmenson, I., Peterson, L. C., and Kluft, C.,** Purification and characterisation of a novel oligomeric plasminogen kringle binding protein from human plasma: tetranectin, *Eur. J. Biochem.,* 156, 327, 1986.

399. **Barrett, A. J.,** Which enzymes degrade cartilage matrix, in *Cellular Interactions,* Dingle, J. T. and Gordon, J. L., Eds., Research Monographs in *Cell and Tissue Physiology,* Vol. 6, Elsevier, Amsterdam, 1981, 185.

400. **Woessner, J. F. and Howell, D. S.,** The enzymatic degradation of connective tissue matrices, in *Scientific Foundation of Orthopaedics and Traumatology,* Owen, R., Goodfellow, J., and Bullough, P., Eds., William Heinemann Medical Books, London, 1980, 232.

401. **Barrett, A. J. and Saklatvala, J.,** Proteinases in joint disease, in *Textbook of Rheumatology,* Vol. 1, Kelley, W. N., Harris, E. D., Ruddy, S., and Sledge, C. B., Eds., W. B. Saunders, Philadelphia, 1981, 195.

402. **Taylor, T. K. F., Ghosh, P., Bushell, G. R., and Stephens, R. W.,** The scientific basis of the treatment of intervertebral disc disorders, in *Scientific Foundations of Orthopaedics and Traumatology,* Owen, R., Goodfellow, J., and Bullough, P., Eds., William Heinemann Medical Books, London, 1980, 387.

403. **Ehrlich, M. G., Houle, P. A., Vigliani, G., and Mankin, H. J.,** Correlation between articular cartilage collagenase activity and osteoarthritis, *Arthritis Rheum.,* 21, 761, 1978.

404. **Ehrlich, M. G.,** Degradative enzyme systems in osteoarthritic cartilage, *J. Orthop. Res.,* 3, 170, 1985.

405. **Etherington, D. J.,** Proteinases in connective tissue breakdown, in *Protein Degradation in Health and Disease,* Ciba Found. Symp., *Excerpta Medica,* 75, 1980, 87.

406. **Roughley, P. J., Poole, A. R., and Mort, J. S.,** The heterogeneity of link proteins isolated from human articular cartilage proteoglycan aggregates, *J. Biol. Chem.,* 257, 11908, 1982.

407. **Chandrasekhar, S., Kleinman, H. K., and Hassell, J. R.,** Interaction of link protein with collagen, *J. Biol. Chem.,* 258, 6226, 1983.

408. **Poole, A. R., Pidoux, I., Reiner, A., and Rosenberg, L.,** An immunoelectron microscope study of the organisation of proteoglycan monomer, link protein, and collagen in the matrix of articular cartilage, *J. Cell Biol.,* 93, 921, 1982.

409. **Poole, A. R., Reiner, A., Mort, S., Tang, L.-H., Choi, H. U., Rosenberg, L. C., Capito, C. B., Kimura, J. H., and Hascell, V. C.,** Cartilage link proteins: biochemical and immunochemical studies of isolation and heterogeneity, *J. Biol. Chem.,* 259, 14849, 1984.

410. **Jahnke, M. R., Donahue, I., and Caterson, B.,** Human intervertebral disc proteoglycans and link proteins resemble those from older articular cartilage, *Trans. Orthop. Res. Soc.,* 10, 317, 1985.

411. **Fife, R. S., Myers, S. L., Hook, I. G. L., and Caterson, B.,** Characterisation of link proteins and a related 70k protein in synovial cell cultures and articular cartilage, *Clin. Res.,* 32, 757A, 1984.

412. **Roughley, P. J., Poole, A. R., Campbell, I. K., and Mort, J. S.,** The proteolytic generation of hyaluronic acid binding regions derived from the proteoglycans of human articular cartilage as a consequence of ageing, *Trans. Orthop. Res. Soc.,* 11, 209, 1986.

413. **Roughley, P. J., White, R. J., and Poole, A. R.,** Identification of a hyaluronic acid binding protein that interferes with the preparation of high-buoyant-density proteoglycan aggregates from adult human articular cartilage, *Biochem. J.,* 231, 129, 1985.

414. **Pearson, J. P. and Mason, R. M.,** Proteoglycan aggregates in adult human costal cartilage, *Biochim. Biophys. Acta,* 583, 512, 1979.

415. **Treadwell, B. V., Mankin, D. P., Ho, P. K., and Mankin, M. J.,** Cell free synthesis of cartilage proteins: partial identification of proteoglycan core and link proteins, *Biochemistry,* 19, 2269, 1980.

416. **Weiss, A. P. C. and Dorfman, H. D.,** The distribution of S-100 protein in human cartilage lesions, *Trans. Orthop. Res. Soc.,* 10, 48, 1985.

417. **Choi, H. U., Tang, L. H., Johnson, T. L., Pal, S., Rosenberg, L. C., Reiner, A., and Poole, A. R.,** Isolation and characterisation of a 35,000 molecular weight subunit cartilage matrix protein, *J. Biol. Chem.,* 258, 655, 1983.

418. **Niyibizi, C., Wu, J. J., and Eyre, D. R.,** A trimeric protein associated with proteoglycans in young cartilage and nucleus pulposus, *Trans. Orthop. Res. Soc.,* 11, 417, 1986.

419. **Paulsson, M. and Heinegard, D.,** Non-collagenous cartilage proteins: current status of an emerging research field, *Collagen Relat. Res.,* 4, 219, 1984.

420. **Paulsson, M., Sommarin, Y., and Heinegard, D.,** Metabolism of cartilage proteins in cultured tissue sections, *Biochem. J.,* 212, 659, 1983.

421. **Aletras, A. J. and Tsiganos, C. P.,** In situ interaction of cartilage proteoglycans with matrix proteins, *Biochim. Biophys. Acta,* 840, 170, 1983.

422. **Von Der Mark, K., Mollenhauer, J., Muller, P. K., and Pfaffle, M.,** Anchorin CII a type II collagen binding glycoprotein from chondrocyte membranes, *Ann. N.Y. Acad. Sci.,* 460, 214, 1985.

423. **Mollenhauer, J., Dee, J. A., Lizarde, A., and Von Der Mark, K.,** Role of anchorin CII, a 31,000 molecular weight membrane protein in the interaction of chondrocytes with type II collagen, *J. Cell Biol.,* 98, 1572, 1984.

424. **McDevitt, C. A., Torelli, R., Amadio, P., Arnoczky, S., and Warren, R.,** A 160 K Da protein is present in fibrillated OA but not normal cartilage, *Trans. Orthop. Res. Soc.,* 10, 46, 1985.

425. **Manicourt, D. H., Pita, J. C., and Howell, D. S.,** New glycoproteins associated with proteoglycan aggregates, *Arthritis Rheum.,* 26 (Suppl.) S23, 1983.

426. **Rosenberg, L. C., Pal, S., and Beale, R. J.,** Proteoglycans from bovine proximal humoral articular cartilage, *J. Biol. Chem.,* 218, 3681, 1973.

427. **Bowness, J. M.,** Comparison of cartilage structural glycoproteins with matrix proteins and fibronectin, *Can. J. Biochem.,* 59, 181, 1980.

428. **Kleine, T. O. and Singh, A.,** Isolation and characterisation of glycoproteins in proteoglycan aggregates of calf rib cartilage, *Connect. Tissue Res.,* 9, 145, 1982.

429. **Chaminade, F., Stanescu, V., Stanescu, R., Maroteaux, P., and Peyron, J. G.,** Non-collagenous proteins in cartilage of normal subjects and patients with degenerative joint disease, *Arthritis Rheum.,* 25, 1078, 1982.

430. **Stanescu, V., Chaminade, F., Stanescu, R., and Maroteaux, P.,** Gel electrophoresis of non-collagenous proteins extracted from normal and arthritic cartilages, *Trans. Orthop. Res. Soc.,* 6, 151, 1981.

431. **Paulsson, M. and Heinegard, D.,** Matrix proteins bound to associatively prepared proteoglycans from bovine cartilage, *Biochem. J.,* 183, 539, 1979.

432. **Paulsson, M. and Heinegard, D.,** Purification and structural characterisation of a cartilage matrix protein, *Biochem. J.,* 197, 367, 1981.

433. **Paulsson, M. and Heinegard, D.,** Radioimmunoassay of the 148 kilo dalton cartilage protein. Distribution of the protein among bovine tissues, *Biochem. J.,* 207, 207, 1982.

434. **Fife, R. S. and Brandt, R. D.,** Identification of a high molecular weight (>400,000) protein in hyaline cartilage, *Biochim. Biophys. Acta,* 802, 506, 1984.

435. **Fife, R. S., Hook, G. L., and Smith, G. N.,** Interaction of the 550,000 Dalton cartilage protein with collagen, *Trans. Orthop. Res. Soc.,* 11, 71, 1986.

436. **Fife, R. S., Hook, G. L., and Brandt, K. D.,** Topographic localisation of a 116,000 Dalton protein in cartilage, *J. Histochem. Cytochem.,* 33, 127, 1985.

437. **Fife, R. S., Hook, G. L., and Brandt, K. D.,** Immunologic and quantitative studies of the 400 kilo Dalton protein in hyaline cartilage, *Clin. Res.,* 32, 463A, 1984.

438. **Fife, R. S. and Hook, G. L.,** Non-collagenous proteins of meniscal cartilage, *Trans. Orthop. Res. Soc.,* 10, 45, 1985.

439. **Jander, R., Troyer, D., and Rauterberg, J.,** A collagen-like glycoprotein of the extracellular matrix is the undegraded form of type VI collagen, *Biochemistry,* 23, 3675, 1984.

440. **Naylor, A., Happey, F., and Macrae, T.,** The collagenous changes in the intervertebral disc with age and their effect on its elasticity, *Br. Med. J.,* 2, 570, 1954.

441. **Shikata, T., Sanada, H., Yamamuro, T., and Takeda, T.,** Experimental studies of the elastic fibre of the capsular ligament: influence of ageing and sex hormones on the hip joint capsule of rats, *Connect. Tissue Res.,* 7, 21, 1979.

442. **Johnson, E. F., Berryman, H., Mitchell, R., and Wood, W. B.,** Elastic fibres in the annulus fibrosus of the adult human lumbar intervertebral disc. A preliminary report, *J. Anat.,* 143, 57, 1985.

443. **Eulitz, M. and Linke, R.,** Amyloid fibrils derived from V-region together with C-region fragments from a lambda II immunoglobulin light chain (HAR), *Hoppe-Seyler Biol. Chem.,* 366, 907, 1985.

444. **Benson, M. D., Dwulet, F. E., and Dibartola, S. P.,** Identification and characterisation of amyloid protein AA in spontaneous canine amyloidosis, *Lab. Invest.,* 52, 448, 1985.

445. **Johnson, K. H., Westermark, P., Nilsson, G., Sletten, K., O'Brien, T. D., and Hayden, D. W.,** Feline insular amyloid: immunohistochemical and immunochemical evidence that the amyloid is insulin related, *Vet. Pathol.,* 22, 463, 1985.

446. **Husby, G., Ranlov, P. J., Sletten, K., and Marhaug, G.,** The amyloid in familial amyloid cardiomyopathy of Danish origin is related to pre-albumin, *Clin. Exp. Immunol.,* 60, 207, 1985.

447. **Gejyo, F., Yamada, T., Odani, S., Nakagawa, Y., Arakawa, M., Kunimoto, T., Kataoka, H., Suzuki, M., Hirasawa, Y., Shirahama, T., Cohen, A. S., and Schnid, Y.,** A new form of amyloid protein associated with chronic hemodialysis was identified as Beta-2-microglobulin, *Biochem. Biophys. Res. Commun.,* 129, 701, 1985.

448. **Dwulet, F. E. and Benson, M. D.,** Structural studies of an amyloid forming pre-albumin, *Arth. Rheum.,* 26(Suppl.)S23, 1983.

449. **Di Bartola, S. P., Benson, M. D., Dwulet, F. E., and Cornacoff, J. B.,** Isolation and characterisation of amyloid protein AA in the Abyssinian Cat., *Lab. Invest.,* 52, 485, 1985.

450. **Pras, M., Prell, F., Franklin, E. C., and Frandione, B.,** Primary structure of an amyloid pre-albumin variant in familial polyneuropathy of Jewish origin, *Proc. Natl. Acad. Sci. U.S.A.,* 80, 539, 1983.

451. **Costa, P. P., Figueira, A. S., and Bravo, I. R.,** Amyloid fibril protein related to pre-albumin in familial amyloidotic polyneuropathy, *Proc. Natl. Acad. Sci. U.S.A.,* 75, 4459, 1978.
452. **Benson, M. D.,** Partial amino acid sequence homology between an heredo-familial amyloid protein and human plasma prealbumin, *J. Clin. Invest.,* 67, 1035, 1981.
453. **Skinner, M. and Cohen, A. S.,** The pre-albumin nature of the amyloid protein in familial amyloid polyneuropathy, *Biochem. Biophys. Res. Commun.,* 99, 1326, 1981.
454. **Rowe, I. F., Jensson, O., Lewis, P. D., Candy, J., Tennant, G. A., and Pepys, M. B.,** Immunohistochemical demonstration of amyloid P component in cerebro-vascular amyloidosis, *Neuropathol. Appl. Neurobiol.,* 10, 53, 1984.
455. **Cole, T., Melrose, J., and Ghosh, P.,** Cysteine proteinase inhibitors of the canine intervertebral disc, *Biochim. Biophys. Acta,* in press, 1988.

INDEX